CURE YOUR LETHAL LIFESTYLE!

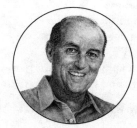

www.jerrybaker.com

Other Jerry Baker Books:

Jerry Baker's Top 25 Homemade Healers
Healing Fixers Mixers & Elixirs
Grandma Putt's Home Health Remedies
Nature's Best Miracle Medicines
Jerry Baker's Supermarket Super Remedies
Jerry Baker's The New Healing Foods
Jerry Baker's Amazing Antidotes!
Jerry Baker's Anti-Pain Plan
Jerry Baker's Oddball Ointments, Powerful Potions, and Fabulous Folk Remedies
Jerry Baker's Giant Book of Kitchen Counter Cures

Jerry Baker's Solve It with Vinegar!
America's Best Practical Problem Solvers
Jerry Baker's Can the Clutter!
Jerry Baker's Cleaning Magic!
Jerry Baker's Homespun Magic
Grandma Putt's Old-Time Vinegar, Garlic, Baking Soda, and 101 More Problem Solvers
Jerry Baker's Supermarket Super Products!
Jerry Baker's It Pays to be Cheap!

Grandma Putt's Green Thumb Magic
Jerry Baker's The New Impatient Gardener
Jerry Baker's Supermarket Super Gardens
Jerry Baker's Dear God . . . Please Help It Grow!
Secrets from the Jerry Baker Test Gardens
Jerry Baker's All-American Lawns
Jerry Baker's Bug Off!
Jerry Baker's Terrific Garden Tonics!
Jerry Baker's Backyard Problem Solver
Jerry Baker's Green Grass Magic
Jerry Baker's Great Green Book of Garden Secrets
Jerry Baker's Old-Time Gardening Wisdom

Jerry Baker's Backyard Birdscaping Bonanza
Jerry Baker's Backyard Bird Feeding Bonanza
Jerry Baker's Year-Round Bloomers
Jerry Baker's Flower Garden Problem Solver
Jerry Baker's Perfect Perennials!

To order any of the above, or for more information on Jerry Baker's
amazing home, health, and garden tips, tricks, and tonics, please write to:

Jerry Baker, P.O. Box 1001, Wixom, MI 48393

Or visit Jerry Baker online at

www.jerrybaker.com

CURE YOUR LETHAL LIFESTYLE!

2,149 Jaw-Dropping Discoveries, Fix-It-Fast Formulas, and Remarkable Remedies for a Longer, Happier Life!

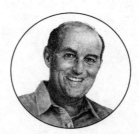

www.jerrybaker.com

Published by American Master Products, Inc.

Executive Editor: Kim Adam Gasior
Managing Editor: Cheryl Winters-Tetreau
Writer: Vicki Webster
Copy Editor: Nanette Bendyna
Production Editor: Debby Duvall
Interior Design and Layout: Sandy Freeman
Indexer: Nan Badgett

Publisher's Cataloging-in-Publication
(Provided by Quality Books, Inc.)

Baker, Jerry.
    Cure your lethal lifestyle! : 2,149 jaw-dropping discoveries, fix-it fast formulas, and remarkable remedies for a longer, happier life! / Jerry Baker.
    pages cm
    Includes index.
    ISBN 978-0-922433-68-1

    1. Self-care, Health--Popular works.   I. Title.

RA776.95.B348 2015   613
                        QBI14-600198

Printed in the United States of America
2 4 6 8 10 9 7 5 3   hardcover

Contents

Part 1   Are You Making Yourself Sick?

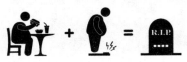

• •

Part 3   Is Your Home Toxic Territory?

Introduction

➔ I know what you're thinking: "There's nothing 'lethal' about my lifestyle. I have a simple, perfectly safe desk job. And I don't have dangerous hobbies like mountain climbing, scuba diving, or running the rapids on rain-swollen rivers. My idea of an action-packed adventure is an all-day shopping spree with my girlfriends. This book can't possibly apply to me."

Wrong you are, my friend. In fact, you could be dead wrong! Take a moment to ponder your daily routine and ask yourself the seven questions below. If any one of your answers is yes, then guess what?—you're living a lethal lifestyle. And if you give an affirmative nod to more than one query, you're on a fast track to big trouble.

50 to 70 million Americans **suffer** from **sleep disorders** that affect health and longevity.

1. Do you frequently have trouble getting a good night's sleep (as 7 out of 10 Americans do)? You may be shortening your life by as much as 8 to 10 years (see page 17).

2. Do you talk on a cell phone for 30 minutes or longer at least once a week? According to a recent study by the World Health Organization (WHO), those seemingly innocent chats could be upping your risk of a deadly brain tumor by 40 percent (see page 22).

3. Do you buy your meat and poultry at your neighborhood supermarket? Then there's a 50-50 chance that you're consuming staph bacteria, possibly including the potentially deadly MRSA strain (see page 103).

4. Do you use common commercial cleaning products in your home? If so, then you're exposing yourself to chemicals that might increase your risk for fatal cancer by as much as 54 percent (see page 247).

5. Are you overweight or obese (as two out of every three Americans are)? You're a sitting duck for literally every health problem under the sun (see page 124).

6. Do you routinely watch television for more than four hours a day? That makes you 80 percent more likely to die from cardiovascular disease than folks who spend fewer than two hours in front of the boob tube every night (see page 162).

7. Worst of all, do you smoke? This disgusting habit is the number one cause of preventable death, killing more Americans each year than alcohol, car accidents, suicide, AIDS, homicide, and illegal drugs *combined* (see page 8).

The good news is, it's never too late to clean up your act—and you can actually have fun doing it! This book is crammed full of terrific tips and tricks for improving your health, boosting your happiness, and lengthening your life. For instance, you'll learn how to break bad habits like excessive drinking and overeating, get off your butt and get moving, and nix the noxious chemicals and invisible toxins that can impair your immune system and bring on health woes, ranging from constant colds to deadly diseases.

But that's not all! You'll also find fantastic features like **Jaw-Dropping Discoveries**, which contain the latest mind-boggling findings from top-notch medical researchers. For example, studies show that owning a cat can reduce your risk of suffering a heart attack by as much as 60 percent (see page 160), and simply by switching to dinner plates that are 2 inches smaller, you can lose 2 pounds in 30 days—without changing a single food in your diet (see page 133)!

Jaw-Dropping DISCOVERY

In **Yikes!** I'll share some seriously sobering facts guaranteed to jolt you into mending your ways—that is, if you want to spend more quality time on this planet. Sneak preview: People who drink two or more sodas a day—regular or diet—raise their risk for pancreatic cancer by a whopping 87 percent (see page 148)!

Remarkable Remedies deliver astounding (and sometimes unbelievable-sounding) treatments for physical and psychological woes of all kinds. Here's just one oddball—and highly versatile—cure: Giving bushels of big ol' bear hugs to your favorite people releases a hormone that banishes the blues; enhances your ability to handle stress; lessens addictive cravings for drugs, alcohol, and sweets; and even helps reduce inflammation and speed up wound healing (see page 60).

Finally, **Fix-It-Fast Formulas** are super-duper recipes that can help you solve or prevent health problems of all kinds. A case in point: Toodle-oo Tick Spray will keep you and your family free of disease-spreading ticks, with none of the potential health hazards of chemical insect repellents (see page 335).

While this book is chock-full of sensational strategies for taking charge of your own health and well-being, none of this information is intended to replace professional medical care. The CALL 911 features spell out—loud and clear—when you need to forgo the DIY measures and hightail it to your doctor's office or the closest emergency room.

Also, always consult with your health-care provider before you use any of the remedies presented in these pages. That's especially crucial if you are suffering from a chronic medical condition, are taking drugs of any kind, are a nursing mom, or are pregnant or think you might be pregnant.

PART 1

Are You
Making Yourself Sick?

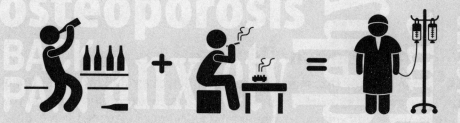

Let's face it: When it comes to deciding how long—and how well—you live, *you* call the shots. Granted, heredity plays a role in determining your health and longevity to some degree, and you could fall victim to a freak accident, natural disaster, manmade catastrophe, or raging pandemic. But for most of us, it's our bad habits that do us in. In this section, we'll take a cold, hard look at some of the ways you may be all but begging for trouble that could make you bow out before your time—or greatly impair your ability to lead a full, happy, and productive life.

Your Deadly Daily Routine

Unless you have a dangerous occupation, like fighting wildfires or serving in a military combat unit, chances are you rarely stop to think that you may be putting your life on the line every day. Believe it or not, many of the choices you make, day in and day out, can spell the difference between a long, healthy, active life—and a shorter, sicker one that you wouldn't wish on your worst enemy.

Will Liquor Be Your Downfall?

 While it is true that moderate consumption of alcohol isn't likely to hurt you, and can even be beneficial to your health, overdoing it can do you in big-time. If you find yourself reaching for an alcoholic beverage to calm down, relax, sleep better at night, or summon up the courage to tackle an unpleasant task, you may have more of a problem than you think.

Dying for a Drink

For many of us, alcohol, in one form or another, is such an integral part of our cultural and family traditions that it can be hard to know when we're lifting the glass too often. But medical gurus suggest cutting back if you fall into one of these two categories:

▶ A woman who routinely has more than three drinks at one time or more than seven drinks per week

▶ A man who routinely has more than four drinks at one time or more than 14 drinks a week

NOTE: *A "standard drink" is defined as one can or bottle of beer, one glass of wine, or one mixed cocktail.*

Booze: Good, Bad—and Ugly

Moderate drinkers (folks who have one or two drinks a day) tend to have lower levels of heart disease and LDL (bad) cholesterol than teetotalers do. And some studies indicate that people who drink occasionally may live longer than nondrinkers. On the other hand, hitting the bottle too hard too often can lead to increased risk for life-threatening problems, ranging from cancer and liver damage to obesity, an impaired immune system, and just about every infectious disease under the sun.

The Myth of the Happy Drunk

True or false? Drinking is a dandy way to drown your sorrows.

A resounding false! Although sharing a few cocktails with your pals can make for some jolly good times, long-term, excessive intake of alcohol has been proven to cause major depression and other serious mental problems, including severe anxiety, panic attacks, hallucinations, delusions, and psychotic disorders.

The Trouble with Tippling

There are scads of unhealthy habits that can shorten your life, but in most cases, the damage occurs gradually over many years. Not so with alcohol. The sobering truth is that you don't even have to be a problem drinker. In fact, just one beverage too many can cut your reaction time, impair your mental processes, and lower your inhibitions enough that you suffer— or cause—deadly consequences. And while the most likely scenario is getting slapped with a hefty fine for DUI, you don't even have to get behind the wheel of a car to land yourself in hot water. You could stagger in front of one. Or you could accidentally start a fire, mishandle your lawn mower, or take a daredevil risk on a ski slope. The possibilities are endless. But your life isn't.

Fix-It-Fast
FORMULA

One for the Road

Wish your guests "safe home" (as the Irish like to say) by ending the evening with booze-free beverages, like this delicious, energizing cocktail.

3½ oz. of apple juice

1¾ oz. of pear juice

⅔ oz. of lemon juice

Small chunk of fresh ginger

Crushed ice

Ginger ale

Apple wedge (optional)

Maraschino cherry (optional)

Fill a cocktail shaker with ice, and add the apple, pear, and lemon juices. Grate the ginger to taste into the shaker. Shake it vigorously so the juices soak up the ginger flavor. Strain the mixture into a highball glass filled with crushed ice. Fill the balance of the glass with ginger ale. If desired, garnish with the apple and cherry, impaled on a toothpick, and serve with a straw.

NOTE: *To serve a crowd, multiply the recipe as needed, and stir the ingredients in a pitcher.*

Alcohol has adverse interactions with literally hundreds of prescription drugs, over-the-counter medications, and even some natural and herbal remedies. The nature and severity of the interactions vary, depending on the meds in question and the amount of alcohol consumed, but—and this is scary, folks—the problem is on the rise. There are two reasons:

1. Due in large part to the obesity epidemic, Americans of all ages are taking more drugs to control related conditions such as diabetes, high blood pressure, and high cholesterol.

2. The older you get, the more likely you are to suffer from chronic health conditions. As our population ages, more folks are taking more prescription medications—often as many as 10 different kinds each day.

Problematic Prescriptions

Dozens—if not hundreds—of alcohol-med combos can cause relatively mild reactions, like drowsiness, headache, and nausea, but when you combine alcohol with any of these widely used prescription drugs, you're asking for serious trouble:

Blood-thinning medications can lead to internal bleeding.

Heart meds can cause rapid heartbeat and sudden changes in blood pressure.

Nonsteroidal anti-inflammatory drugs (NSAIDs) increase the risk of ulcers and abdominal bleeding.

Sleep preparations can result in impaired breathing, decreased motor control, and even some unusual behavior.

Over-the-Counter Catastrophes

Combining alcohol with the popular pain reliever acetaminophen (a.k.a. Tylenol®) ranks among the most common causes of severe liver damage. Some cases even require a liver transplant. OTC antihistamines and herbal remedies, including kava kava, chamomile, lavender, St. John's wort, and valerian, are also potentially hazardous partners for booze.

The Noxious Nighttime Toddy Trap

Having a glass of wine or a cocktail before you hit the sack may seem like a good way to lull yourself to sleep, and every once in a while it won't hurt you (especially in the form of a hot drink when you're battling a bad cold or the flu). But if you make it a habit, you can seriously damage your health. That's because drinking even a little alcohol within three hours of bedtime can disrupt your most restful period of sleep, the rapid eye movement (REM) stage. And, as I'll explain coming up, ongoing failure to get enough sound, soothing sleep is one of the surest routes to an early grave.

Every minute of every day, **someone is injured** by a drunk driver.

Don't Be the Death of the Party

Whenever your social plans involve alcohol—whether you're a host, a guest, or part of a happy-hour gathering—plan ahead. Taking a few commonsense precautions could save your life, and the lives of others. For example:

Before you head out with a group, assign a designated driver.

Anytime you've been drinking, snag a ride home or call a taxi, even if that means going back the next day to retrieve your car.

When you're throwing a party, always have nonalcoholic beverages available. Make sure everyone leaves with a sober driver. And just to cover all the bases, be prepared to have guests bunk down overnight if they don't have safe travel plans.

Dollars Down the Drain

Besides putting your life and the lives of others at risk, heavy drinking can take a huge toll on your bank account. Of course, the cost of the liquor itself will vary wildly, depending on whether you fancy cheap beer, fine wine, or something in between. But regardless of their choice of libations, overindulgers can expect to pay much higher premiums for both health and life insurance than either non- or moderate drinkers. Then there's the matter of drinking and driving, or DUI, as it will appear on your police citation. Even a single incident will send your car insurance premiums soaring to the strato-sphere—that is, unless you lose your license, or even land in jail, in which case auto insurance costs will be the least of your worries!

12 Steps to Broken Habits

Since its founding in 1935, Alcoholics Anonymous (AA) has helped so many problem drinkers overcome their addiction that people with just about every unhealthy behavior you can name have adopted AA's famous 12-step approach to cleaning up their acts. This system is not everyone's cup of tea, but if you're battling an obsession of any kind, or have a loved one who is, it's well worth investigating. You'll find a complete listing of programs at www.12step.org, but here are some of the most popular:

Alcoholics Anonymous (AA):
www.aa.org

Marijuana Anonymous (MA):
www.marijuana-anonymous.org

Narcotics Anonymous (NA):
www.na.org

Nicotine Anonymous (NicA):
www.nicotine-anonymous.org

Overeaters Anonymous (OA):
www.oa.org

3 Crazy Cures for the Morning-After Miseries

Almost everyone who drinks at all gets a little carried away once in a while. For that reason, there are more hangover remedies than there were "champagne" bubbles on Lawrence Welk's TV stage set. But not to worry—any of these winners should put you back in the land of the living in no time at all.

1. Mix 1 teaspoon of freshly squeezed lime juice and a pinch of cumin in a glass of freshly squeezed orange juice, and drink up.

2. Eat 1 teaspoon of raw honey every hour until you feel better. You can take it straight from the spoon, stirred into milk or tea, spread on toast or English muffins, or mixed with yogurt.

3. Drink a tall, cold glass of buttermilk.

Addiction Advisory: 7 Signs That You May Be Hooked

Here are a Baker's half-dozen clues that your drinking (or pot-smoking—see page 13) habit may have crossed the line from social pastime, with perhaps an occasional overindulgence, to full-blown addiction:

Increased tolerance. You have to continuously drink more to produce the same effects.

Having more than you intended—more often. You frequently start out having only one cocktail but wind up having more.

Inability to cut down. You've tried and tried to decrease your consumption, but you just can't.

Becoming dependent on it for relaxation. You simply can't chill out unless you've got a drink in your hand.

Curtailed agenda. You no longer take part in activities you once enjoyed because you're too busy catering to your habit.

Trouble at work. The effects of your "hobby" are hindering your job performance.

Failure to learn from experience. You've harmed your health, or you've suffered other consequences—such as damaged relationships or an arrest for drunk driving—but you still can't stop or cut back.

NOTE: *These indicators can also apply to potentially obsessive behaviors like texting or talking on your cell phone, watching television, playing cyber games, and even compulsive shopping and gambling.*

Weird Ways to Head Off Trouble

A hangover may not be a life-threatening condition, but it sure can feel like one. Fortunately, there are ways to avoid that "I just want to die—*now!*" feeling. Here's a trio of the best:

Before you leave for an event where you'll be drinking, swallow a tablespoon of olive oil. It'll help prevent an upset stomach.

Chemicals Cause Hangovers

Jaw-Dropping
DISCOVERY

Chemicals called congeners are used to add color and flavor to alcoholic beverages, and the more congeners a drink has, the more likely it is to give you a hangover. According to the folks at the Mayo Clinic, these are the worst culprits:

▶ Bourbon ▶ Red wine

▶ Brandy ▶ Scotch

▶ Dark-colored beers ▶ Tequila

Conversely, colorless libations such as gin, vodka, and light rum, as well as lighter-colored beers and white wine, are less likely to produce unpleasant aftereffects. Of course, there is one caveat: If you toss back too many drinks of *any* color, you're going to feel miserable the next morning.

Alternate a glass of water with every cocktail or glass of vino. The H_2O will keep you hydrated and fill you up, so you'll drink less alcohol.

As soon as you get home, drink at least 8 ounces of Gatorade® or similar sports drink. It'll replace the electrolytes the alcohol depleted from your system.

Time to Ditch the Deadly Habit

➡ Attention, smokers! According to the American Cancer Society, every year smoking cigarettes kills more Americans than alcohol, car accidents, suicide, AIDS, homicide, and illegal drugs combined. Furthermore, unlike many other causes of death, death from smoking is entirely preventable. So, are you ready to quit yet?

Each year, about **1** out of every **5 deaths** in the U.S. is caused by **cigarette smoking**.

The Cruelest Killer

Chronic obstructive pulmonary disease (COPD) is a long-term lung ailment that combines emphysema and chronic bronchitis. It's the third-leading cause of death in the United States, and in 90 percent of cases, the blame lies squarely on cigarettes. COPD most often starts in young smokers, and it generally reaches a critical level before it's diagnosed. In fact, the Centers for Disease Control and Prevention estimates that as many as 12 million people in the United States have COPD and don't even know it. Now for the *really* scary part: There is no cure for COPD, and the late stage, which makes people gasp for breath and feel as if they're drowning, is one of the most agonizing of all illnesses.

Now for the good—or at least better—news: While it is true that COPD cannot be cured or reversed, swearing off cancer sticks can help control symptoms and slow their progress.

9 Unheralded Hazards of Smoking

We all know that smoking is the quickest road to lung cancer. What you may not know is that smoking also puts you at high risk for developing cancer in every other part of your body. Plus, it paints a huge target on your back for stroke and coronary heart disease. But that's not all! This deadly practice can cause, contribute to, or worsen just about every health problem under the sun, including these—and they're only the tip of the iceberg!

1. Aneurysms

2. Asthma, bronchitis, emphysema, pneumonia

3. Cataracts, macular degeneration

4. Gum disease

5. Impaired immune system

6. Osteoporosis

7. Peripheral artery disease

8. Sexual impotence

9. Vitamin deficiencies

3 Sinister Signs of COPD

The sooner you realize that your smoking habit has ushered in this hit squad, the better chance you'll have to stem the advancing menace. Toss your smokes in the trash and see a doctor if you experience any of these symptoms:

▶ Wheezing, rattling, or whistling sounds in your chest

▶ Shortness of breath during any kind of physical activity

▶ Coughing up mucus

Sorry, Ladies!

Although middle-aged smokers of both sexes are at equal risk for mental problems, the effects of smoking on feminine hormones invariably lead to these three catastrophic consequences for women:

1. Female smokers, especially those who started as teenagers, tend to reach menopause two to three years earlier than their nonsmoking counterparts do, and they experience more severe side effects.

2. Because smoking reduces estrogen levels, it leads to premature bone loss and, in turn, to the early onset of osteoporosis.

3. Postmenopausal women who smoke, or used to smoke, have a higher risk of breast cancer than nonsmokers have.

Will Your Mind Go Up in Smoke?

In addition to the physical damage that smoking causes, it has been proven to elevate your stress level, impair your cognitive function, and increase your chance of developing a variety of mental problems.

The outlook is especially dire for people who smoke heavily during middle age. Studies show that smoking two packs a day in midlife more than doubles the likelihood that you'll develop Alzheimer's disease or another form of dementia. Folks who smoke less than two packs a day reduce their risk—but not much.

Your Money or Your Life?

Make that your life *and* your money. Every smoker knows that cigarettes don't come cheap, but figuring out how much your habit is costing you in dollars and cents should be a powerful incentive to give it up for good. The cost of the cancer sticks themselves varies, depending on local prices and your own consumption. But it's a snap to do the math. If you're, let's say, a pack-a-day smoker, and the stores in your area charge $5 per pack, you're spending $1,825 per year for the privilege of killing yourself.

Costly Collateral Damage

If you think you're shelling out a lot of dough for cigarettes, just consider these three other budget categories where you're sending your financial future up in smoke:

More than **480,000 Americans die** each year from smoking and from exposure to secondhand smoke.

Health-care costs. Just about all health insurance companies, and many employers, charge smokers considerably higher premiums—as much as double the ones that nonsmokers pay. That's in addition to whatever out-of-pocket expenses you're paying to treat smoking-related medical conditions.

Life and property insurance. Life insurance companies typically charge smokers more than twice as much as they do nonsmokers. Likewise, smokers usually pay more for homeowner's or renter's insurance.

Keeping up appearances. It's no secret that smoking can make a mess of your teeth, hair, skin, and fingernails. And making those body parts pretty again (or at least trying to) can cost you a pretty penny. On top of that, your clothing demands more frequent dry cleaning or laundering to banish the nasty smell of smoke.

A Pack of Lethal Lies

Thanks to the creativity of tobacco companies' marketing gurus—not to mention the potent power of denial—a lot of smokers have some major misconceptions about the true danger of the noxious weed. Here's a trio of the deadliest:

Lie #1: "Light" cigarettes are not as harmful to your health as "regular" brands are.

FACT: Light or ultralight cigarettes deliver the same amounts of tar, nicotine, and carbon monoxide as their full-strength counterparts. To make matters worse, a lot of folks who favor these supposedly safer alternatives tend to smoke more cigarettes and inhale harder, which drives the killing smoke deeper into their lungs.

Lie #2: As long as you don't smoke it, tobacco won't hurt you.

FACT: While it is true that smokeless varieties like snuff, spit, and chewing tobacco are not as lethal as cigarettes, they're far from harmless. Because the juice from smokeless tobacco is absorbed directly through the lining of your mouth, you're a sitting duck for cancer of the mouth, throat, and esophagus, as well as gum disease, tooth decay, and jaw-bone loss. Users also increase their risk for high blood pressure and heart disease.

Lie #3: Smoking is only dangerous if you inhale.

FACT: Even if you don't inhale a single puff, you can't help but breathe in secondhand smoke, thereby increasing your chances for

Going Down!

In addition to the direct costs incurred by smoking, the resale value of everything you own plummets in value when it's been exposed to tobacco smoke. That includes your car, your furniture—and even clothes that you might consign to a resale shop. But the biggest hit will likely come when it's time to sell your home. According to real estate agents, the vast majority of their clients simply will not buy a house that smells of smoke. That means you'll have to ante up for a thorough cleaning, most likely painting and recarpeting, and possibly at least a partial refurnishing. Just think of the dent that'll put in your profit margin!

developing lung cancer and all the other effects of smoking. What's more, pipe and cigar smokers, who tend not to inhale, are prime candidates for lip, mouth, and tongue cancer.

3 to Get Ready, 4 to Go!

There's no getting around it: If you're like the vast majority of smokers, giving up the habit will be the hardest thing you've ever done or ever will do. Nothing can make it easy, but these stage-setting steps can help ensure that you'll achieve your goal.

Step 1. Mark your calendar. Get ready by choosing the day you will quit smoking. Many ex-smokers found that making the date meaningful, such as a loved one's birthday or anniversary, helped them take this first big step.

Step 2. Set up a smoke-free environment. Get rid of all ashtrays, and clean your home and car(s) from top to bottom—or treat yourself to professional cleaning services. Also, declare a strict no-smoking policy for family members, visitors, and vehicle passengers. When your surroundings are spic-and-span, you'll be less tempted to sully the air.

It's no secret that smoking is one of a half-dozen risk factors for heart disease, which is the number one cause of death in the United States. But here's a shocking factoid you may not know: The *single biggest* risk factor for sudden death from a heart attack is cigarette smoking. To be precise, a smoker who has a heart attack is more likely to die within 60 minutes of the episode than a nonsmoker is.

Step 3. Pinpoint your personal craving times and triggers. Often, the urge to light up is strongest first thing in the morning, after your body has been without nicotine for hours. As for triggers, picking up the phone, sitting down with a cup of coffee, or being in a stressful situation may all scream, "I need a cigarette—*now*!"

Step 4. Now go! Tell your family and friends that you're quitting. They'll be delighted to join your booster squad—guaranteed! Find friends or coworkers who also want to quit, and tackle the project together. Consider joining a formal support group (see "12 Steps to Broken Habits" on page 6), and line up a smoking-cessation hotline that you can call in a pinch (you'll find dozens of them on the Internet).

Weighing In on "Weed"

Some states have legalized the recreational use of marijuana, and others are easing the penalties for possession. These actions have sparked strenuous debate about how safe "weed" really is. Most medical pros agree that when used medicinally (generally in extract form), it can be effective in easing pain and treating other symptoms of life-threatening conditions, such as cancer and AIDS. But, like any other drug, marijuana has potentially dangerous side effects, and experts differ in their opinions on whether, and under what circumstances, the benefits outweigh the risks.

Enjoy an Occasional Joint? Proceed with Caution!

As far as recreational use is concerned, the American Cancer Society says that marijuana smoke contains carcinogens similar to those found in tobacco smoke. The jury is still out on the exact degree of harm involved, but researchers caution that pot use may lead to many of the same results as smoking cigarettes, including cancer of the lungs, mouth, and tongue, as well as increased propensity for various respiratory diseases and heart attacks.

3 Potent Perils of Pot

While marijuana does not pose the same deadly dangers as "hard" drugs like heroin and cocaine (for instance, there have been no reported incidents of people dying from an overdose of pot), it does carry its fair share of hazards, including this trio:

1. Studies indicate that it suppresses your body's ability to fight infections of all kinds. For people whose immune systems are already weakened, that can lead to a truckload of trouble.

2. Regular marijuana use can cause psychological problems, including severe anxiety, paranoia, and depression.

3. Pot hampers coordination, perception, reaction times, and judgment, just as alcohol does, thereby leaving you (and innocent victims) vulnerable to all manner of unsafe behaviors and accidents, both vehicular and otherwise.

E-Cigarettes Are Not A-OK

Like just about every other activity on the planet, smoking has entered the electronic age with the advent of the e-cigarette. Proponents claim that these gadgets offer all of the psychological comforts of lighting up without any of the physical dangers. But if you want to live to a ripe old age, don't buy into that hype. Tests show that while these pseudo-cigs don't produce smoke—the greatest danger from tobacco—they do deliver a full load of nicotine. Not only is it damaging in its own right, but it is also highly addictive. When you stop imbibing it, you usher in major withdrawal symptoms, including anxiety, restlessness, and depression. What's more, these cutting-edge gadgets have been shown to harm your arteries, and they pose particular peril for people with heart problems.

The Marvels of Multitasking

Jaw-Dropping DISCOVERY

Traditionally, most mental health pros have deliberately ignored their patients' smoking habits. Their reasoning was that psychiatric issues can be extremely challenging to resolve and that a simultaneous smoking-cessation project would hinder the complex game plan. But now, research at the Washington University School of Medicine in St. Louis has found that just the opposite is true: Patients who either quit cold turkey or reduce their daily cigarette consumption by half actually lower their propensity for mood disorders like depression and anxiety, as well as for alcohol and drug abuse.

The Power of Positive Addiction

Giving up a long-standing habit is hard for anyone, but for folks with obsessive personalities, it's essentially impossible to shed one fixation without latching on to another one. If you even suspect that you have obsessive tendencies, get counseling help for your withdrawal process and also choose a healthier focus to replace the one you're dropping. Here are some suggestions:

- Plunge into a sport, or other physical activity.
- Go back to school and study a subject that fascinates you.
- Take up painting, gardening, woodworking, or quilting.
- Become an active volunteer in your community, perhaps at the local zoo, animal shelter, museum, library, or hospital.

9 Helpful Hints from Successful Quitters

There is no single best way to quit smoking. A strategy that works like a charm for one person may be a total dud for someone else. But here's a smorgasbord of tips, tricks, carrots, and sticks that have helped legions of folks ditch the horrible habit, and could help you, too.

1. Opt for acupuncture. Studies show that nearly 80 percent of people who try the narrow-needle treatment are able to quit.

2. Plan for hands-on success. Find a cigarette stand-in to occupy your hands. For example, keep pads and pencils handy so you can doodle. Or take up needlepoint, knitting, or cross-stitch, and stash your gear close at hand.

3. Get a job where you can't smoke. Many companies have strict no-smoking rules. A give-it-up-or-get-fired policy can be a mighty powerful incentive to puff no more.

4. Frequent no-smoking zones. In your free time, hang out in places where smoking is not allowed, like theaters, shopping malls, restaurants, museums, libraries, and churches.

5. Camp without your cigs. Exploring the great outdoors for a few days, smoke-free, should make you realize how much better you feel (and breathe!) without them.

6. Gross yourself out. Cruise the Internet for pictures of long-time, heavy smokers and cancer-infested body organs, so you'll have clear visual proof of the damage your smoking habit is doing to your body.

7. Make a bet. Challenge a fellow smoker to join you in a quitting competition, with the one who crosses the finish line first claiming the agreed-upon stakes.

8. Dangle a prize ahead of you. Promise yourself that when you quit for good, you'll do something you've always dreamed about—maybe taking an exotic vacation or spending a week at a fancy spa. Better yet, plan on having family or friends join you—you won't want to disappoint them!

9. Try, try again. If your first effort fails, don't give up. Most smokers quit as many as five times before they're able to swear off cigarettes for good.

The Wacky Weight-Gain Myth

There's a rampant misconception that when you quit smoking your weight automatically skyrockets. Baloney! While it is true that smokers who kick the habit tend to put on weight, the average gain is 5 to 15 pounds, and many folks lose it within six months to a year after quitting. Furthermore, you'll be a darn sight healthier toting a little extra baggage and *not* smoking than the other way around. So if you're using the thought of a ballooning waistline as an excuse to keep on puffing, forget it!

Nonsmokers live **10+ years** longer than smokers do.

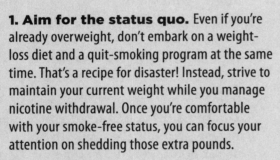

2 Simple Strategies for Staying Slim . . .

Or at least as slim as possible.

1. Aim for the status quo. Even if you're already overweight, don't embark on a weight-loss diet and a quit-smoking program at the same time. That's a recipe for disaster! Instead, strive to maintain your current weight while you manage nicotine withdrawal. Once you're comfortable with your smoke-free status, you can focus your attention on shedding those extra pounds.

2. Ditch temptation. Toss out all the junk food in your house, and stock your larder with nutritious, low-calorie—but delicious—snacks like apples, carrots, and sweet-pepper sticks. That way, when you feel the need for oral gratification, you can satisfy your urge and give your health a boost at the same time. (For more on foods that can help you quit smoking, see "Terrific Tricks for Tossing Cancer Sticks" on page 77.)

4 Freaky Reasons Former Smokers Gain Weight

If you want to pack on as few surplus pounds as possible, it helps to understand the connection between smoking cessation and weight gain.

Reason #1. Nicotine helps keep your weight down in two ways: by acting as an appetite suppressant and revving up your metabolism. When it's gone from your system, your desire for food increases (surprise!), and your body burns calories less efficiently.

Reason #2. Once the aromas of tobacco and smoke are no longer all around you, you'll begin to notice that food smells and tastes a whole lot better—so, of course, eating becomes more enjoyable.

Reason #3. Most folks who give up cigarettes miss the hand-to-mouth gratification they provide. Food makes a dandy substitute.

Reason #4. Ex-smokers who routinely reached for a cigarette in stressful situations frequently turn to food to help them calm down.

Picture This

Every time you get the urge to light up, visualize your family and/or pets suffering from smoking-related diseases. Not only are you serving them heaping helpings of secondhand smoke, but when it comes to your kids, you're also increasing the odds that they'll follow in your footsteps. In fact, the offspring of smoking parents are four times more likely to take up the habit than children in nonsmoking households are.

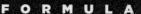

Fix-It-Fast
FORMULA

Craving-Kickin' Oil Mix

This triple-oil blend will not only help you stop cigarette cravings cold but will also help detoxify your system and heal the damage smoking has done to your body.

3 parts lemon essential oil

2 parts geranium essential oil

1 part *Helichrysum* (a.k.a. immortelle or everlast) essential oil

Mix the three oils in a small bottle, and carry it in your pocket, purse, or briefcase. Then, whenever you crave a smoke, open the bottle and take a deep sniff. Or, if you prefer, use a spray bottle and spritz the blend into the air around you.

NOTE: *All of these oils are available in health-food stores, herbal-supply stores, and online.*

Good Health—Sleep on It!

➲ A sleepless night every now and then won't do anyone any long-term harm. If it did, very few parents would survive their children's infancies, much less live to see them graduate from college! But study after study has shown that consistently poor sleep can reduce your life span by (are you ready for this?) as much as 8 to 10 years. So don't just sit there—get ready to start some serious snoozin'!

3 Deadly Dangers of Too Little Shut-Eye

According to the National Sleep Foundation, at least 7 out of 10 Americans have frequent sleeping problems. If you're one of those

YIKES! If you think your tossing and turning puts only your own health at risk, consider these findings, courtesy of a National Sleep Foundation survey: Every morning, nearly 100 million admittedly sleepy Americans hop into their cars and drive off to work. Their drowsiness has been directly implicated in causing accidents galore, not only on the road, but also in the air, in hospitals, in factories, and even in nuclear power plants. What's more, each year drivers who fall asleep at the wheel cause more than 100,000 motor vehicle crashes—many of them with fatal results.

folks, you're at increased risk for a trio of killers, namely these:

Colon cancer. A recent study published in the journal *Cancer* found that people who sleep less than six hours a night, on average, were 50 percent more likely to fall victim to colorectal adenomas than folks who got at least seven hours of sleep each night.

Diabetes. Researchers at Harvard Medical School found that women who get fewer than five hours of sleep each night are one-third more likely to develop diabetes than their better-snoozing counterparts are.

Heart disease. Studies at both Harvard and the University of Chicago have found a direct correlation between too little sleep and a higher risk of heart disease—possibly because sleep deprivation can raise both blood pressure and blood sugar levels and pump extra stress hormones into the bloodstream.

6 Signs That You Need More (or Better) Sleep

Here are a half-dozen hints that you're sleeping either too little or not soundly enough:

1. You've become accident-prone.

2. You're often grumpy and irritable.

3. You doze off while watching TV or reading.

4. You fall asleep in public places, like church, movie theaters, or waiting rooms.

5. You get drowsy in a car, whether you're the driver or merely a passenger.

6. You can't remember the last time you woke up without the aid of an alarm clock.

About **1/3** of Americans get an average of **6 hours or less** of sleep each night.

Beyond the Big 3 Killers

When it comes to negative effects of sleep deprivation, colon cancer, diabetes, and heart disease are only the beginning. Spending too little quality time between the sheets can also lead to or worsen a host of other physical and mental problems, including age-related disorders, depression, obesity, stroke, a weakened immune system, decreased memory retention, and impaired decision-making abilities.

Sleep Less, Die Sooner

Doctors who specialize in sleep and sleep disorders tell us that getting the right amount of sound, restful sleep has been scientifically proven to be the single most important factor in predicting a person's longevity—even more than diet, exercise, or heredity. Yet, in our round-the-clock, squeeze-it-all-in society, sleep is often viewed as a waste of time. In fact, some famous motivational authors actually advise readers to shave hours of shut-eye time from their schedules in the interest of working more "accomplishments" into their days. The amount of sleep necessary to ensure peak health and performance varies from one person to the next, but the average adult needs seven to nine hours of good z's each night. If you haven't been getting your full allotment, now's the time to start!

Fix-It-Fast FORMULA

Snoozefest Punch

Whether you suffer from chronic insomnia or simply have trouble falling asleep once in a while, treat yourself to this milky formula about half an hour before bedtime. Then, when your head hits the pillow, you'll be in the land of nod before you know it.

8 oz. of milk

2 tsp.–1 tbsp. of raw honey to taste

$1/8 - 1/4$ tsp. of ground nutmeg to taste

Warm up the milk until it's hot, but not boiling, and pour it into a mug. Stir in the honey, and sprinkle the nutmeg on top. Let the potion cool to a drinkable warmth, and sip it slowly while you ease into sleepy-time mode.

2 Serious Slumber Blunders

Occasional failure to get a good night's sleep may be caused by factors beyond your control, like a backache, a nagging cold, or a loud party next door. But if you suffer from ongoing sleeping difficulties, the problem—and therefore the solution—may lie with your own routine. Here are two ways you may be keeping yourself awake when you should be snoozing soundly:

Blunder #1: Keeping an erratic schedule. The human body thrives on regularity. If, like many folks, you either stay up late on holidays and weekends, or use those mornings to catch up on sleep that you lost during the workweek, you're throwing your internal clock out of whack.

SOLUTION: Establish a routine and stick to it as best you can. By going to bed and rising at roughly the same times, day in and day out, you'll develop a consistent rhythm that tells your brain when to release the hormones that alternately play *taps* and *reveille*.

Blunder #2: Grinding to a screeching halt. Asking your body to go abruptly from full steam ahead to blissful slumber is a formula for failure. Your system needs time to produce enough neurotransmitters so that your brain knows when the hour has come to haul out the old bedroll.

SOLUTION: Let yourself gear down. Turn off the television set, talk radio, and all electronic devices at least two hours before bedtime. Otherwise, the potent load of stimuli they send to your brain may keep it in fast-action mode for hours after you hit the hay. An hour or so before bedtime, start setting your mind and body at ease by dimming the lights and doing whatever activities you find most relaxing, whether it's taking a warm bath, listening to calming music, or reading (but, please, don't read on your cell phone, laptop, or tablet, and steer clear of work material, action-packed thrillers, and newspapers!).

Lights Out!

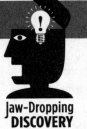

Jaw-Dropping DISCOVERY

Believe it or not, that bedside alarm clock that wakes you up in the morning could also be keeping you from getting the deep, healthful sleep you need at night. That's because, in order to ensure the necessary quantity *and* quality of sleep, your body needs a steady supply of the hormone melatonin, which your pineal gland only produces sufficiently in intense darkness. Even the glowing numbers on your clock and the tiny lights on your cell-phone charger or cordless telephone disrupt melatonin production and disturb your sleep cycle. Your action plan: Remove all electronic devices from view or mask their lights, and install light-blocking window coverings. If those measures are not possible, wear an eye mask.

Bedtime TV:
A Deadly Deception

If you're like a great many people, you may think that because you so frequently doze off in front of the TV set in the living room, watching television in bed is a dandy way to lull yourself to sleep at night. Wrong! While it is true that staring at the boob tube may cause you to conk out quickly, it's all but guaranteed that you'll wake up later on. What you're actually doing is establishing a pattern of poor sleep that can easily lead to chronic insomnia. The simple solution: Get the TV out of the bedroom—*now*!

Is Your Bedroom Sabotaging Your Health?

The design and decor of your sleeping quarters may be hindering your ability to get an effective 40 winks each night. Why? Because regardless of personal taste, there are some hard-and-fast rules of physics that influence the way your eyes, and therefore your mind, perceive your surroundings. Here's a duo of handy hints that can make your bedroom more conducive to rejuvenating downtime:

Color it restful. Get rid of any bedding, curtains, or wallpaper in bold colors or busy prints. No matter how much they appeal to you aesthetically, they deliver a resounding wake-up call to your brain just when you need to relax. Replace the visual chaos with solid colors in soft, soothing tones. If you absolutely must have some pattern, make it muted, and confine it to one element, like the curtains or bed cover.

A Lovely Lavender Lullaby

REMARKABLE REMEDY

For centuries, the soothing scent of lavender has been helping people drift off to dreamland, with none of the toxic side effects of commercial sleeping aids. Whether you're a genuine insomniac, or you only have occasional nights when you just can't summon the sandman, try one of these fragrant options:

▶ Keep a vase of fresh or dried lavender on your bedside table.

▶ Fill a small fabric pouch with dried lavender, and tuck it under your pillow.

▶ On laundry day, put some dried lavender into a small, zippered pillowcase or tightly closed cheesecloth bag, and toss it into the dryer with your bed linens. They'll emerge with a delicate, sleep-inducing aroma.

▶ Pour cooled, strong lavender tea into a plastic spray bottle, and spritz your pillowcase. (Be sure you give it time to dry before you hit the sack.)

Can the clutter. Keep stuff—especially small furnishings and tiny trinkets—to an absolute minimum in your sleeping area. As psychologists know, a space that contains just a few large objects looks and feels more restful and serene than one that's filled with scads of little things, no matter how beautiful or treasured they may be.

Too Much of a Good Thing

Craving excessive amounts of shut-eye can be a side effect of a medication you're taking, it could mean that you're depressed, or it might be that you simply enjoy sleeping. Or it may indicate an underlying health condition. Whatever the reason, sleeping too much can result in many of the same issues as snoozing too little. If you average more than nine hours of sleep a night, ask your doctor about changing or eliminating the problem-causing meds. Or, if you're not taking any drugs, have a thorough checkup to determine the cause of your problem.

The Dangers of Constant Connection

The electronic age has ushered in communication miracles that we never dreamed of even 10 or 15 years ago. Unfortunately though, for many—if not most—of us the devices that were intended to be useful helpers have become unrelenting taskmasters that impose never-ending workweeks. Much worse, when used improperly, these digital marvels can be true killers.

Can Your Wireless Wonders Give You the Big C?

Debate has raged about whether cell phones and other wireless devices, like laptop computers, cordless phones, iPads, and baby monitors—all of which produce nonionizing radiation—can cause cancer. Well, guess what? A study called Interphone, conducted by the World Health Organization (WHO) in 13 countries over a 10-year period, found that people who used cell phones for as little as 30 minutes a day were 40 percent more likely to develop a glioma (a deadly type of brain tumor) than their less-connected counterparts were. This comes on top of earlier studies that linked heavy cell-phone use to cancer of the salivary glands and auditory nerves.

3 Approaches to Avoiding Emissions

Even if you're skeptical that your mobile may be emitting dangerous levels of radiation, it can't hurt to take a few precautions.

Precaution #1. Hold the phone as far away from your ear as you can (cell-phone manuals generally recommend a minimum distance of ⅞ inch). Better yet, use the speakerphone mode whenever you can.

Precaution #2. If reception isn't good, hang up. Those annoying crackly sounds and broken-up voices indicate that your phone's antenna has latched on to a distant satellite or tower. The farther away it is (and, therefore, the more trouble you have understanding the conversation), the more radiation your phone is cranking out.

Precaution #3. When you're not using your phone, turn it off. Why go to the bother? Because every few minutes, a powered-up cell

 Based on the findings of the Interphone study (at left), here are four reasons why your wireless devices may be slowly killing you:

1. Normally, brain tumors cannot be detected by any medical tests until they've been growing for 20 to 30 years. Yet the malignant growths found in the Interphone study were large enough to appear after only 10 years of cell-phone use.

2. The study defined "heavy" users as those who used their cell phones for just 30 minutes or so a day—a fraction of the time that hordes of people spend chatting.

3. Researchers classified people as "regular" users even if they only tapped into their cell phones once a week for six months. The fact that these folks were exposed to far less radiation than more frequent callers were diluted the data, making the cancer rates appear artificially low. It's like doing a lung-cancer study that lumps pack-a-day smokers in with those who light up once a week.

4. The study examined only adults, not adolescents and children, who tend to be die-hard cell-phone users, whose thinner skulls offer less brain protection than those of grown-ups, and who face decades of radiation exposure.

By far, the most effective way to guard yourself from harmful radiation is to opt for an old-fashioned landline telephone whenever that's possible. But dodging cancer is far from the only health-related reason to maintain an active traditional phone line. In "An Unseen Danger" (see page 305), I'll open your eyes to many more ways that relying on a cell phone as your only conversational option could easily endanger your life and the lives of your loved ones.

phone sends out signals to locate the closest tower—whether you're talking or not. And if you want to check your calendar, watch videos, listen to music, or do whatever else it is that you do on your phone, switch the device to non-irradiating airplane mode.

The Devastating Automotive Equation

According to police accident reports, drivers who use cell phones (even in hands-free mode) cause thousands of deaths and hundreds of thousands of injuries each year. But the danger doesn't stop there. Whether you're behind the wheel or not, anytime you have a drive-time phone chat, you expose yourself to higher levels of radiation than you'd get elsewhere. The same goes if you're in a train, bus, warehouse, or any other metallic structure. The reason is twofold: Your phone's signal must be stronger in order to break through the metal, and some of those more potent rays are reflected back onto you. Your best defense: Keep the phone turned off or set to airplane mode. Every now and then, check for messages, and return them later.

At least **1.5 million auto crashes** a year are caused by **drivers** who are talking or **texting** on cell phones.

Get Your Laptop Off Your Lap

As of this writing, there have been no studies exploring possible links between cancer and the use of laptop computers, iPads, or other e-tablets. But as the old saying goes, it's better to be safe than sorry. Medical pros advise that, given the fact that carrying a cell phone at your waist or hip area has been shown to cause cancer and other health problems, you should not hold any portable WiFi device on your lap for an extended length of time.

Suicide by Sitting

If you think that's an exaggeration, consider this: On average, Americans spend 56 hours or more per week planted on their butts, either at work, in their cars, or slouched in front of a television set. In the process, they're increasing their risk for cardiovascular disease, diabetes, chronic back pain, depression, and severe stress, as well as breast and colon cancer. For that reason, a whole new field of medicine, called inactivity physiology, has sprung up to explore a deadly new epidemic that researchers have dubbed "sitting disease."

Hey, That's NEAT!

The good news is that to save yourself from sitting disease, all you need to do is move your body every chance you get or, as the inactivity physiologists put it, ramp up your daily non-exercise activity thermogenesis (NEAT). That's a fancy term for the calories you burn doing everything *but* exercising—like folding laundry, feeding the dog, or strolling to the watercooler. Here are six simple ways you can NEATen up your day:

AT WORK

1. Stand up at least every 30 minutes, and grab every chance you get to walk around your cubicle—while reading, on the phone, or with a visitor.

2. Rather than phoning or e-mailing a coworker, step down the hall for a face-to-face chat.

3. Instead of holding sit-down meetings, gather your colleagues for a walking conference in the corridors or (better yet) outdoors.

ON YOUR OWN TIME

4. Whenever you have the option of standing up or sitting down to do a chore—whether it's opening the mail, peeling potatoes, or writing checks—opt for upright.

5. When you arrive for an appointment and find that you'll need to wait, don't plop into a chair. Instead, stroll around the block, down the hall, or however far time permits.

6. Practice intentional inefficiency. For example, if you need to carry a couple of boxes from your car to the house, make separate trips, even if you could easily do it in one.

Plugged-In Perils

It's not only wireless electronics that pose health risks. Spending too much time at any kind of computer can take a big toll on your physical, mental, *and* emotional well-being. For starters, typing on a keyboard and sliding a mouse around for hours on end often lead to repetitive stress injuries, like carpal tunnel syndrome (CTS). Furthermore, sitting at a computer desk for long periods is all but begging for back problems. (For the scoop on treating backaches, see Save Your Spine from Back and Neck Pain! on page 183.) Last, but not least, experts predict that by 2020, 1 in 3 people will be nearsighted, thanks to time spent staring at computer screens.

92.5%
of scientific studies confirmed that **cell-phone radiation** exposure creates imbalances that are known to cause **cancer**.

3 Diabolical Dangers of Computer Addiction

Too many hours at the computer can be just as damaging—if not more so—to your mental and emotional health than it is to your body. Here's a sampling of the wreckage that can occur in your life if you become hooked on your beloved screen:

Danger #1: Damaged relationships. As die-hard users spend more and more time at the keyboard, they withdraw from family and friends and avoid social gatherings. Eventually, relationships wither, and marriages often fail.

Danger #2: Trouble at work. The combo of late nights on the computer at home and personal computer use at work can lead to impaired performance and job loss.

Danger #3: Altered reality. In extreme cases, users withdraw into an artificial world where their emotions center on events in computer

2 More Wired Woes ⬇

Excessive computer use plays right into two of the major health problems we discuss in this chapter:

▶ Late-night keyboard sessions cut into much-needed sleep time.

▶ All those sedentary hours make you a sitting duck for all-too-real sitting disease.

games and warped sexuality on pornography sites. People whose best "pals" are screen names in online chat rooms can become all but inept at face-to-face communication. In short, they let their electronic existence override their human one, and that opens the door to a whole host of mental and physical complications.

YIKES! Computer-game addiction appears to be reaching epidemic proportions in parts of Asia. In both South Korea and China, people have actually died after playing games nonstop for several days. Both countries have established special counseling centers to handle gaming addictions, and China has enacted strict laws limiting access to Internet cafés.

The Terrors of Texting

When you send or receive a text message, there is an initial burst of radiation, but after that, it becomes less intense than it is during a phone conversation. That makes texting somewhat safer than talking on a cell phone (unless you're driving, of course, in which case the hazard is multiplied enormously), but you still need to keep your phone as far away from your body as possible to avoid potentially deadly damage.

Dying for Beauty

➡ It's only natural to want to look your best. But there's a good chance that some of the products or procedures you're using to achieve that end, from skin treatments to nail care, could be undermining your health—or even putting your life at risk.

A Killer Cosmetic

Since Botox® first appeared on the cosmetic scene in 1989, tens of millions of people have shelled out anywhere from a few hundred dollars to $1,000 a pop for injections that temporarily erase facial lines without the potent dangers of plastic surgery. But are Botox and recent copycat products truly safe alternatives? Not by a long shot! In technical terms, Botox is a neurotoxin—a killer of nerve cells. It's made from the botulinum toxin, the same bacterium that causes botulism. Although it's lethal in large doses or when administered improperly, in smaller quantities, injected by an expert (preferably a cosmetic surgeon), botulinum won't kill you. It merely paralyzes the nerve endings in your face, immobilizing the muscles that make you frown, squint, or smile. Your face remains essentially frozen, so it's unable to create lines and crow's-feet. The results last for three to six months. Then you'll need another treatment to keep life's souvenirs at bay.

NOTE: *The FDA recently approved two other products, Dysport® and Xeomin®, that work the same way as Botox. But, like Kleenex® and Vaseline®, the big B brand has become so familiar that it's almost universally used as a generic term.*

There have been **16** recorded **deaths** resulting from **Botox**® treatments.

The Hidden Horrors of Vanity

Each year, Americans spend more than $10 billion on cosmetic surgery procedures, ranging from eye tucks and nose bobs to liposuction, breast augmentation, and full-blown face-lifts. But when you choose to go under the knife for the sake of improving your looks, you're not only putting a dent in your bank account—you're also leaving yourself wide open to the same dangers you'd face in other kinds of surgery. These are just some of the possible, and sometimes fatal, complications:

- Blood clots
- Brain damage or stroke
- Heart attack
- Infection at the incision site
- Nerve damage
- Permanent scarring
- Pneumonia
- Serious bleeding

Just Say, "No Way!"

If you smoke, do yourself a favor, and don't even think of having cosmetic surgery! Not only will you be at higher risk for complications, but your body will also take longer to heal. Obese folks, those who have diabetes, and those with a history of cardiovascular or lung disease are also more apt to suffer major adverse side effects of surgery.

The Nasty Not-So-Fine Print

Aside from shelling out a pretty penny for Botox or similar products, regular users wind up resembling zombies in old-time horror movies. But, unfortunately, those are far from the worst possible side effects of these wrinkle removers. Even the Botox website cautions that in some cases the botulinum toxin may stray beyond the injection site and cause symptoms of botulism, including these:

- Blurred vision, double vision, and drooping eyelids
- Hoarseness or change or loss of voice
- Loss of bladder control
- Muscle weakness and loss of strength throughout the body
- Trouble breathing or swallowing
- Trouble enunciating clearly

CALL 911

If you've had Botox injections, and you experience any signs of botulism—which could appear at any time within hours or weeks after treatment—hightail it to the ER *immediately*! (see "The Nasty Not-So-Fine Print," above). Likewise, if you start wheezing or launch into an asthma attack (other possible reactions to the botulinum toxin), get medical help pronto.

Other Menacing Side Effects

Chances are that a shot or two of Botox or its kin will not give you botulism. Most likely, the physical price you'll pay for trying to trick Father Time will come in the form of nonlethal issues, such as pain at the injection site, skin rashes, dry mouth, tiredness, headache, neck pain, and eye problems ranging from dry eyes or swollen eyelids to (according to some reports) glaucoma.

Who Needs It?!

You say you'd just as soon not go through all that discomfort and potential danger for the sake of ditching a few signs of experience? I don't blame you! Fortunately, there are plenty of safer, cheaper, and longer-lasting ways to make your skin smoother and younger looking. Here's a quartet of the best and simplest:

Use a cream or lotion. Choose one containing alpha-hydroxy acids (AHAs). These natural substances, which come from fruit, milk, and

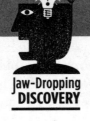
sugarcane, work their magic in two ways: They remove dead cells from the surface of your skin, and they boost the growth of collagen, which fills in wrinkles. **NOTE:** *Although AHAs are harmless, they can irritate your skin, so test the product on a small area. If it hasn't turned red by the next day, you're good to go.*

Hit high C. Pack your diet with fruits and vegetables that deliver megadoses of vitamin C, and for good measure, use a face cream that contains at least 5 percent vitamin C. It boosts collagen production and, according to recent research, can help minimize signs of aging after six months of use.

Exercise daily. Aim for 20 to 30 minutes of activity every day, or as close to it as you can (a brisk walk is perfect). It'll send nourishing, beautifying blood and oxygen flowing to the capillaries in your face and throughout your body.

Quit smoking! Besides destroying your health, smoking damages the capillaries in your skin, which is why smokers develop wrinkles years before nonsmokers do.

1 out of every **500** **"tummy-tuck"** procedures results in **death**.

Get Egg on Your Face

Here's another easy wrinkle-reducing trick that's a darn sight safer and less painful than either going under the knife or getting "shot" in the face: Let an egg warm up to room temperature, separate it, and whip the white just enough to make it easily spreadable. Then smooth it over your face, and lie down (with no pillow under your head) for 15 to 20 minutes. As the egg white hardens, it'll pull your skin back, just as a plastic surgeon would do in a face-lift. When the mask has hardened completely, rinse your face with cool water. (Whatever you do, don't perform this maneuver sitting up, or gravity will drag the egg whites down and take your skin with it!)

Screen Out Wrinkles

We hear it over and over again, but it bears repeating: Always apply sunscreen to your face, neck, and other exposed skin before you go outdoors. But when you do, keep these two guidelines in mind:

- To achieve optimal protection, choose a product with a sun protection factor (SPF) that's between 30 and 50.

- Always buy sunscreen labeled "full-spectrum," which means it's been proven to protect against both UVB rays, which burn your skin and increase your risk for skin cancer, and UVA rays, which damage collagen and accelerate the aging process.

A Grape Way to Smooth Your Skin

Anti-wrinkle routines don't come any simpler than this one: Every day, slice a few green, seedless grapes (preferably organic) in half. Crush them slightly, and rub the cut sides over your face, paying attention to the lines in your forehead and around your eyes and mouth. Leave the pulp and juice on your skin for 20 minutes, then rinse gently and follow up with a good moisturizer. The secret to success: Grapes contain a potent load of the same AHAs found in expensive facial creams. And, unlike many commercial products, this treatment will not irritate sensitive skin.

Fix-It-Fast FORMULA

A Honey of a Wrinkle Reducer

Let's face it: Nothing can make you look 25— or even 45—forever. But this mask has been known to keep women's skin looking soft, smooth, and firm well into their senior years.

2 tbsp. of heavy cream
1 tbsp. of raw honey
400 IUs of vitamin E oil*

Pour the ingredients into a bowl, and stir until the mixture has a smooth, creamy consistency. Spread it onto your face and neck, and go about your business for at least 30 minutes—the longer, the better. (The mask takes just seconds to dry, and you won't even notice it's there.) Rinse it off with lukewarm water, and pat dry. Repeat every day, or as close to it as you can, storing any leftover formula in the refrigerator. Before long, your friends will be demanding to know where you discovered the Fountain of Youth!

* Or substitute the contents of one capsule.

3 Sobering Sunscreen Additives

The jury is still out on how damaging chemical-based sunscreens really are, but with scads of highly effective natural products on the market, why take chances? These three culprits have been shown to be especially damaging to your health and your looks. (And the higher the SPF is, the more chemicals a product contains.)

1. Oxybenzone. This is an active ingredient in most commercial sunscreens. It can cause skin irritation and allergies, and (worse) it reacts with UV rays to create cell-damaging free radicals, which are linked to hormone disruption and increased cancer risk.

2. Parabens. These are synthetic preservatives that disrupt hormones and may stimulate cancerous tumors. In small quantities, they pose little or no risk. The problem is that they're used in so many beauty and personal-care products, including deodorants, shampoos, shaving creams, makeup, and sunscreens, that you can give yourself a dangerous dose without knowing it. Fortunately, they're easy to spot because they generally appear last on ingredient lists. Look for methylparaben, propylparaben, and/or butylparaben.

3. Retinyl palmitate (a.k.a. vitamin A). When exposed to UV rays, it breaks down into toxic free radicals, causing premature aging and raising cancer risk.

Shades of Loveliness

REMARKABLE REMEDY

Whenever you go outdoors in the daytime, even in overcast weather, wear dark sunglasses—the bigger and darker the better. When Ol' Sol is shining, the lenses will prevent you from squinting. In dimmer weather, they'll protect your skin from wrinkle-causing rays, which float through the atmosphere even when you can't see the sun. (Just make sure you get glasses that are guaranteed to block 100 percent of the sun's UV rays.) At worst, the shades will help fend off more lines than you have now. And if you're only starting to develop crow's-feet, they just may vanish after several months of consistently wearing your eye gear.

Nail Salon Nightmares

Most of us assume that getting a professional manicure or pedicure is a terrific way to indulge in some feel-good fun. But here's the shocking truth: If the salon you choose isn't spotlessly clean and hygienic—

and many are not—your relaxing, beautifying treat could turn into big-time trouble. Here are four freaky horrors that may be lingering in even the fanciest-looking salon or spa:

Horror #1: H1N1 virus (a.k.a. swine flu). Like any other flu virus, it attacks when you make contact with someone who has it, or with a surface he or she has coughed on, sneezed on, or touched with a germ-laden hand. The difference is that, because H1N1 is fairly new, most people have no immunity to it.

Skin Cancer Alert!

A new study at Georgia Regents University shows that regular visits to the nail salon could increase your risk for skin cancer as a result of the UVA rays emitted by the drying lamps. While an occasional treatment isn't likely to cause harm, researchers recommend using a full-spectrum sunscreen or wearing UVA-protective gloves that leave only your nails exposed. Either precaution will help reduce any cancer danger and prevent signs of premature skin aging.

Horror #2: MRSA. This staph infection can lead to severe scarring, amputation, and even death. And it's resistant to all known antibiotics. Although it's not common, it is known to spread in nail salons through improperly sanitized tools and soaking vessels.

Horror #3: *Mycobacterium fortuitum*. It produces large boils and/or open sores on toes, feet, or legs. The wounds can be lanced by a doctor and treated with potent antibiotics, but may cause permanent, heavy scarring.

Horror #4: Hepatitis. Both the B and C strains of this vicious virus are on the rise in nail *and* hair salons. The cause: sloppy hygiene practices that leave tiny specs of infected blood on razors, nail clippers, cuticle sticks, and other implements.

Nails *Not* to Die For

Fortunately, you can enjoy attractive finger- and toenails without risking life and limb to get them. Here's a fistful of simple precautions you can take:

- Make sure the salon is fully licensed and that the aestheticians' licenses are posted.
- Look for a UV sterilizer tool that disinfects all instruments.

- Ask the manager or a technician to describe the shop's general hygiene practices. Between uses, all workstation surfaces and soaking vessels should be thoroughly sterilized with disinfectants labeled "germicidal."

- Go the extra mile, and take your own tools, soaking bowl, and/or foot basin (or plastic liner) to the shop.

- Before the procedure begins, ask the technician whether she's washed her hands after working on her previous client. If the answer is no, say, "Do it now, please."

75% of nail salons do not comply with local hygiene regulations.

2 Noxious Nuisances

Aside from the fearsome foursome listed on page 33, unsanitary nail salons frequently hand out two less serious, but still highly unwelcome, "souvenirs." Both athlete's foot (a.k.a. the tinea pedis fungus) and warts (caused by the human papillomavirus) can spread like crazy when infected folks stroll in for manicures or pedicures.

4 Wily Ways to Bar the Door on Germs

Bacteria, fungi, and viruses can weasel their way into your body through even the teeniest-tiniest entryways. For that reason, even if your chosen salon meets the highest hygienic standards, don't take chances. Lock the doors using these four no-fail defenses:

1. If you have any open cuts, cracks, scratches, bug bites, or rashes—no matter how small—on your hands or feet, postpone your appointment until after they've healed.

2. Wait at least 24 hours after shaving, waxing, or using a hair-removal cream on your legs before getting a pedicure.

3. Nix fake nails. They can lift up from the base of your natural nail, providing a dandy entry point for dangerous germs.

4. Never let anyone cut into your skin, using either a cuticle clipper or a credo blade (which many salons use to remove calluses, even though it's illegal in most states).

2

Malevolent Matters of Mind

Until not so long ago, the medical community assumed that mental problems and physical problems were separate deals altogether, and doctors treated their patients accordingly. Well now we, and they (at least a great many of them), know better. For better *and* for worse, your brain and your body work as a single, intertwined, and highly sophisticated unit. Yes, that means your thoughts and feelings can literally make you sick—or even kill you. On the other hand, if you play your cards right, your marvelous, miraculous mind can help you fend off, recover from, or lessen the effects of almost any physical ailment you can name.

Toxic Tension—The Agony of Anxiety

➲ Everyone feels tense, nervous, or fearful from time to time—for example, when you're facing surgery or you're preparing for a cross-country move after decades in your family home. But if you have a constant feeling of dread, you panic every time the phone rings, or you're so tense that you often break out in a cold sweat, then you've moved from everyday nervous tension to the hair-raising realm of anxiety. And left untreated, it can lead to depression and chronic stress, with all their potentially lethal health consequences.

Worry or Anxiety? The Devil Is in the Details

Not sure whether you've got a genuine anxiety disorder, or you're simply as worried as all get-out? Here's how to tell for sure:

Worry is a natural response to any distressing situation, say, when your child has a serious illness, or your company is set to downsize and your job could be on the chopping block.

Anxiety, on the other hand, generally stems from what folks used to call "borrowed trouble." Anxious people are forever fretting about disasters that may never happen and imagining worst-case scenarios in all their gory detail.

GADzooks!

Generalized anxiety disorder (GAD) is by far the most common type of anxiety. Fortunately, it is also the most responsive to the kind of gentle, natural treatments presented in this chapter—in conjunction with care from a doctor or natural-health-care pro. Here are four clues that you've got GAD:

1. You're constantly worried, impatient, irritable, and restless.

2. You have difficulty sleeping.

3. Your nonstop fretting is giving you physical woes, such as headaches, indigestion, and muscle pain or tightness.

4. Your relationships are suffering because your family and friends are getting fed up with your incessant bellyaching.

CALL 911

Physical signs of anxiety often include chest pressure, tightness or heaviness in the throat, headaches, and shortness of breath. But if you experience chest discomfort and/or shortness of breath accompanied by nausea or sweating, you may be having a heart attack—so call 911 pronto!

The Deadly Drug Dilemma

The most commonly prescribed anti-anxiety drugs are in the benzodiazepine class, which includes such brand names as Ativan®, Klonopin®, Valium®, and Xanax®. Because they work quickly—typically providing relief within 30 to 60 minutes—they can literally save your life when they're taken during a panic attack or other dangerous situation. But continued over time, they can produce dire, even fatal, consequences. The reason: These meds reduce brain activity. Even low doses can make people feel so foggy and sleepy that they have trouble functioning at work, at school, or behind the wheel of a car. And, of course, the higher the dose, the more serious any problems are likely to be.

10 Appalling Effects of Anti-Anxiety Drugs

Benzodiazepine drugs are metabolized slowly, so over time they build up in the body. Oversedated people often look—and act—as if they're drunk. Call your doctor immediately if you experience any of these common side effects:

- Blurred or double vision
- Clumsiness and slowed reflexes
- Confusion and disorientation
- Depression and suicidal urges
- Dizziness and light-headedness
- Forgetfulness and memory loss
- Impaired thinking and judgment
- Indigestion and nausea
- Sexual dysfunction
- Slurred speech

Research shows that at least 25 percent of people whose doctors prescribe anti-anxiety drugs have not been diagnosed with any type of anxiety disorder. Rather, these folks are given the meds simply to help them sleep better or to suppress general mood issues. This fact is especially alarming given the results of a seven-year study by the University of Warwick in England, recently published in the *British Medical Journal*. It found that participants who took anti-anxiety medications such as Valium and Xanax or the sleep aids Ambien®, Lunesta®, and Sonata® were more than twice as likely as members of the nondrugged control group to die prematurely during the study.

Benzodiazepines Can Backfire—Big-Time!

Sometimes anti-anxiety meds perform exactly the opposite of what they're supposed to do. Medical pros refer to these "Whoops!" occurrences as "paradoxical effects." The most common ones are increased anxiety, irritability, and agitation. But some folks experience dangerous reactions, including aggressive or impulsive behavior, hallucinations, hostility and rage, and manic episodes. Fortunately, these severe effects are rare and most often occur in children, the elderly, and people with developmental disabilities.

Anti-anxiety drugs may double your **risk** for **premature death**.

Fish for Anxiety Relief

Did you know that watching fish swim around in a home aquarium is every bit as effective as biofeedback and meditation for easing anxiety and stress and lowering blood pressure? It's true—at least according to researchers at the University of Pennsylvania's Center for the Interaction of Animals and Society. So what are you waiting for? Put a few goldfish or guppies in a tank, pull up an easy chair, and feel your jitters float away!

4 Fundamentals for Fending Off Anxiety

Coming up, you'll find an arsenal of amazing anxiety-axing remedies that carry no adverse side effects whatsoever. But tapping into that bag of tricks won't get you very far unless you also heed your body's need for these four essentials:

1. Fresh air and exercise

2. Good, wholesome food

3. High-quality sleep

4. Plenty of pure, clean water

By paying attention to these bottom-line basics (as Mom always told you to do), you'll relieve anxiety at its root by reducing stress hormones in your body and raising your levels of such soothing brain chemicals as serotonin and gamma-aminobutyric acid (GABA).

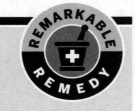

Oniony Tension Tamer

Believe it or not—as bizarre as it sounds—this simple topical treatment works like a charm to eliminate nervous anxiety: Grate a large raw onion, and divide the gratings between two pieces of gauze or cheesecloth about 12 inches square. Fold the sides over to form pouches. Then sit back in a chair, prop your legs up, and place a poultice under each calf. Relax for 30 minutes or so, and you'll feel your tension drain away.

The Myth of Mellow Yellow

Myth: Painting your walls yellow gives you a cheery environment in which to relax and cast off your anxiety and tension.

REALITY: According to experts, the color yellow—even in its palest shades—actually activates the anxiety center of your brain. Numerous studies show that because of this nerve-irritating effect, infants cry more in yellow nurseries, couples fight more in yellow kitchens, and divas throw more temper tantrums in yellow dressing rooms.

Anxiety disorders are the most **common** form of **mental illness** in the U.S.

Calm Down with Color

If you want to create an atmosphere—indoors or out—that will *really* set your mind and spirit at ease, keep these rules of physics in mind:

- The colors of water—such as blue, violet, mauve, and green—make you feel calm and relaxed.

- A room, or an outdoor living space, with a limited color palette (especially white with one or two pastels) imparts peace and restfulness.

- Conversely, an area that features walls and furnishings (or flowers) in a Joseph's-coat mixture of colors can send your stress and anxiety into overdrive, no matter how visually attractive the technicolor decor may be to you.

3 Foolproof Fret Fixes

Anxiety relievers don't come any easier—or safer—than this terrific trio of tips:

1. Pinch your fingers. Grab a handful of clip-type clothespins. Attach one to each fingertip on your left hand, so that they're pressing down on your nails, and leave them in place for seven minutes. Then repeat the process on your right hand. The pressure exerted on the nerve endings will relax your whole nervous system. Perform this routine as needed, first thing in the morning and before, during, or immediately after any especially tense situation.

2. Serve yourself some seaweed. Kombu (available in health-food stores and Asian markets) is a type of seaweed that has a remarkable ability to calm tense nerves. All you need to do is put a 3-inch strip of the stuff in a quart of water, boil it for 10 minutes, and then strain it into a heat-proof container. Drink ½ cup of the tea at a time, either warmed up or at room temperature, throughout the day.

3. Take a stroll on a beach. If that's not possible, just turn on a sink faucet in your kitchen or bathroom. Better yet, install a simple foun-

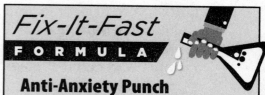

Fix-It-Fast
FORMULA

Anti-Anxiety Punch

Whether you're battling chronic anxiety, or your stress level is soaring toward the stratosphere, this relaxing (and tasty) beverage can help calm your turbulence.

10 raw almonds

Water

1 cup of warm milk

1 pinch of ginger

1 pinch of nutmeg

Put the almonds in a bowl with enough water to cover them, and let them soak for six to eight hours. Then liquefy them in a blender with the milk and spices, and drink the potion just before you go to bed. It should help you sleep soundly and wake up ready to face the day on a more even keel.

tain on your deck or in your living room. (You can find both indoor and outdoor versions, in all price ranges, online and in many garden centers.) It's long been known that listening to the sound of waves or running water almost magically reduces anxiety and stress.

A Kooky Cukey Crutch to Keep Your Cool

Studies have shown that the scent of cucumbers helps you calm down during tense situations. So the next time you're anticipating a stressful experience—say, a job interview, medical tests, or a speech that you have to give—wash your hair with cuke-scented shampoo. Then, so you'll have calming help at the ready, put a dab of the shampoo on a cotton ball or a piece of cloth, and take it with you.

25% of the **people taking** potentially dangerous anti-anxiety **drugs don't need them**.

Incredible Calming Cream

As weird and wacky as it sounds, this potent, penetrating, but oh-so-gentle cream can send your anxiety level plummeting—with none of the dangerous side effects of prescription drugs. Here's how to make it in four simple steps:

Step 1. Round up ½ cup of wheat germ oil, 1 ounce of beeswax, ¼ cup of unflavored yogurt, four 400 IU vitamin E capsules, and 10 drops of juniper essential oil. You'll also need a double boiler, a blender, and a glass jar with a tight-fitting lid.

Step 2. Heat the wheat germ oil and beeswax in the top of a double boiler until the wax melts, but the mixture is still cool enough to touch. (Don't let it get too hot, or you'll damage the healing compounds in the oil.)

Step 3. Put the yogurt and vitamin E oil (squeezed from the capsules) in the blender, and turn it on its lowest setting. With the motor running, slowly pour in the warm wax and oil mixture, and add the juniper oil. Continue blending until you've got a smooth cream.

Step 4. Pour the cream into the jar, and let it cool to room temperature before putting the lid on. Store it in the refrigerator, where it will keep for about 30 days.

Several times a day, rub the cream onto your hands to keep stress away.

All Stressed Out

→ **What's that? You say your long work hours, traffic-clogged commute, a 24-hour stream of distressing news, and a mile-long to-do list have you climbing the walls? Welcome to the 21st century! So start finding ways to ease your stress load now, because this inescapable bugaboo of modern life has been proven to cause or complicate just about every physical and mental health problem you can name.**

Fight-or-Flight Can Be Fatal

During any stressful situation, your body reacts in three ways:

1. Your endocrine system churns out a stream of hormones with such tongue-twisting names as epinephrine, norepinephrine, and adrenocortico-tropic hormone (ACTH).

2. As these hormone levels rise, your blood pressure and heart rate climb, and more cholesterol is released into your bloodstream.

3. Once the stressful event has passed, your internal system returns to normal.

This automatic reaction—commonly referred to as the fight-or-flight response—was essential for our ancient ancestors, who had to either battle or run away from bears, boars, and saber-toothed tigers on a regular basis. Those hormonal outpourings are just as valuable to us when we need to handle genuine emergencies, such as auto accidents, physical attacks, and natural disasters. But when the fight-or-flight

A Couple of Bum Raps

While it is true that stress triggers more than its fair share of health problems, it is commonly blamed for two woes for which it is *not* responsible:

Inflammatory bowel disease (IBD). This is a term used to describe several disorders, including Crohn's disease and ulcerative colitis. The jury is still out on the exact cause, but it is not stress, anxiety, or any other psychological problem. Researchers say that, most likely, the culprit is a virus or bacteria that trigger a reaction in the immune system, causing the intestines to become red and swollen.

Ulcers. These infamous pains in the belly are brought on by the *Helicobacter* bacterium, not—as assumed for decades by doctors and sufferers alike—by stress, anxiety, or a hard-charging type A lifestyle. Having said that, it *is* true that stress can intensify your pain and/or hinder the healing process.

response becomes a constant fact of life, whether it's needed or not, your body stays in red-alert mode for prolonged periods of time. And your health suffers, too—big-time!

The Wily Ways of Chronic Stress

Your **heart attack risk triples** within 2 hours of a very **stressful** event.

Long-term stress works its vile deeds in two ways:

Constant surges in blood pressure and cholesterol damage blood vessels and greatly increase your risk for heart disease.

The overload of stress hormones damages your immune system, thereby hindering your ability to fend off and recover from all kinds of diseases. It causes, contributes to, or worsens health problems, ranging from acid reflux and backaches to insomnia, psoriasis, and stroke. It also aggravates allergic reactions and makes your skin age faster.

2 Hairy Tales about Hair Loss

Tale #1: Stress and worry make your hair turn gray.
FALSE! Pigment-producing cells called melanocytes are genetically programmed to stop manufacturing hair pigment when you reach a certain age, and there's not a blasted thing that any of your emotions have to do with it.

Tale #2: Stress can make your hair fall out.
TRUE! Both chronic stress and specific stressful events, such as childbirth or a death in the family, can trigger the loss of hair—sometimes as much as 70 percent of your "crop." The good news is that in nearly all cases, your mane will grow back once you've fully recovered from the experience.

A Messy, Stressy Mouthful of Maladies

Chronic stress can take an especially large toll on your teeth and gums. For starters, when you're operating under a constant state of pressure, it's all too easy to ignore two crucial elements of oral health: a good diet and proper dental hygiene. Those factors and other effects of stress can lead to more problems, including this quartet:

- Canker and cold sores
- Clenching or grinding your teeth
- Chewing your nails, ice cubes, pencils, or other objects
- Periodontal disease

The Tense Truth about Exercise and Stress

Common assumption: Folks who run marathons, climb mountains, or hit the golf links and tennis courts on a regular basis are cleaning stress clear out of their lives.

FACT: While it is true that exercise is a top-tier de-stressor—and absolutely essential for good health—in some cases, it can actually raise stress to dangerously high levels. That's because for many people, engaging in competitive sports or goal-oriented recreational pursuits activates their "inner cavemen," who, by necessity, viewed life as an ongoing battle in a hostile, winner-take-all world. When these folks lose a match or fall short of whatever performance standards they've set for themselves, the "defeat" generates frustration, raises their blood pressure, and produces all the other ill effects of stress.

NOTE: *If you have a naturally competitive personality, make sure that you balance your sporting endeavors with plenty of noncompetitive stress-reducing techniques, tonics, and toddies.*

10 Sobering Signals That You're Sinking Fast

Stress overload can reveal itself in a myriad of ways that vary greatly from one individual to another. But if you're experiencing several of these symptoms, it's a good bet that you're stressed to the breaking point and you need to mend your ways—*NOW*!

1. Change in appetite (either heightened or lowered)
2. Digestive problems
3. Dry heaves or vomiting
4. Frequent headaches
5. Inability to concentrate or make decisions
6. Inability to cope with even minor setbacks
7. Increased susceptibility to colds and flu
8. Rapid breathing
9. Sleeping problems
10. Tingling in your hands and feet

80% of doctors' **patients** have **stress**-related symptoms.

Fix-It-Fast FORMULA

De-Stressing Bath Blend

The next time you feel your stress level rising, take it sitting down—in a bathtub filled with this calming combo.

4 cups of dry whole-milk powder

2 cups of cornstarch

4 or 5 drops of your favorite essential oil*

Mix all of the ingredients in a blender or food processor. When it's time to unwind, add ½ cup of the mixture to hot bathwater, sink into the tub, and relax. Store the remaining blend in an airtight container at room temperature. (The recipe makes enough for about 12 baths.)

* Geranium, jasmine, lavender, orange, and vanilla are all good stress-busting choices.

A Trio of Triple-Treat Calming Champs

No matter what's pushing your stress buttons, any of these three unlikely sounding helpers can calm you down in a hurry. What's more, it'll also lift your spirits and boost your energy at the same time.

Cayenne pepper. Start by drinking ⅛ teaspoon of the pepper in 8 ounces of warm water once a day. Stick with that dosage until you've gotten used to its firepower, then increase the amount of pepper to ¼ teaspoon, then ½ teaspoon. Continue this "drinking habit" until your stress level goes down.

Coconut oil. Put a few drops on your fingertips and massage it onto your forehead and temples using circular motions. The soothing aroma of the oil combined with the gentle pressure of your fingertips will have you feeling better in no time at all.

Eucalyptus oil. Simply mix 15 to 20 drops of eucalyptus oil per ounce of distilled water in a plastic spray bottle, and mist yourself whenever you're feeling anxious, down, or stressed out.

Sock It to Stress

Looking for stress relief? It's in your sock drawer. At least it can be if you try this terrific trick: Mix up equal parts of dried lavender, dried rosemary, and broken cinnamon sticks, all of which have aromas that are highly effective at lowering stress levels. Stuff a handful or so of the mixture into a clean sock until you have a lump that's about the size of a baseball, and tie the top closed with yarn or ribbon. Then anytime you feel on edge, repeatedly squeeze the ball to release a blast of calming scent. And if you keep your stress buster in your sock drawer, it'll remind you to start off every morning on an easygoing foot!

You Can't Fool Mother Nature!

Jaw-Dropping DISCOVERY

In a recent study at the University of Washington, researchers had volunteers perform mildly stressful tasks for 40 minutes in two *almost* identical office settings. The only difference: One had a window overlooking a pleasant grassy area with trees and a fountain. In the other work space, the window was fitted with a 50-inch plasma-screen HDTV showing the same bucolic scene.

The researchers recorded the subjects' heart rates before, during, and after each task. They also noted when each worker looked out the window, at the screen, or at a wall. The result: The folks who had the real deal to gaze upon recovered from their stress faster—and the more time they spent looking at the view, the more quickly their heart rates dropped to normal. Meanwhile, the pretty picture on the screen had no effect whatsoever on anyone's stress level. Heart rates of volunteers in the TV room fell at the same slower pace whether they looked at the screen or at a blank wall.

5 Effortless Ways to Up Your Outdoor Time

You don't have to visit a nature preserve or take a hike in the woods to lower your stress level. Simply spending time outdoors—anywhere, at any time, doing anything (or nothing) will do the trick. You say that sounds nice, but your busy schedule just doesn't allow it? Poppycock! Weather permitting, lots of activities that you perform

Can the Cantankerous Clutter

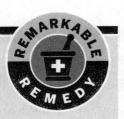

If there is any doubt in your mind that clutter is a major contributor to stress and tension, just think of the gazillion books, magazine articles, and websites devoted to the subject. There are even scads of professional organizers whose full-time job is helping folks de-clutter their homes and offices. You can get detailed advice from any of those sources, but the essence of making and keeping your surroundings clutter-free is to follow this single simple guideline with every object you own: If you don't need it, love it, and/or use it, get rid of it.

The same goes for your jam-packed to-do list. Keep the real essentials and the things you love to do, but weed out the marginal stuff. Your mind and your body will thank you!

in your house or office every day can be done just as well on a deck, porch, patio, or park bench. Here's a handful of examples:

- Complete your regular exercise or yoga routine.
- Eat meals or snacks.
- Pay bills, check e-mail, or cruise the Internet on your laptop.
- Read books, the newspaper, or work materials.
- Return calls on your cell phone.

You get the idea. Now go out and do it!

Clutter Kills

Well, not directly. But it does send your stress-hormone producers into overdrive, and, as we've seen throughout this chapter, that can do you in fast. Need more convincing that it's time to go on a lifesaving sorting spree? Then consider these half-dozen horrific ways that clutter clobbers your mind and, in turn, your body:

1. It bombards your brain with excessive stimuli, forcing your senses to work overtime and often disturbing your health-giving sleep.

2. It distracts you from things that you need to focus on.

3. It makes it harder to relax, both mentally and physically.

4. It constantly whispers to your subconscious that your work is never—and can never be—done.

5. It triggers feelings of guilt and embarrassment, especially when unexpected visitors drop by your home or office.

6. It sends your frustration skyrocketing when things such as keys, bills, or important documents get buried in piles of junk.

Fix It or Forget It

Whenever you find yourself in a spot that's sending you into a frenzy, ask yourself these four questions:

1. Is this issue really important to me?

2. Would a reasonable person be this upset?

3. Is there anything I can do to change the matter?

4. Would the fix be worth the time, energy, and possibly money it would cost?

If the answer to all four questions is yes, then leap into action, whether that means challenging your boss about a major work issue, demanding that your teenager start keeping more regular hours, or telling your philandering spouse to shape up or ship out. On the other hand, if you responded no one or more times, then it's best to simply ride out the situation.

Stress can trigger the **loss** of up to **70% of your hair**.

'Tis the Season to Be SAD

➡ No one is quite sure why some folks are troubled by seasonal affective disorder (SAD) while others are not, but we do know what triggers it: The absence of light during winter's gray days and long nights causes the pineal gland in your brain to turn the hormone serotonin into melatonin. This reduction in serotonin makes the chilly months miserable—and if you don't face the problem head on, the symptoms can lead to major trouble down the road.

5 Sinister Signs of SAD

For many folks, SAD, a.k.a. winter depression, is far more serious than a simple case of cold-weather blahs. Like any other type of depression, it can affect your whole life and well-being. Symptoms vary greatly in their intensity from one person to another, but these are the most common signs that SAD has struck:

- Craving for sweets and starches
- Depression
- Intense desire to hibernate
- Permanent jet-lagged feeling
- Sleep disturbances

Here Comes the Sun!

Even many folks who don't suffer from SAD find it hard waking up on dark winter mornings. The simple solution: Get what's called a dawn simulator (available from catalogs and online). Essentially it's a lamp that increases its glow gradually from dim to more intense light, mimicking a natural sunrise in mid-May. All you do is program the show to begin one to three hours before wake-up time, and your body detects the increasing light through your closed eyelids.

NOTE: *At any time of the year, this gentle wake-up call can be a lot more pleasant than a buzzing alarm clock!*

SAD affects **half a million** people **every winter**.

3 Simple SAD Solutions

A few of the most effective ways to turn your SAD woes into glad wows are also the easiest—namely these:

Flee your cave. Force yourself to get outdoors for part of every day, even on dim, overcast days. Exposure to the sun's rays ups your levels of vitamin D, which in turn increases your serotonin supply.

NOTE: *Even during the darkest downpour, there is 30 times more light outdoors than in.*

Tipple some tea. Whenever you feel a craving for carbohydrates, sip a nice cup of chamomile tea instead. It'll divert your attention from food and give your immune system a boost at the same time.

Tipple some more tea. To curb your overall appetite—and, therefore, avoid packing on pounds—buy a bottle of fennel essential oil at a health-food store or on the Internet. Then before each meal, add two drops of the oil to a cup of warm water, and drink up.

When Sacking SAD Is Not a Solo Project

If your SAD symptoms are so severe that they're hindering your ability to function through the winter, don't rely on home remedies alone. Ask your doctor to refer you to a psychiatrist or psychologist who can evaluate your condition and recommend medication if it's necessary.

Feeling Blue? Think Orange!

Orange essential oil has an almost magical knack for lifting low spirits. Here's a sampling of ways you can put it to work for you:

- Add a few drops of the oil to your favorite hand and body lotions.

- Dab the oil onto a few lightbulbs around your house. (Make sure the bulbs are turned off and cool to the touch.)

- Fill a plastic spray bottle with water and a few drops of orange oil, and spritz the air in your home or office.

- Mix a few drops of orange oil with your dishwashing liquid and household cleansers.

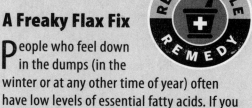

A Freaky Flax Fix

People who feel down in the dumps (in the winter or at any other time of year) often have low levels of essential fatty acids. If you take 1 tablespoon of flaxseed oil once or twice a day during the winter, there's a good chance you'll stop SAD in its tracks.

Whatever you do, never use orange—or any other—essential oil directly on your skin. It can be very irritating.

A BLT to Beat the Blues

No, not the sandwich. In this case, BLT is a remarkably simple, yet highly effective, treatment called broad-spectrum light therapy. All you do is sit in front of a desktop light box equipped with special high-intensity bulbs for a certain period of time each day. The usual R_x is 30 minutes every morning. The timing and length of exposure are highly individual though, so ask your doctor for guidance.

3 out of 4 SAD sufferers **are women**.

Take a Chill Pill

When you don't have a compelling need to be out and about on a cold winter's day—heading to work, for example—it's all too easy to hunker down under a cozy blanket and stay there. Well, don't do it! It'll only make the situation worse. Instead, before any chilly winds begin to blow, plan a passel of pleasant things that'll get you out of the house. If at all possible, take your annual vacation in the winter, and head straight for the sun. But don't stop at that. Make firm commitments with family and friends to attend plays or concerts, go on day or weekend trips, or throw birthday or holiday parties. With fun times to look forward to, you'll breeze through the blue days.

Follow Every Rainbow . . .

Right into your house. How? Simply buy as many full-spectrum lightbulbs as your budget allows, and install them in lamps and ceiling fixtures throughout your home. Because they include all the colors of the rainbow, these bulbs are much more like natural daylight than their ordinary counterparts are, and they'll give a big lift to your mood.

Shake, Shake, Shake

Shake your booty—and lose those dark clouds hanging over your head. If you're not up to joining winter sports lovers on the slopes or frozen ponds, or even taking brisk walks around your neighborhood, head for an indoor skating rink or the warmth and light of your local fitness center. Getting 30 minutes of exercise each day, in whatever form you like (even dancing in your living room!), will keep your system pumping out endorphins that will help you battle the blahs of a long, cold, dark winter. Just be sure to begin your exercise routine while the weather is still mild, so you have habit on your side when the gloomy-doomy season sets in.

Fix-It-Fast FORMULA

Rekindle-Your-Fire Bath

Even in its mildest forms, SAD (like any other type of depression) robs your body of essential electrolytes. So recharge those energizers—and soothe your spirit at the same time—with this terrific tub-time mixer.

2 cups of Epsom salts

2 cups of sea salt

2 tbsp. of potassium

1 tbsp. of vitamin C crystals

Pour all of the ingredients into the tub while the water is running (at a temperature of your choice). Then ease yourself in and soak your troubles away for as long as you like.

Cravings for **starchy** and **sweet** foods are **common** for SAD sufferers.

The Funky Facts about SAD

True or false? SAD only strikes in the wintertime.

FALSE! While SAD commonly peaks from December to February, half a million people experience SAD symptoms starting as early as September and continuing into April. A milder form, the "winter blues," affects even more people.

. . . .

Don't Lose Your Mind

➡ As medical science finds more and more ways to prolong our lives, for nearly all of us, one fear looms ever larger: that our minds will flicker and die long before our physical bodies give out. The good news is that there *are* things you can do to help ensure that your brain stays active and alert your whole life long.

By 2050, **16 million** Americans could have **Alzheimer's disease**.

. . . .

2 Wicked Whoppers about Alzheimer's

Whopper #1: Dementia equals Alzheimer's disease (AD).

THE HIGHLY HOPEFUL TRUTH: Many factors can cause the severe memory loss, confusion, and chronic disorientation that are commonly identified as AD. Furthermore, it is impossible to make a definitive diagnosis of AD in a living person. Only a postmortem biopsy of the brain can detect the clumps and tangled strands of protein (amyloid and tau in medical lingo) that are the slam-dunk indicators of Alzheimer's.

Whopper #2: If you do have AD, you're probably in for an unavoidable downhill slide.

THE HIGHLY HOPEFUL TRUTH: Medical science has found many people who have retained their full, or nearly full, intellectual capacities well into old age—even, in some cases, close to the century mark. Only when these "escapees," as researchers call them, finally died of causes unrelated to their minds did autopsies show that their brains were actually riddled with the unmistakable plaques and shrinkage of Alzheimer's.

The Chat That Could Save Your Life . . .

Or at least your sanity. If you're starting to feel confused, disoriented, or forgetful, and you're taking multiple prescription medications, ask your doctor to join you in some detective work. It could be that the root of the problem is one, or more likely a combination, of the drugs. Cutting back some dosages, or even weaning you off some of the meds entirely, could revive your mental clarity without doing you any physical harm.

4 Secrets to Sidestepping Dementia

Your daily lifestyle can go a long way toward keeping you mentally fit as you enter your senior years. These four factors hold the key to a sane success:

Mental workouts. Stimulate your brain every day by reading, playing word games, engaging in crafts or hobbies, and doing puzzles—especially crosswords. Recent studies show that working crossword puzzles at least four days a week cuts your dementia risk by 47 percent.

 YIKES! If this isn't frightening news, I don't know what is: We are now finding out that in a great many cases, people who die in nursing homes, having been diagnosed with Alzheimer's disease, don't have it—or any other form of dementia. Rather, these folks had been suffering from severe confusion brought on by the multiple drugs they'd been prescribed to take for various physical conditions.

Physical exercise. Physical activity—even if it's a stroll around the block—helps keep blood flowing to your brain and encourages the formation of new brain cells.

Social engagement. People who remain actively connected with friends, family, and colleagues are less likely to succumb to dementia than those who avoid social gatherings or confine their interactions to texting, sending e-mail, or spending hours on social networking sites.

Weight control. Obesity in middle age doubles the odds that you'll develop dementia in later life. (For more on the importance of staying trim—and tips on how to achieve that goal—see Chapter 5, "The Fatal Fat Factor.")

How-To Help for Harried Caregivers

More than 10 million Americans (mostly women) are caring for family members who have dementia—and that's often on top of running busy households and holding down demanding jobs. If you're one of those heroes, you know that it's all too easy to get so caught up in the daily whirlwind that you neglect your own health. Well, don't do it! Remember, if you don't take good care of yourself, you can't do much for anyone else. So consider this section your own personal Tender Loving Tool Kit.

Do what Mom always told you. Eat right, get a good eight hours of sleep each night, don't smoke, and get plenty of fresh air and regular exercise. (If you think you don't possibly have time to work that last item into your day, check out the "Move It!" section, starting on page 142.)

Take a mental health day. Everyone needs a break every now and then. If you work, call in sick. If you're based at home, simply devote the day to yourself—even if that means calling in a substitute caregiver. And what should you do with your very own day?

Whatever you want. Go to a movie or an art exhibit. Take a walk in the park. Curl up on the couch and read a murder mystery. Or simply sit around and do nothing. Then, when stressful moments come up, think back to that quiet time. **NOTE:** *When remembering your mental health day no longer re-energizes you, it's time to take another one!*

Stay connected. Having friends and other supportive people around you is crucial to good mental and physical health. In fact, you may find that being under a lot of strain makes you feel the need to be more social, even if you're the solitary type by nature. According to recent scientific research, stress causes your body to produce a hormone called oxytocin, which promotes a desire to connect with other people. Granted, when you're caught up in a whirlwind of caregiving activity, it's hard to remain socially active. But whether you volunteer in your community, join a bridge club, or become more involved in your church, the lift to your health and spirits will pay off in big dividends for you *and* your loved one.

A Breathtaking Way to Boost Your Brainpower

Numerous studies indicate that inhaling the aroma of cinnamon in any form can enhance your overall brain function and improve both your long- and short-term memory. So what are you waiting for? Try one—or all—of these terrific tricks:

- Bake a batch of spicy cinnamon cookies (or whip up any other cinnamon-rich recipe).

- Toss broken cinnamon sticks into one of your favorite potpourris.

- Dab a spot of cinnamon extract onto a few lightbulbs around your house. (Just make sure the bulbs are turned off and completely cool to the touch before you anoint them!)

50%
of people age
85 and older
have
dementia.

NOTE: *As a bonus, the scent of cinnamon also makes you feel calmer and more relaxed!*

Revealed: The Big Hormone Hoax

If you're a woman heading toward menopause, and you're thinking about—or already are—taking hormone-replacement therapy (HRT) because you've heard that it'll keep your mind sharp, I have two words of advice: Forget it! Numerous studies have found no difference in memory function between postmenopausal women who did or did not use HRT. (If you're feeling mentally muddled, it could just be that all those hot flashes that wake you up at night are making you too tired to think straight.)

Trip the Light Fantastic

REMARKABLE REMEDY

A recent study, published in *The New England Journal of Medicine,* found that regular ballroom dancing—the kind that requires you to move in sync with a partner—can reduce your risk for dementia by 76 percent. That's a greater success rate than that of any other activity studied. So haul out your dancing shoes and cut a rug!

Time to Dial the Doc

It's one thing to forget where you put your keys. But when you look at a bunch of keys and think, "What are these things?" it's time for a thorough medical checkup. Also see a doc in any of these instances:

- You have trouble performing the steps of a familiar task, such as making a pot of coffee.
- You suddenly can't remember where you are or what month it is.
- You've forgotten the names of close friends or family members.

CALL 911

Hightail it to the ER if your memory loss is accompanied by a headache, dizziness, balance problems, or loss of coordination in your hands or feet. These could be signs that you've suffered a stroke or have a brain tumor.

2 Sneaky Strategies to Corral Your Meandering Mind

As you well know if you're of a certain age, there comes a time when it's all too easy to get on a path to distraction and forgetfulness. These two tricks can help you stay on task (as the efficiency gurus like to say):

1. Whenever you're tackling a long project, keep your mind focused by taking a five-minute break every 30 minutes.

2. Never try to do several things at once. Instead, make it a point to finish one task before you start another.

Happiness Is Next to Healthiness!

➡ For decades, science has known that chronic unhappiness contributes mightily to all forms of mental and physical illness. Now medical science is finding that it's not simply the absence of negative emotions that helps us stay well. Happiness itself actually makes people healthier. Happy folks have stronger immune systems, which makes them more resistant to ills ranging from life-threatening cardiac disease to the common cold. They handle stress better, and they're far less likely to suffer from anxiety or depression. Believe it or not, they even have fewer accidents.

The Awful Aura of Unhappiness

No one except a performer in an old MGM musical can possibly go around singing, dancing, and smiling *all* the time. But if you're

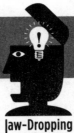
The Born-Happy Humbug

True or false? Happiness is hereditary.
THE ANSWER: True *and* false. Recent research at the University of California, Riverside, suggests that about 50 percent of your capacity for happiness is determined by your genes. Circumstances in your living environment account for another 10 percent. But—and this is the clincher—*you* control the remaining 40 percent. In other words, you have the power to take charge of your outlook on life and create a happier, healthier you!

4 Surprising Secrets of Happy People

Happiness cuts across all occupations, geographic regions, and socioeconomic categories. But invariably, the folks who rank highest on happiness surveys and tests (including those conducted year after year by the famous Pew Research Center) share four common traits:

They read newspapers (yes, actual *printed* newspapers!).

They go to church regularly and are active in their congregations.

They routinely socialize with family and friends (in person—not simply on Facebook or by e-mail).

They accentuate the positive, habitually viewing their personal "glass" as half full rather than half empty.

Go with the Flow

A great many happy, contented people have a major habit in common: They frequently flow. In psychological terms, "flow" is a state in which you're so focused on what you're doing that you become one with the task. Nothing distracts you, and your emotions—whether anger, anxiety, fear, or sorrow—simply vanish. For a lot of folks, running is a flow experience. For others, it may be bird-watching, painting a room, digging a garden bed, or working a jigsaw puzzle. Give it a try. Even if you're already as happy as a clam, flowing is a great way to get some deep-down relaxation after a long week at work or a traffic-clogged drive home!

Boost Your Mood with Random Acts of Kindness

Optimists have **19% longer life** spans than pessimists.

This idea was all the rage a number of years ago, when bumper stickers, buttons, and posters urged us all to get out there and do nice things for strangers—for instance, put a quarter in an expired parking meter before a cop got there, pay a bridge toll for yourself and the car behind you, and so on. Well, guess what? It works just as well now as it did then. Only now it's been proven in scientific studies. But your good deeds don't have to be anonymous. Giving a gift, helping a neighbor, or simply offering someone a sincere compliment makes you *and* the recipient of your kindness happier.

It can be difficult to hear that happiness and health go hand in hand if you are one of the millions of people who suffer from depression. According to the World Health Organization (WHO), depression rates in the United States and other developed countries are skyrocketing. What's more, depression is being fingered as a major contributor to obesity and diabetes, as well as other serious health conditions, including chronic pain and some forms of cancer. Worst of all, as many as 80 percent of depressed people are not getting treatment of any kind.

7 Dastardly Depression Triggers

Unlike a passing case of the blues, clinical depression is caused by chemical changes in the brain. These may be triggered by malfunctioning genes, traumatic events, or a combination of both. Some types of depression run in families. Certain medications, such as steroids, and some medical conditions, including cancer, hormonal imbalances, or chronic pain, can spur the onset of symptoms. So can any of these seven factors:

1. Alcohol or drug abuse
2. Chronic unhappiness
3. Inactivity
4. Insufficient sunlight
5. Nutritional deficiencies
6. Sleeping problems
7. Social isolation

The Depressing Truth about Antidepressants

Every year, American doctors write about 200 million prescriptions for antidepressant drugs such as Paxil®, Prozac®, and Zoloft®. For those who are severely depressed and potentially suicidal, these meds can be literally lifesaving. But four out of five people who are diagnosed with depression have it in a mild or moderate form. And according to a recent study published in *The Journal of the American Medical Association*, for those folks, antidepressants were no more effective than placebos.

For help with depression, visit www.depressionanonymous.org.

Forgive and Flourish

When hurtful or downright nasty things happen to happy people, they don't deny their hurt and anger. They feel it to the core—but then they find a way to release those emotions and feel compassion toward themselves and the perpetrator of the dirty deed. Don't get me wrong! Forgiving does not mean that you condone or excuse the action in question. Nor is it easy. It takes time, honest reflection, and sincere effort, but the reward is a big benefit to your body and soul.

Don't Worry, Be Happy!

Even when you're feeling down in the dumps, it pays to fake it till you make it. As show biz pros have known since Will Shakespeare was a pup—and behavioral scientists have confirmed—if you go around acting as if you're cheerful, positive, and joyful, before long you *will* be. So smile, smile, smile!

Pessimists have a **30% higher** risk for **dementia** than optimists have.

The Shocking Impact of Shaking Hands

Believe it or not, a simple, firm handshake—whether it's with your best pal or a total stranger—can deliver a joyful jolt to your subconscious mind. That's because any friendly human touch activates the reward center in your central nervous system, automatically giving you a cheery lift. A quick hug, a pat on the back, or a kiss on the cheek can perform the same fabulous feat. And the more often you make physical contact with others, the happier you'll be!

4 Steps to Happiness

The first step to achieving real happiness is accepting the fact that no one else can make you happy. Only you can do it. Here's a primer to get you started on that DIY project:

1. Do the things you love. For example, throw dinner parties, plunk out your favorite tunes on the piano, putter in your garden, or simply chill out with a good book.

2. Hang around with happy people. Happiness is contagious. Seek out people who can "infect" you with their joyful outlook on life.

3. Have faith—and live it to the hilt. Establishing a connection with the source of all creation can give you a deep sense of purpose, which is a hallmark of happy—and successful—people. Plus, attending church is a guaranteed way to connect with positive, upbeat folks.

4. Laugh. It releases torrents of feel-good brain chemicals that boost your spirits. Every day, make it a point to share jokes, watch a funny movie, or read a funny story.

A No-Fail Formula for Nixing Negativity

Many moons ago, one of our most masterful songwriters, Johnny Mercer, offered up the surest route to a happy life when he advised us to "Accentuate the positive, eliminate the negative." Easier said than done, you say? Not necessarily. Simply follow this basic guideline: Never engage in a conversation that is neither pleasant nor productive. And how, you ask, can you pull *that* off without moving into a cave? Just use either of these two tactics:

Tactic #1. Let's say you're speaking with a neighbor who starts complaining about litter on the streets. Instead of joining in an "Ain't-it-awful?!" groan fest—or denying that a problem exists—take the comment as a call to action. Say something like, "Yes, it is mushrooming. Let's organize a neighborhood cleanup next weekend."

Tactic #2. In situations where nothing you say will steer the

Hooray for Hugs!

REMARKABLE REMEDY

Looking for a really simple way to make your spirits soar? Then start giving out bushels of big bear hugs to your favorite people. The simple act of hugging, or being hugged by, someone close to you (or hugging a beloved pet) triggers your pituitary gland to release a hormone called oxytocin, a.k.a. the "cuddle chemical," which automatically elevates your mood. Engaging in sex with your spouse also sends heaping happy helpings of oxytocin into your bloodstream.

But this heroic hormone does more than make you more cheerful. It also enhances your ability to handle stress; lessens addictive cravings for drugs, alcohol, and sweets; and even helps reduce inflammation and speed up wound healing. So what are you waiting for? Get out there and hug up a storm!

discussion in a more positive direction, just glance at your watch and "remember" an urgent engagement elsewhere. Then hightail it outta there!

Just Say, "Thanks!"

If you've spent your life gazing at clouds and ignoring silver linings, it's not likely that you'll change that habit overnight. But there is one surefire way to get the ball rolling in a more positive direction. Instead of fretting about what you *don't* have, be grateful for what you *do* have. Here's a foolproof plan to help you cultivate an attitude of gratitude:

Don't Let Strangers Drag You Down

Unfortunately, there are lots of cranky people out there. Well, don't let 'em spoil your day. The next time (let's say) a driver cuts you off in traffic or makes an ugly gesture, simply grin back at him. Your cheerful reaction just may make him realize what a jerk he's being. At best, it'll keep your spirits up while he fights his own demons.

Count your blessings. Each evening, list (preferably in writing) five things that happened that day for which you're grateful. Think back over the past 24 hours. Did you see a beautiful sunset or a patch of colorful flowers? Have a pleasant chat with a neighbor? Open your mailbox to find no bills inside? You get the idea.

Say grace. Even if it's only a short, silent prayer when you're grabbing lunch on the run, giving thanks for abundant, healthy food is a powerful reminder of a blessing that most of us take for granted.

Send thank-you notes. And not just to friends who've given you a gift or entertained you in their home. When people have helped or encouraged you in some way—even if they don't know it—write and mail them letters of gratitude. Your expression of thanks will benefit you as much as it pleases the recipient.

Express your appreciation—often. Make a point of saying a sincere "Thank you!" to everyone who gives you a compliment, does you a favor, or performs any service for you, even if it's part of their job. Not only will you feel good about yourself—it just might make that person's day.

CHAPTER 3

Dietary Dangers

As the old adage says, you are what you eat. Well, you're also what you *don't* eat. Unfortunately, these days, what a whole lot of folks are eating—and failing to eat—is making them tired, sick, fat, unhappy, and old (or even six feet under) before their time. The good news is that as long as you're alive and kicking, it's never too late to clean up your act—and it's a lot easier and more pleasant than you might think.

The Perils of Poor Nutrition

➔ The modern American diet (known in nutritional circles as MAD) is infamous for its role in launching our country's obesity epidemic and mushrooming rates of related ills, such as diabetes. But that's far from the only damage caused by poor eating habits. Nutritional deficiencies and overloads of junk food not only trigger or worsen scads of specific conditions, ranging from carpal tunnel syndrome to cancer, but also wreak havoc on your immune system. That, in turn, makes you a sitting duck for literally every health problem—major or minor—that comes barreling down the pike.

What You Don't Eat Will Do You In

Remember the old days, when your mother was always hounding you to eat your fruits and vegetables? Well, as much as we might have squawked back then, as adults we know how right she was: Those nutritional gold mines are an absolute must for maintaining good health. Yet somehow, without Mom on the scene to prod us, most of us have forgotten her loving words of wisdom—at least judging from these alarming figures in a recent report by the Centers for Disease Control and Prevention (CDC):

• Only 33 percent of adults eat fruit two or more times a day.

• Just 27 percent of the grown-up population eats vegetables three or more times a day.

If you're one of those shirkers, shape up already!

3 Reasons Why We're Deficient in Vitamins and Minerals

Much of the blame for our malnourished state lies in the fact that we're getting an excessive amount of these three diabolical demons:

Demon #1: Sugar and white flour. Roughly one-third of the typical American diet is composed of these two substances—which happen to be almost totally devoid of nutrients.

Demon #2: Processed food. Processing guts food of its natural nutrients and, in most cases, adds gobs of health-destroying sugar, sodium, trans fats, and synthetic chemicals. (For more about the stupefying stuff in processed food and the mess it makes of your system, see Chapter 4, "Fearsome Food Fallacies.")

Demon #3: Modern life. Commercial farming methods deplete the soil, and therefore crops growing in that soil, of their life-giving vitamins and minerals. On top of that, stress, anxiety, air pollution, and the chronic use of antacids and other drugs (both OTC and prescription versions) either drain your body of essential micronutrients or block their absorption.

Sugar Shrinks Your Brain

Yes, literally. Medical science has found that eating a diet high in sugar and other refined carbohydrates reduces your supply of a protein called brain-derived neurotrophic factor (BDNF). Scientists

Bypass the Drive-Through Brain Drain

Jaw-Dropping DISCOVERY

Fast food can bust your mood—and not just by eating it. It's no secret that the crud in fast food is as bad for your brain as it is for your body. Well, researchers now tell us that just looking at a fast-food restaurant or its associated icons can put a serious damper on your spirits. How so? Think about it: The avowed mission of fast-food chains is to get you in the door and out again in a flash. So those big corporations spend millions of dollars quizzing focus groups and developing graphics, symbols, and architectural elements that convey a "Gotta hurry!" message to your subconscious mind. And, boy, do they work! Studies have found that living in an area that has a lot of fast-food restaurants can actually impair your ability to slow down and savor such simple joys as a beautiful sunset or a fragrant flower. That, in turn, can lead to unhappiness, stress, and anxiety—real fast.

have dubbed it "Miracle-Gro® for the brain" because of its astounding ability to help generate new cells and produce new connections—especially in the areas that regulate mood, memory, and cognitive skills. To put it another way, when you're low on BDNF, you're blue, stressed out, forgetful, and slow on the mental uptake. But when you increase your BDNF—bingo! You're primed for good moods, clear thinking, and learning new things, no matter how old you are.

The secret to filling up your mental "tank" is regular exercise and a diet low in processed foods and high in natural chow that's rich in these three nutrients:

Folate, in asparagus, avocado, beans, broccoli, leafy greens, oranges, spinach

Vitamin B$_{12}$, in beef, eggs, fish, milk and other dairy products, poultry

Omega-3 fatty acids, in Brussels sprouts, eggs, fish, kale, milk, peanut butter, pumpkin seeds, spinach, walnuts, yogurt

---

Fix-It-Fast
FORMULA

Marvelous Multinutrient Smoothie

With this simple formula at your fingertips, there's no excuse for shortchanging yourself out of essential nutrients, no matter how much your action-packed agenda keeps you on the go. Believe it or not, this tasty beverage delivers almost all of the vitamins and minerals that you need each day for tip-top health.

1 banana, peeled

1 cup of green grapes

1 cup of vanilla yogurt (preferably full-fat)

½ apple, chopped (but not peeled)

1½ cups of fresh spinach

1 tbsp. of flaxseeds

1 cup of ice cubes

Add all of the ingredients to a blender in the order listed, and blend for 30 to 45 seconds, or until the contents are thoroughly liquefied and freely circulating. Then drink up, or pour the mixture into a travel cup and take it with you.

Sugar Substitutes: Boon or Boondoggle?

Artificial sweeteners let you satisfy your sweet tooth with no calories whatsoever. That's just about the biggest win-win situation on the planet, right? Wrong! While these sugar substitutes can prove useful in cutting calories and managing diabetes, they do have their fair share of drawbacks. For that reason, they've been mired in controversy among nutritional scientists since 1878, when saccharin was accidentally discovered by a chemist working with coal tar. Although it and a handful of other sweeteners have been approved for use by the U.S. Food and Drug Administration (FDA), researchers are finding plenty of evidence that what marketers pitch as weight-loss miracle workers do not live up to their promise—and pose undue health risks to boot.

3 Threats from Fake Sugar

If you routinely use artificial sweeteners (either alone or in sugar-free foods and beverages) because you think they're better for you than sugar, think again. Here are three ways these great pretenders could be harming your health:

They pull the wool over your taste buds. Artificial sweeteners are hundreds, even thousands, of times sweeter than sugar. Studies suggest that bombarding your taste buds with these super-strength stand-ins makes them less receptive to the natural sweetness of fruits and certain vegetables. As a result, you're more likely to seek out sweeter and sweeter treats.

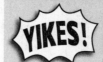

A recent study published in *The American Journal of Clinical Nutrition* found that fewer than 5 percent of the folks surveyed were getting the recommended dietary allowances (RDAs) of essential minerals. That statistic is especially sobering given the fact that a whole lot of the study's subjects had every reason to know that their sloppy eating habits were sabotaging their health. Why? Because they worked at one of the world's foremost dietary think tanks: the U.S. Department of Agriculture's Human Nutrition Research Center in Beltsville, Maryland. The moral of this story: Even people who work every day on nutritional research don't always practice what they preach, so that can help explain why we mere mortals often fail to lead a healthy lifestyle!

The **average American** will consume more than **5 tons** of **sugar** by age 65.

They trick your tummy. Besides messing up your metabolism and your hormones, artificially sweetened foods can lure you into overeating because of the way they feel in your mouth. Why? Foods that are high in fat and sugar taste dense, as well as sweet, which sends a signal to your brain that you're eating something substantial. On the other hand, foods that are artificially sweetened tend to have a thinner consistency, which makes them less satisfying to your subconscious mind. As a result, you may not feel as though you've eaten enough, so it's much more likely that you'll keep on noshing long after you should have stopped.

You may be consuming genetically modified organisms (GMOs). Some artificial sweeteners, including aspartame, neotame, and sucralose, can be made from corn, soy, or sugar beets, and the vast majority of those crops are genetically altered—to the great detriment of our health. (For the full scoop on GMOs and what they're doing to your mind and body, see Chapter 4, "Fearsome Food Fallacies.")

The Shocking Truth about Diet Soda

Statistics show that half of all Americans drink diet soda on a regular basis, consuming (brace yourself) 4 billion gallons of the stuff each year! Well, if you're one of those dedicated guzzlers, here are four facts you absolutely need to know:

1. According to a recent study at the University of Texas, diet soda drinkers were 65 percent more likely to be overweight than non-soda drinkers. What's even more surprising, they were more likely to be overweight than folks who drank regular soda.

2. Numerous studies have found that diet soda drinkers are at increased risk of developing type 2 diabetes. The jury is still out on the exact cause. It may be hormonal reactions triggered by the chemicals in the sweeteners, or it could be that people eat unhealthy foods that undo any calorie-saving effects of the no-cal drinks.

3. A study at the University of Iowa Hospitals and Clinics found that women who drank two or more diet drinks a day were 30 percent more likely than non-diet-pop drinkers to have a heart attack or similar cardiovascular "event" and 50 percent more likely to die from the experience.

4. Even though they don't contain sugar, diet sodas can still put you at risk for dental problems. That's because they contain phosphoric acid and citric acid, which, according to the American Dental Association, can damage the enamel on your teeth, leaving them more vulnerable to decay.

Diet soda increases your **risk** of a fatal **heart attack**.

Stevia's Not So Sweet After All

Many folks assume that because stevia is a natural substance, it has none of the drawbacks of artificial sweeteners. Not so! While stevia is derived from the leaves of an herb, and it does appear on the FDA's GRAS list, it pulls all the same tummy- and mind-fooling tricks that other ultra-sweet sugar substitutes do. In addition, here are some other factoids you need to keep in mind before you start dousing your food with stevia:

- It can cause unpleasant side effects, the most common of which are bloating and nausea.

- Its interaction with medications used to control blood pressure and diabetes can cause hypotension or hypoglycemia.

- Only powdered, processed forms of the sweetener carry the FDA seal of approval. Both fresh stevia and whole-leaf stevia extract can damage your heart and kidneys and cause problems with blood sugar control.

The Lethal Low-Fat Fable

For decades, dietary gurus have urged us all to opt for low-fat or nonfat dairy products. Well, that's changing. A growing number of experts now say that it's healthier to eat and drink dairy products with all their natural fat left in, as everyone routinely did until the 1950s, when flawed research connected animal-derived saturated fat with an increased risk of cardiovascular disease and coronary heart disease. Recent studies show no such connection and, in fact, those in the know tell us that the only types of fat that really hurt you are the man-made varieties, such as trans fats, and the refined polyunsaturated fats found in canola and other vegetable oils.

Here's another kicker: During the manufacturing process, low-fat dairy products are stripped clean of a key health-giving ingredient in whole milk: conjugated linoleic acid (CLA), a fat that's been proven to fight cancer and help fend off abdominal fat deposits. (For more on the deadly dangers of belly fat—and how to banish it—see Chapter 5, "The Fatal Fat Factor.")

Artificial Sweeteners Can Make You Fat

Jaw-Dropping DISCOVERY

A growing body of scientific evidence from such key academic players as Yale, Purdue, and the Harvard School of Public Health (to name just a few) is showing that, far from stemming our obesity epidemic, sugar substitutes may actually be fueling it. Studies indicate that there are two reasons:

1. Regular consumption of artificial sweeteners, particularly in beverages, slows down your metabolism, which makes it easier to pack on pounds and harder to lose them.

2. In nature, there is no such thing as sweetness without calories. When you consume zero-calorie sugar substitutes that are anywhere from 200 to (yes!) 7,000 times sweeter than the real deal, it triggers hormonal processes that ramp up your brain's craving for real food. Research suggests that artificial sweeteners actually prevent your body from producing GLP-1, a hormone that controls your blood sugar levels and feelings of fullness. As a result, you can easily wind up eating a whole lot more than you would if you allowed yourself to enjoy moderate amounts of sugar.

A Fat-Free Diet Will Kill You

Notice that I said "will," not "can." How? By depriving you of four vitamins that are necessary for life. Although vitamin C and the entire B group are soluble in water, your system cannot absorb and use vitamins A, D, E, and K without the presence of dietary fat. And if these key players can't do their jobs, your days are numbered— possibly in triple digits. If that statement sounds extreme, consider these biological facts: Your immune system and your eyesight depend upon a steady supply of vitamin A. Vitamin D works with calcium and other minerals to build and maintain your bones. Vitamin E is a key player in limiting the formation of free radicals that wreak havoc on every cell in your body, and vitamin K makes your blood clot as it should (thereby preventing you from hemorrhaging to death).

The Great Gluten Rip-Off

In supermarkets all across the country, products labeled "gluten-free" (usually in big, bold letters) are multiplying like rabbits—and selling to the tune of more than $2 billion a year. But here's the real shocker: Although shunning gluten is essential for people with celiac disease, statistics show that most of the folks who buy gluten-free products don't have that condition—or even a mild sensitivity to wheat. Somehow, it seems, the notion has spread that eliminating gluten from your diet will make you healthier. Well, it ain't so, Joe! Here are three facts you need to know about this freaky food fad:

Fact #1. While gluten itself does not offer any particular health benefits, the whole-grain foods that contain it deliver heaps of them. Their rich assortment of vitamins, minerals, and fiber has been proven to lower your risk of developing heart disease, type 2 diabetes, and some forms of cancer. In addition, their nutrients keep your internal "plumbing" functioning smoothly.

Galloping Gluten Marketing Hype

Pricey, gluten-free chow is selling like hotcakes these days, even to folks who don't need it (see "The Great Gluten Rip-Off," at left). And a lot of unscrupulous food marketers are making hay from that trend by pitching their wares as gluten-free, even if nothing in the whole product category ever contained the stuff—like meats, cheeses, and even fruits and vegetables. Well, friends, keep this fact in mind as you stroll the supermarket aisles or belly up to the deli counter: Gluten is found *only* in wheat, rye, barley, and foods that are made with those grains. So don't be taken in by jacked-up prices on hoaxes like "gluten-free" chicken or frozen strawberries.

NOTE: *While it is true that all grains contain some form of gluten, the kind in wheat, rye, and barley is the only type that poses problems for people with celiac disease.*

Fact #2. It makes no sense to cut back on your gluten intake. If you have celiac disease, even trace amounts of the stuff can cause major damage. Otherwise, you can eat it till the cows come home, and it won't hurt you.

Fact #3. Gluten-free pasta, cereals, breads, and other baked goods cost two to three times more than their standard counterparts. So whenever you buy these high-ticket items—unless your health hangs in the balance—you're throwing big buckets of your hard-earned bucks right down the drain.

Frightening Facts about Low-Carb Diets

Talk about food fads that have stayed the course! Low-carb diets have been with us since 1972, when Dr. Robert Atkins introduced his famous (some would say infamous) Atkins Diet Plan, which all but prohibits the consumption of carbohydrates such as bread, pasta, rice, and starchy vegetables. Since then, a number of variations have appeared on the scene, but they all work on the same basic theory: Normally, your body burns carbohydrates as fuel. When you drastically cut your carb intake, your body goes into a metabolic state called ketosis and begins to burn its own fat instead. And when your fat supply becomes your primary energy source, bingo—you lose weight.

Granted, this eating plan does have its share of proponents—many of whom just happen to be the authors of low-carb diet books or manufacturers of low-carb processed foods. On the other side of the debate are scads of nutritionists, medical doctors, and health-care pros who claim that these ultra-low-carb diets are unhealthy at best. At worst, their combination of too much protein, too little fiber, and a short supply of vitamins and minerals can kill you.

A Dieter's Dream: The Easy-Way-Out Enticements of Low-Carb Diets

Desperate folks who have tried and failed to lose weight with every other diet under the sun often flock to Atkins and other low-carb, high-protein plans for three reasons:

1. Rich treats such as steak, bacon, butter, and cream, which are blacklisted on most low-calorie or low-fat diets, are not only permitted but also encouraged on the Atkins plan.

2. As long as you stick to "permitted" foods, you can eat as much as you like, so you can toss calorie counting out the window. What's more, curtailing carbohydrates helps stabilize blood sugar levels, so between-meal hunger pangs go poof!

3. Folks who follow these diets report significant weight loss during the first, most carb-restrictive phase. This instant gratification motivates them to stay on course—at least for a while.

The Catastrophic Consequences of Ketosis

Folks who promote low-carb, high-protein diets make ketosis sound as though it's a perfectly harmless trade-off—like burning oak instead of maple logs in your fireplace. In reality, it's a whole different story. Ketosis occurs when your supply of carbohydrates drops below a critical level, and your body has to rely on protein and fat to produce the energy it needs to function. That fuel exchange puts a huge burden on your liver and kidneys. Most nutritionists and medical pros caution that if you stay on one of these highly unbalanced diets for more than 14 days, you can pay a serious—even fatal—penalty.

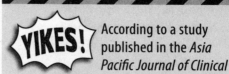

According to a study published in the *Asia Pacific Journal of Clinical Nutrition*, following a low-carb diet may increase your risk for abnormal heartbeat, kidney damage, lipid abnormalities, osteoporosis, and even sudden death.

Another study that appeared in the journal *Cell Metabolism* found that if you're on a high-protein ketogenic diet and you're under age 65, you could be upping your chances for diabetes, cancer—and premature death.

The bottom line: The surest, and only truly healthy, way to lose weight and keep it off is to adopt a healthier lifestyle, following commonsense guidelines, such as the ones you'll find in Chapter 5, "The Fatal Fat Factor."

Words to the Wise about Water

We all know that to maintain your good health (and good looks), you should drink eight glasses of water a day, right? Wrong! While it is true that a steady supply of H_2O is essential for your well-being, no scientific research supports the magic number eight. On the contrary, according to a study in the *American Journal of Physiology*, here's the truth of the matter:

1. There's no need to count. Your body will tell you when it's time to drink up. Clue: You'll feel thirsty (surprise!). Just to play it safe, though—because your busy mind may ignore that wake-up call—look at your urine output. If it's brown or dark yellow, that indicates that you're dehydrated, and you need to chug more liquid. On the other hand, if that bodily fluid is clear or close to it, you're doing just fine.

2. You don't have to guzzle water to keep your body sufficiently hydrated. Beverages of all kinds, including juice, milk, tea, and (yes, nutritionists now tell us) coffee, deliver the elixir of life. So do fruits, vegetables, and plenty of other foods.

Fabulous Fuel: Nutrition 101

You don't need a degree in nutrition science to build yourself a better diet. All it takes is a basic understanding of what makes your body tick. These are the three key elements:

Macronutrients come in three types: protein, fats, and carbohydrates. These are the nutrients you need the most of, because they provide your body with energy; promote growth, development, and tissue repair; and regulate your bodily functions.

Micronutrients are the vitamins and minerals, from A to zinc. If you don't get enough of them, you can land in *big* trouble because these hard workers coordinate and fine-tune *all* of your internal systems.

Phytonutrients, a.k.a. phytochemicals, are not vital for maintaining life itself, but a deficiency can cause significant weight gain and major difficulty shedding the extra pounds. The best known of this bunch are in fruits and vegetables (for example, the beta-carotene in carrots and sweet potatoes), but equally valuable are those in herbs and spices, whole grains, beans, and nuts.

5 Fantastic Feats of Phytonutrients

In Mother Nature's scheme of things, the mission of phytonutrients is guarding plants against diseases. And those power-packed chemicals can do the same thing for you. That's why it's important to include a variety of fruits, vegetables, and herbs in your diet. Here's a fistful of deeds this fix-it team can perform:

1. Boost your body's ability to repair damaged cells and expel waste products and toxic compounds

2. Enhance your immune system, thereby shoring up your defenses against illnesses of all kinds

3. Fight off free radicals and reduce the oxidation that causes Alzheimer's and other degenerative diseases

4. Help prevent damage from such cancer-causing agents as ultraviolet rays, secondhand smoke, and environmental pollutants

5. Reduce inflammation throughout your body

4 Vicious Vitamin Deficiencies

A serious lack of certain vitamins can result in some truly gruesome diseases, the most infamous being beriberi (vitamin B_1, a.k.a. thiamine), pellagra (vitamin B_3, a.k.a niacin), rickets (vitamin D), and scurvy (vitamin C). Fortunately, those horrors are all but extinct in the United States and other developed countries, but less severe underdoses of vitamins can— and routinely do—cause trouble for

The Magic of Magnesium

REMARKABLE REMEDY

Magnesium is essential for maintaining crucial bodily functions, such as muscle control, tissue healing, the elimination of harmful toxins, and the processes that control your heart and circulatory system. But most of us don't get enough magnesium in our daily diets, and popping supplements could easily give you a toxic overdose. What to do? Three times a week, pour 2 cups of Epsom salts into a tub of warm water, and soak for 12 to 20 minutes. If you like, add ½ cup of your favorite bath oil. But don't use soap of any kind—it'll interfere with the action of the salts. Besides improving your blood circulation, lowering your stress level, and relieving general aches and pains, this powerful soak can help alleviate a truckload of major and minor health conditions, including these:

▶ Arthritis   ▶ Hives

▶ Bruises   ▶ Kidney stones

▶ Gout   ▶ Sciatica

hordes of Americans who could easily mend their ways. Just consider these four sobering examples:

A low intake of vitamin A can lead to major intestinal and lung infections, and night blindness.

Too little vitamin B$_2$ (a.k.a. riboflavin) can produce a multitude of woes, ranging from digestive problems to slowed mental processes, dizzy spells, insomnia, cataracts, skin rashes, and hair loss.

A diet that's low in vitamin C has been found to increase your likelihood of developing high blood pressure, diabetes, heart disease, and certain forms of cancer, as well as memory loss, urinary tract infections, and muscle soreness after exercise—and that's just for starters.

A shortage of vitamin D can contribute directly to bone diseases, hypertension, and certain forms of cancer.

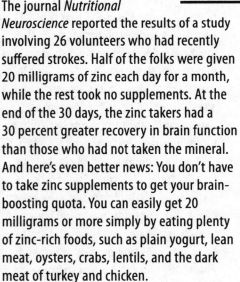

Zinc Speeds Up Stroke Recovery

Jaw-Dropping DISCOVERY

If you've had a stroke or know someone who has, this news will be music to your ears: The journal *Nutritional Neuroscience* reported the results of a study involving 26 volunteers who had recently suffered strokes. Half of the folks were given 20 milligrams of zinc each day for a month, while the rest took no supplements. At the end of the 30 days, the zinc takers had a 30 percent greater recovery in brain function than those who had not taken the mineral. And here's even better news: You don't have to take zinc supplements to get your brain-boosting quota. You can easily get 20 milligrams or more simply by eating plenty of zinc-rich foods, such as plain yogurt, lean meat, oysters, crabs, lentils, and the dark meat of turkey and chicken.

Mighty Minerals Demystified

Medical science has identified 28 minerals that perform specific, essential functions in the body and 12 others that are just as crucial to our health but whose roles are not yet fully understood. As you might expect, there are hundreds of mineral supplements for sale, and like most folks, you are probably confused about what kinds, if any, are necessary for your diet. So let's set the record straight.

Misconception #1: Minerals are solo performers.
FACT: While it is true that, for instance, calcium builds strong bones and iron gives you strong blood, neither one does its job alone. In

reality, minerals team up with vitamins, enzymes, and other minerals to carry out these and other highly complex processes.

Misconception #2: If you show signs of a deficiency, all you need to do is pump more of the lacking mineral into your body.
FACT: A short supply of any mineral is rarely the only cause of an abnormal condition exhibited by your body. In fact, very often, you may have plenty of the needed mineral, but your system can't use it effectively because one of its essential teammates is AWOL.

Misconception #3: You should always take the standard RDA of every mineral.
FACT: Individual mineral requirements vary tremendously, depending on scads of factors, including your age, sex, size, metabolism, health condition, activity level, and (yes) even your personality, the type of work you do, and the climate you live in.

Misconception #4: To correct a mineral deficiency, you need to take one or more supplements.
FACT: Sometimes, yes, depending on the nature and severity of the problem, you may need a supplemental boost, at least temporarily. But in many, if not most, cases, eating more of the right foods will do the trick just fine.

Make Your Food Work for You

➡ Hippocrates, the Father of Medicine, routinely advised his patients to "Let food be thy medicine and medicine be thy food." Well, he wasn't just blowing them off so he could flee his office and spend the day on the golf course! He knew then what we're beginning to learn now: that the answer to curing everyday ills and fending off or alleviating even the most serious diseases may be as close as your kitchen—or your local supermarket.

Say "Nuts!" to the Blues

Feeling down in the dumps? Whether the problem is caused by your monthly bout with premenstrual syndrome (PMS), an attack of winter depression, or a simple case of the blahs, nuts can help. Best of all, because nuts

Nuts
beat the blues
**better than
Prozac®**.

are food, and not drugs, they solve the problem at its root rather than just temporarily relieving your symptoms. These three types can perform highly effective "funkectomies." Plus, the only side effect you'll have will be better health!

Brazil nuts are one of Mother Nature's best sources of selenium, a mineral that is likely to be lacking in your system if you're feeling depressed, anxious, irritated, and tired for no apparent reason. (Studies show that most people today are deficient in selenium.) Simply eating three Brazil nuts a day will provide your recommended daily dose of this essential nutrient.

Cashews have been shown to work just as well as, if not better than, prescription antidepressants such as Prozac®. The secret lies in tryptophan, an amino acid that helps boost your mood, stabilize your thoughts, and produce a generally mellow feeling. A large handful of cashews contains 1,000 to 2,000 milligrams of tryptophan.

The Astonishing Deeds of Sunflower Seeds

To look at a sunflower seed, you'd never take it for a nutritional superstar. But it is! Believe it or not, eating just a handful of the unsalted seeds every day can help you quit smoking, lower your LDL (bad) cholesterol levels, relieve constipation, prevent tooth decay, improve your memory—and much more.

Walnuts are high in serotonin, which helps lift your spirits when you're suffering from seasonal affective disorder or wallowing in a funk. The easy R$_x$: During a blue phase, eat a handful of walnuts every day or so.

The Truth about Tea: 3 Myths Debunked

Study after study has shown that tea, whether black, green, white, or oolong (all of which are made from the leaves of the *Camellia sinensis* shrub), can fight inflammation, boost your immune system, preserve your brainpower, and help prevent diabetes, osteoporosis, and many types of cancer—and that's just for starters. Unfortunately, a few misconceptions have arisen about this bracing beverage, so let's set the record straight right now.

Tall tale #1: Adding milk to tea destroys its health benefits.
THE TRUTH: Although some reports a while back suggested that was

the case, recent research, including a study published in the *Journal of Agricultural and Food Chemistry*, has found that tea offers up about the same potent load of antioxidants whether it's laced with milk or not.

Tall tale #2: To get the biggest health boost from tea, you should drink it plain.

THE TRUTH: There are a couple of additives that actually increase the health-giving properties of tea. When you're brewing it ahead, say for iced tea, squeezing some lemon, lime, or orange juice into the pitcher helps preserve the flavonoids that deliver many of tea's health benefits. Furthermore, drinking tea with honey stirred into it seems to enhance your ability to work more productively—apparently by activating the areas of your brain that control concentration.

Tall tale #3: Tea never goes bad.

THE TRUTH: While it's true that tea does not spoil in the way that meat or produce does, after about six months, its antioxidant supply starts to diminish. To maintain full potency for as long as possible, always store tea (whether it's loose or in bags) in a sealed container in a cool, dark place. Mark the date you bought the tea on the container, and toss the contents into your compost pile after a year.

> # The Unsavory Scoop on Nondairy Creamer
>
> Attention, coffee drinkers! Thanks to its brimming boatload of antioxidants, your beloved bracing beverage can be a powerful part of your health-care arsenal. That is, unless you add nondairy creamer to your cup. A study published in *The Journal of Nutrition* found that these dairy stand-ins may block the absorption of the phenolic acids that give java its disease-fighting firepower. On the other hand, neither milk nor half-and-half disrupts your body's antioxidant uptake. So do yourself a favor: Drink your coffee either black or with the real deal mixed into it.

Terrific Tricks for Tossing Cancer Sticks

Trying to quit smoking? Congratulations! Nothing can make that process pleasant, but this trio of tricks can help ease your constant desire for hand-to-mouth gratification. Whenever you crave a smoke, try one of these healthy alternatives:

Grab a raw carrot, and chomp away. It'll give you a big antioxidant boost and satisfy your craving at the same time.

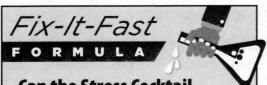
Reach for a cinnamon stick, and suck on it (or brew a cup of cinnamon tea and sip it slowly) until the urge to smoke passes.

Suck on a lime. Besides curbing your desire for tobacco, it will replace some of the vitamins, phosphates, and calcium that smoking may have drained from your system.

7 Startling Secrets about Carrot Juice

In many parts of the world, folks consider carrot juice to be the "king of juices," and for good reason: Drinking an 8-ounce glass of this golden treasure several times a week can work wonders for your health and well-being. Like these, for instance:

1. Balance your blood sugar levels

2. Cleanse your liver

3. Fortify your blood and help prevent anemia

4. Guard against the effects of secondhand smoke

5. Help fend off asthma attacks and other respiratory ailments

6. Prevent water retention

7. Strengthen your immune system

NOTE: *You can get all of these benefits from bottled 100 percent carrot juice, but the kind you make in your own home juicer or buy fresh from the machine at your local juice bar is far more potent.*

Spicy Help for Body and Mind

Curcumin, the active ingredient in turmeric, is of one the most powerful, naturally occurring anti-inflammatory substances ever identified— and, therefore, one of your most potent weapons in the fight against chronic diseases. What's more, turmeric has also been shown to have strong anti-cancer properties and to reduce the buildup of plaque in your brain that causes Alzheimer's and cognitive decline. Your R$_x$ for good health: Simply add turmeric to your favorite soups, stews, and other foods as often as you can—the more, the merrier!

An Unlikely Lift for Your Liver

Horseradish is one of the most potent sources of glucosino-lates—compounds that increase your liver's ability to detoxify carcinogens. Not only does that action help lessen your risk of developing cancer, but studies show that it may suppress the growth of existing tumors. The recommended dose: as little as ¼ teaspoon a day, either freshly ground or bottled. How you take it is your call. You can slurp it straight from a spoon, spread it on sandwiches, mix it into salad dressings, or—for a tasty, tangy dip—stir it into plain yogurt, and eat it with crackers or raw veggies.

Facts vs. Fiction about Fresh Food

True or False? Fresh fruits and vegetables are far superior to frozen and canned versions. **A RESOUNDING FALSE—WITH ONE EXCEPTION:** When you pick fully ripe, organic fruits or veggies fresh from your own garden or buy them, fresh-picked, from a local organic farmer and eat them that day, then yes, they are more nutritious (and delicious) than canned or frozen produce. But the picture-perfect stuff that's piled up at your local chain

Eye-Opening Facts about Tomato Nutrition

Jaw-Dropping DISCOVERY

Before you reach for fresh tomatoes at your local supermarket, bear in mind that those red orbs were probably picked when they weren't nearly so rosy—and that could make them much less valuable dietary allies than you might think. Studies have proven that vine-ripened tomatoes contain almost twice as much vitamin C and beta-carotene as their green counterparts. And don't be hoodwinked by signs saying "vine-ripened." Unless it's high tomato season and they were grown locally (which in a big store is highly unlikely), they won't be up to snuff. It is true that tomatoes can be ripened on the vine in greenhouses, but they aren't as nutritious as the ones raised in the fresh air and hot summer sun.

supermarket has some serious nutritional shortcomings—even if it was grown organically. There are two major reasons:

1. The vast majority of the produce that you see in big stores has traveled a long way to get there. In the process, those tender plant parts have been exposed to extreme temperatures and other conditions that deplete important nutrients. (Vitamins A and C are especially prone to going AWOL during long road trips from farm to market.)

Cooked and **canned tomatoes** are **healthier** than fresh ones.

2. Fruits and vegetables pack their full nutritional punch only when they've ripened completely. But by necessity, most produce that will be shipped a considerable distance is harvested before the vitamins and other nutrients have had a chance to fully develop. Be especially wary of anything that is out of season in your area, or that can't even grow there—for instance, papayas in Vermont or peaches in January almost anywhere.

The Real Facts about Frozen Food

While it is true that frozen produce is often healthier than its fresh counterparts—especially when you have a choice between, let's say, a bag of frozen organic blueberries and a box of fresh ones that have been treated with pesticides and herbicides—there is one caveat: When frozen food is allowed to thaw and refreeze, it loses boatloads of vitamins. So before you toss those packages into your shopping cart, put 'em to the test. Here's what to check for:

- Fruits and veggies that come in individual pieces, such as berries, corn, and peas, should move around loosely or break apart easily in the bag. If you pick up what feels like a solid chunk of ice, put it right back where you got it!

- When you lift a box of pureed squash, spinach, or other greens, the weight should be evenly distributed. If it's all lumped on one side of the package, give it a pass.

Once you've made your way through the checkout line, pack your frozen foods in a thermal bag or small cooler, then hightail it home and stash your bounty in the freezer. Everything should keep all its flavor and goodness for up to six months.

8 Dynamic Dietary Duos

We all know it takes team-work to win a baseball game. Well, guess what? That same strategy can also help you solve a lot of nagging health problems, or simply boost the nutritional arsenal in your diet. Add these synergistic superstars to your dietary roster, and watch 'em light up your scoreboard!

1. Almonds + red wine. Vitamin E in the almonds works with resveratrol in the wine to thin your blood and boost the health of your vessel linings.
THE RESULT: A healthier heart.

2. Bananas + yogurt. Inulin, a fiber in bananas, revs up growth of yogurt's healthy bacteria.
THE RESULT: Improved digestion and a ramped-up immune system.

3. Blueberries + walnuts. Anti-oxidants, called anthocyanins, in the berries guard your brain cells against damage from free radicals, and the omega-3 fatty acids in walnuts boost your brainpower.
THE RESULT: Improved memory, enhanced mental function, and possibly a lowered risk for Par-kinson's disease.

4. Chicken + carrots. The zinc in chicken enables your body to convert the carrots' beta-carotene into vitamin A.
THE RESULT: A rugged immune system, stronger eyes, and healthier skin.

5. Chocolate + raspberries. The catechin in chocolate and querce-tin in raspberries intensify each other's disease-fighting prowess.
THE RESULT: Thinner blood and a healthier heart.

6. Eggs + cheese. The vitamin D in the egg yolks makes the cal-cium in the cheese more readily available to your body.
THE RESULT: Stronger bones, clearer thinking, and a healthier heart—plus reduced PMS symp-toms and easier weight loss.

7. Onions + garlic. Working together increases the potency of their artery-clearing compounds.
THE RESULT: Cleaner blood vessels and reduced risk for arteriosclerosis.

8. Peanut butter + whole-grain bread. The classic peanut butter sandwich packs all nine of the amino acids that your body needs to build muscles, bones, and hormones.
THE RESULT: A stronger, health-ier *you*.

The Bewildering Bashing of Canned Vegetables

Canned fruits and vegetables have gotten a bum rap in recent years. Do they deserve it? In a word, no. Granted, they're rarely photogenic enough to grace the pages of a fancy food magazine. But that's no reason to banish canned foods from your diet. Let's consider the pros and cons of these traditional pantry staples.

First, the highly exaggerated cons:

- During the canning process, vegetables and fruits can lose some of their vitamin C content, but when they're processed quickly—in your kitchen or at the processing plant—the majority of nutrients are locked in and retained, just as they are in frozen foods.

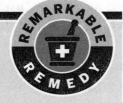

More Is Better— Period!

If you're like most folks, you don't eat nearly as many health-giving fruits and vegetables as you should. So take a tip from top nutritionists: Quit worrying about which form of produce is best. Instead, focus on simply adding more of it to your diet. Calling on a combination of fresh, frozen, and canned fruits and vegetables will help ensure that you meet the ideal intake each day—or at least come a lot closer to your target.

- Many canned vegetables are high in sodium and may have other less than desirable ingredients. Plus, the cans themselves may be lined with BPA, a chemical that's been linked to various health problems (more about both of those issues in Chapter 4). The simple solution to these potential drawbacks: Read labels carefully to avoid harmful additives, and whenever possible, choose organic brands. Also, bear in mind that many soups and other popular canned goods come in low- or no-sodium versions. As for the BPA issue, manufacturers, especially organic ones, are switching to BPA-free can linings, or to glass jars and Tetra Paks®.

The highly practical pros:

- Canned foods have a shelf life of two to four years, compared with six months for frozen types and a week or so, max, for most fresh vegetables. Better yet, unlike their fridge- and freezer-bound counterparts, canned goods sail through even the longest power outages in fine fettle.

- Depending on the season and where you live, canned vegetables and fruits may cost considerably less than fresh versions.
- Because foods must be heated before canning, they're less prone to contamination than fresh vittles can be.
- Foods that are intended for canning (or freezing) are generally picked at their peak of ripeness and processed close to the source, before valuable vitamins have a chance to fly the coop.

7 Dirt-Cheap Superfoods

These days, a couple of exotic berries by the names goji and acai are getting a whole lot of airplay for their potent supplies of antioxidants. For a lot less money though, you can stroll into your local supermarket and pick up a passel of foods that are every bit as effective as those fancy little fruits are in the fight against free radicals. Just pack your diet with heaping helpings of these seven superstars, and you'll fortify your system against everything from cancer and cardiovascular disease to arthritis and Alzheimer's:

1. Apples
2. Black rice
3. Coffee
4. Cranberries
5. Dried beans
6. Sweet potatoes
7. Tea

6 Freaky Food Fixes from the Outside In

It's a fact that what you put on your skin goes into your body—and that's the secret behind these amazing antidotes for a half dozen of your most aggravating health problems.

Banish skin troubles. Stuff a cotton drawstring bag or a panty hose leg with a cup or two of uncooked

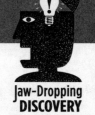

Cabbage Cures Ulcers

Jaw-Dropping DISCOVERY

For centuries, folk-medicine gurus have sworn by cabbage and cabbage juice as top-notch ulcer remedies. Well, it turns out they're right. Recently, numerous medical studies (including one at the Stanford University School of Medicine) have found that drinking 8 ounces of pure cabbage juice four times a day can heal both gastric and duodenal ulcers in anywhere from 2 to 10 days. Eating raw cabbage can perform the same miraculous feat. So if you'd rather not drink a quart of cabbage juice every day, you can substitute a wedge of raw cabbage or about 1 cup of sliced or shredded cabbage for each 8-ounce cup of juice.

oatmeal. Toss it into your tub as you run cool to lukewarm water, then settle in and relax for 15 to 20 minutes. If possible, let yourself air-dry when you're finished, and bid bye-bye to the pain, itch, and inflammation of wind- and sunburn, insect bites, poison-plant rashes, contact allergies, or eczema.

Clear up conjunctivitis. Grate a large, peeled apple, and spread the gratings in the center of a piece of damp cheesecloth that's about 12 inches square. Fold it to form a pouch, lie down, place it over your eyes, and relax for 30 minutes. Within a day or two, all should be well again.

Eradicate athlete's foot. Simply rub plain yogurt directly onto the affected skin. For good measure, eat a cup or two of yogurt each day until the fungus has flown the coop.

Heal cuts. Blend or chop ¼ cup or so of cranberries (either fresh or frozen), apply the mash to the cut, and cover it with a bandage. Change the dressing every few hours until the wound has healed.

Heal hemorrhoids. Chop up a cabbage, lay the pieces on a towel, and sit on them for 30 minutes or so. And don't forget to take your pants off first!

Quell a cold. At bedtime, put a slice of raw onion on the sole of each foot, and hold the slices in place with thick wool socks. Overnight, the curative compounds in the onion will draw out the infection and lower your fever. (Be forewarned: They'll also leave you with onion breath in the morning.)

Take a Trip to Italy

Or at least cook like you're there! Whenever you combine tomatoes and olive oil, a bit of healing magic happens. How? The olive oil helps your body better use the disease-fighting lycopene that's present in tomatoes. The healthy results: improving your ability to prevent cancer and fight heart disease. Buon appetito!

The Hidden Healing Power of Lemonade

For generations of Americans, nothing has shouted "Summertime!" like a tall, cold glass of lemonade. Medical experts now tell us that this sweet and tangy treat can help resolve or prevent a passel of serious health problems. That's because lemons are rich in phytonutrients that are associated with the prevention and/or treatment of at least four of the leading causes of death in Western countries: cancer, cardiovascular disease, diabetes, and hypertension. What's more, although lemons are acidic, they increase the alkalinity of our bodily fluids—and an alkaline system is key to maintaining good health. Here's a sampling of the fabulous feats that a daily glass of lemonade can perform for you:

- Boost your immune system
- Cleanse your system of toxins and impurities
- Conquer cravings for cigarettes, alcohol, and junk food
- Improve your mood
- Increase your energy level
- Prevent kidney stones
- Protect against adult asthma and other respiratory ailments
- Reduce acid reflux
- Speed weight loss

NOTE: *For best results, make your own lemonade from scratch using freshly squeezed lemon juice and sugar (see the Lemonade Twist recipe, at right).*

The Startling Skinny on Apple Skins

Even more than most fruits and vegetables, apples pack their biggest concentration of nutrients in or just under the skin. For example, the antioxidant level is six times higher

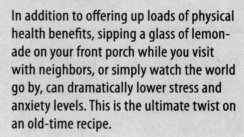

Fix-It-Fast
FORMULA

Lemonade Twist

In addition to offering up loads of physical health benefits, sipping a glass of lemonade on your front porch while you visit with neighbors, or simply watch the world go by, can dramatically lower stress and anxiety levels. This is the ultimate twist on an old-time recipe.

1 cup of water (for simple syrup)

1 cup of sugar (or less to taste)

Zest of 2 lemons

1 cup of freshly squeezed lemon juice (4–6 lemons)

3–4 cups of cold water (to dilute)

1 cup of fresh blueberries, slightly crushed (optional)

Make a simple syrup by heating 1 cup of water in a pan, and then stirring in the sugar and lemon zest until the sugar is dissolved. Mix the syrup and the lemon juice in a pitcher, and add enough cold water to reach the desired strength. Refrigerate, covered, for 30 to 40 minutes. Stir in the crushed blueberries, then take a sip. If the lemonade is too sweet for your liking, add more straight lemon juice, and use less sugar next time. Serve it up in ice-filled glasses, garnished with lemon slices.

NOTE: *This recipe makes 6 servings. Feel free to multiply the ingredients if you're serving a crowd, but stick to the same proportions.*

in the peel than it is in the flesh. Unfortunately, though, apples rank at the very top of the Environmental Working Group's "Dirty Dozen" list of fruits and vegetables that retain huge amounts of pesticides and herbicides. So whenever possible, buy organically grown apples. The benefits and cost of organic foods are discussed in Chapter 4, starting on page 110. And, organic or not, always scrub the skins thoroughly before you eat them. (In Chapter 4 you'll also find the entire Dirty Dozen list as well as the horrifying scoop on pesticides, herbicides, and other dangerous crud in your food.)

A Mind-Boggling Masseuse

R E M A R K A B L E
REMEDY

Nothing relieves tired, stiff muscles like a good massage. But if you don't have time for a rubdown, reach for an avocado seed. Rinse off all of the fruit, and dry the pit. Then rub it over your arms, legs, hips, and as much of your back as you can reach. It'll improve your circulation and make you feel good all over.

4 Wild and Wacky Food Cures

Believe it or not, the solution to a whole lot of nagging health problems may be right in your kitchen—or as close as your local supermarket. Here's a quartet of ultra-common foods that can work wonders for you:

Ease your achin' joints with apples. The next time your knees, elbows, or other joints start hurting—or, better yet, before the pain starts—eat a few apples. Their potent load of boron can relieve joint pain and stiffness and actually seems to protect against arthritis.

Lower your blood pressure with avocados. Their mega-supply of potassium prevents the thickening of your artery walls and also helps regulate your body's fluid levels, which are crucial to controlling your blood pressure.

Rout out gout with cherries. They help clear toxins from your body and clean your kidneys, which puts them at the top of the gout-relief list. Eat 1 to 12 fresh or frozen cherries a day, or a handful of dried cherries. Drinking 100 percent cherry juice will also ease gout pain.

Stave off PMS with pork 'n' beans. This classic combo is rich in thiamine and riboflavin, both of which have been proven to keep monthly miseries at bay. Eating a 3-ounce serving of pork and a cup of cooked beans on a regular basis will do the trick.

Clobber Cancer with Chocolate

Yep—you read that right. Studies have shown that compounds called polyphenols slow the growth of cancer cells. And 1 ounce of dark chocolate contains almost as many polyphenols as a cup of green tea, and twice as many as a glass of red wine (two widely touted sources of the compounds). Just remember that the operative word is *dark*. Look for chocolate that consists of more than 70 percent cocoa. Unfortunately, the lighter milk chocolates that many of us prefer don't cut the mustard when it comes to polyphenol content.

As astounding as chocolate's cancer-fighting power is, that's not this champ's only claim to health-care fame. Compounds in dark chocolate can also perform these fabulous feats:

- Make blood platelets less likely to stick together and form harmful clots, while at the same time promoting normal clotting and improving your circulation

- Decrease inflammation in cardiovascular tissues, thereby reducing your risk for stroke

- Improve cognitive function by increasing the blood flow to your brain

- Lower your risk for tooth decay by hardening your tooth enamel (Of course, you do still need to practice good dental hygiene!)

- Boost your mood by spurring your brain to release feel-good endorphins

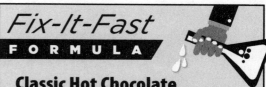

Fix-It-Fast FORMULA

Classic Hot Chocolate

Drinking a frothy cup of hot chocolate made with pure unsweetened cocoa powder does more than stave off winter's chill. Cocoa is rich in flavonoids, which have been shown to prevent oxidation of LDL (bad) cholesterol. When LDL is oxidized, it clings to arteries and increases the risk for heart disease and stroke. Chocolate can also raise levels of beneficial HDL cholesterol, which helps remove LDL from the body. So make a mug and enjoy it without guilt!

2 tbsp. of unsweetened cocoa powder

2 tbsp. of sugar

Dash of salt

1 cup of milk

¼ tsp. of vanilla extract

Mix the cocoa, sugar, and salt in a mug. Heat the milk either on the stove or in a microwave on high for 1½ minutes, or until hot. Gradually pour the hot milk into the mug, stirring constantly until all the cocoa powder is dissolved. Stir in the vanilla.

Give Bruises the Blues

Blueberries are rich in bioflavonoids, which are essential for repairing blood vessels. Eating ½ cup of the tasty fruits each day will not only speed the healing of current bruises but also strengthen your blood vessels so they're better able to fend off future—possibly more serious—damage.

NOTE: *This same vessel-strengthening prowess can also reduce the swelling of varicose veins.*

The Potent Power of Potatoes

The average American eats more than 130 pounds of potatoes each year. Unfortunately, about half of that load comes in the form of potato chips, French fries, and other junk-food treats. For that reason, nutritionists have largely overlooked the nutritional gold mine lurking inside the humble spud. But an article published in *The Journal of Nutrition* has food gurus changing their tune. Specifically, they're now singing the praises of colorful—and far more flavorful—types of taters.

For example, pink, red, blue, and purple potatoes are loaded with anthocyanins, the same phytonutrients that give many berries their potent antioxidant kick. Good choices include All Red, All Blue, and Mountain Rose. And yellow-fleshed potatoes, such as the popular Yukon Gold, contain carotenoids that help boost essential vitamin A action. These colorful characters are turning up in more and more supermarkets and farmers' markets—but it's a snap to grow your own. You'll find ultra-easy gardening directions in "Grow Your Own," starting on page 120.

A **supplement overdose** can **kill** you.

The Monumental Multivitamin Debate

It's probably safe to say that most of us have been taking a multivitamin/mineral pill for years. But do you really need it? The answer depends on whom you talk to. Natural health pros and conventional MDs alike are unanimous in the conviction that it's best to get all of your life-giving nutrients from a wholesome, well-balanced diet. But most of those experts—at least the ones who live on planet Earth—realize that for the vast majority of us, that's highly impractical, if not downright impossible. For that reason, in addition to eating the healthiest diet you can, many doctors generally recommend choosing one of these two options:

Take specific supplements to fill in any known nutritional gaps, for instance, extra vitamin C if you tend to shortchange yourself on C-rich fruits and vegetables, or iron if you eat little or no red meat and other iron-rich foods.

Down a daily multivitamin/mineral blend to make sure all your bases are covered.

NOTE: *If you're on medications or you suffer from a chronic health condition, check with your doctor before you start taking any kind of supplement—even basic multivitamin/mineral pills.*

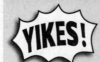 The FDA defines a supplement as an ingestible product containing a "dietary ingredient." And there's the rub. That catchall term includes everything from the standard vitamins, minerals, and herbs to exotic enzymes and ground-up animal glands. To say that hawking these wares has become big business is putting it mildly. There are more than 54,000 dietary supplements on the market, sold under at least 1,000 different brand names. At last count, they were raking in well over $30 billion a year (according to reports from the Government Accountability Office), and sales continue to climb.

Surefire Success with Multis

Taking a multi every day? Good for you! But you may not be getting the most out of your dose. To ensure that your daily vitamin/mineral packs the biggest possible punch, keep these pointers in mind:

1. Choose a product that has 100 percent of the daily values for most of the essential vitamins and minerals.

2. Take it at mealtime. Which meal is your call, but make sure the menu includes a little fat so that your body can absorb the fat-soluble vitamins A, D, E, and K. It doesn't take much: For example, a small handful of nuts, a tablespoon of olive oil in your salad dressing, or full-fat milk on your cereal will do the trick nicely.

3. Chase it with a drink (for instance, a glass of orange or tomato juice at breakfast) to help the pill dissolve.

When Good Food Does Bad Things

The human body is a highly sophisticated mechanism, but on occasion, when you swallow a normally healthy food, your system mistakes it for an alien invader. Then your innards charge to your aid with an onslaught of chemicals, and the ensuing battle can produce some highly unpleasant collateral damage, including any of this quintet:

- Asthma
- Fainting
- Hives
- Itchiness
- Swelling of the lips, mouth, or throat

The Most Unwanted List

When it comes to allergies, the truly deadly demons are peanuts, shellfish, and strawberries, but fortunately, severe reactions are pretty rare. The most common culprits are chocolate, corn, dairy products, eggs, and wheat, all of which can cause nonlethal, though highly bothersome, reactions. Your best defense: common sense! If you know that you're allergic to a food, don't eat it. And when you buy packaged foods, read the labels carefully to make sure your body's "enemies" aren't lurking inside.

The Shocking Shellfish Menace

If you're allergic to shellfish, the problem may not be the fish itself, but the iodine in lobsters, clams, and other crustaceans. So before you have a CAT scan or intravenous X-rays, tell the medical team about your allergy. The dyes used in these procedures contain iodine, and that could do you more harm than the condition the docs are investigating.

Make Peace with Moo Juice

Lactose intolerance is caused by a deficiency of an enzyme that breaks down the sugar in milk. It's not a dangerous health condition, but it can be highly annoying if you love dairy foods such as milk, ice cream, and cheese. Plus, avoiding those foods deprives your diet of sufficient calcium. You can buy lactose-free dairy products marketed under the Lactaid® label. Simpler yet—especially when you're on the go—pick up some Lactaid drops or tablets, and take a dose before downing your favorite treats.

3 Secrets to Safe Supplement Shopping

With literally tens of thousands of nutritional supplements crowding store shelves and streaming across the Internet, how do you tell the real deal from expensive snake oil? Whether you're looking for daily multivitamin/mineral pills or a super-sophisticated health enhancer, follow these simple guidelines:

1. Check the label for a gold stamp that says "USP Verified." This means that the product has been tested and approved by the U.S. Pharmacopeial Convention. Bear in mind, though, that the absence of such a stamp does not necessarily mean the stuff didn't pass muster. It could be that the manufacturer simply chose not to pay for the verification process.

2. Look for a scientific advisory board listed on the company's website.

3. If you have any concerns, pick up the phone and call the manufacturer. **NOTE:** *If you can't reach a human being who can answer your questions—or worse yet, if there is no contact information on the package—don't even think of putting the stuff in your mouth.*

Supplements: Major Danger Ahead?

More and more people are realizing that their diets are lacking in basic nutrients. That's the good news. In a not-so-good response,

You Don't Need Calcium Supplements

Jaw-Dropping **DISCOVERY**

For years, the medical community has promoted the use of calcium supplements to alleviate, prevent, or slow the onset of osteoporosis. But now, bone-health experts are questioning that conventional wisdom for three reasons:

1. Most parts of the world have lower rates of osteoporosis than we have in the United States, and folks in those areas consume less calcium than we do.

2. Studies show that taking calcium supplements cuts your risk of osteoporosis by a mere 1 to 2 percent.

3. It seems highly likely that vitamin D and other nutrients play larger bone-building roles than calcium does.

The new R_X for strong bones: Up your vitamin D intake by spending more quality time in the sun, and shape up your lifestyle to eliminate two factors that deplete calcium from your system: lack of physical activity and a diet that's too high in protein, salt, sugar, and fat.

NOTE: *If you've already been prescribed calcium supplements, check with your doctor before you quit them cold turkey.*

sales of nutritional supplements and fortified foods are soaring off the charts. Unfortunately, some of the vitamins and minerals we need to stay in good shape (or even alive) can cause major problems if we get too much of them. It's all but impossible to develop an unsafe level of any vitamin or mineral from "regular" foods and beverages—with the exception of sodium. But if you take supplements and routinely consume processed foods and drinks that are beefed up with various nutrients, you could easily serve yourself a hazardous—possibly fatal—megadose.

Americans spend **$30 billion** a year on **dietary supplements**.

Revealed: The Shocking Hazards of a Nutrient Overdose

Getting too much of just about any vitamin or mineral is likely to cause bothersome side effects, such as stomach pain, nausea, vomiting, diarrhea, and skin rashes. But in some cases, taking an extra-large dose for a prolonged period of time can have major consequences. Here are five worst-case scenarios a supplemental megadose can cause:

An excess of vitamin A raises the risk for osteoporosis and hip fracture in postmenopausal women, and studies show that it may increase your chance of death from all serious health conditions.

Overdoing it with vitamin E may trigger hemorrhaging and hemorrhagic stroke.

Iron overload (a.k.a. hemochromatosis) can cause fatal damage to your liver, pancreas, and heart.

Massive amounts of magnesium can lead to extremely low blood pressure and ultimately to cardiac arrest and death. The risk of developing this condition (hypermagnesemia in scientific lingo) is greatest for folks with impaired kidney function.

Taking too much potassium can result in potentially deadly cardiac arrhythmia.

The bottom line is—don't OD on supplemental nutrients!

4

Fearsome Food Fallacies

Heaven knows, it's not easy to eat a wholesome, healthy diet these days. Factory farmers are stuffing their livestock with antibiotics and growth hormones, chemical conglomerates are genetically engineering seeds like there's no tomorrow, and giant agribusinesses are dumping mega-tons of pesticides on their food crops. Add to all that a torrent of hype and hoopla from the Big Food industry, and it's enough to make your head spin. Fortunately, with an armload of facts and an arsenal of savvy strategies at your disposal, you and your family *can* eat happily ever after.

Stop Swallowing Poison!

➜ It's no secret that most of the food found in supermarkets and restaurants is loaded with enough crud to kill an elephant. Well, the first step in dodging those deadly demons is knowing exactly what they are and where they're hiding out.

Most of Your Food Comes Fresh from the Factory

Processed food has been on the scene since the early 1900s, when a German chemist named Wilhelm Normann patented the hydrogenation process, which, simply speaking, entails adding hydrogen atoms to vegetable oil. Food manufacturers quickly latched on to the procedure and ran with it, for a two-pronged reason: Hydrogenation increases both the shelf life and flavor stability of foods. That meant their products

YIKES! The synthetic ingredients added to processed foods are not chosen simply to enhance flavor or increase shelf life. Many of these additives are specifically designed to trick your taste buds into wanting more . . . and more . . . and more. Add to this tomfoolery the combo of highly sophisticated marketing tactics, state-of-the-art packaging, and the convenience of meals that are ready to heat and eat, and you've got one staggering statistic: Today as much as 90 percent of the food in your local supermarket is made not by Mother Nature, but by scientists tinkering in laboratories!

would stay fresh and good-tasting far longer than any natural food ever could. Unfortunately, processing also strips out nearly all of the natural nutrients and, in most cases, adds heaps of chemicals that are worthless at best and often dangerous to boot.

2 Appalling Additives in Processed Food

Food manufacturers have Food and Drug Administration (FDA) approval to use more than 3,000 flavorings, preservatives, dyes, and other additives in their products, despite the fact that many of them have been linked to health problems ranging from hormone disruption to cancer. These are two of the most widely used—and most problematic—ingredients:

Fructose, most often used in the form of high-fructose corn syrup (HFCS), is now the number one source of calories in the United States. It contains no vitamins, minerals, or enzymes whatsoever. What's more, it leaches essential micronutrients from your body and has been fingered as a key player in the development of obesity, heart disease, diabetes, osteoporosis, autoimmune diseases, reproductive disorders, and quite possibly premature aging.

Processed food constitutes **95%** of the **American diet**.

Monosodium glutamate (MSG) is added to literally thousands of processed foods as well as to restaurant meals, and for good reason: It really does make food taste fresher and smell better. Unfortunately, this beloved flavor enhancer is what scientists call an *excitotoxin*, which means that it overexcites your cells, sometimes to the point of death, and can cause varying degrees of brain damage. It may even trigger or worsen deadly conditions, such as Alzheimer's, Parkinson's, and Lou Gehrig's diseases.

The Ghoulish, Ghastly Dangers of GMOs

Unless you've been living in a cave for the past 10 years or so, you know that genetically modified organisms (GMOs) are running rampant in just about every kind of processed food on the supermarket shelves. Extensive animal testing has shown that foods containing GMOs cause health problems, ranging from gastrointestinal upsets and infertility to organ damage, immune system impairment, and accelerated aging. Yet, for reasons known only to the bureaucrats in Washington, the FDA not only approves these dangerous ingredients but also, as of this writing, has not even given the green light for human testing. Worse yet, food manufacturers do not have to list GMO ingredients on their labels.

Flee from These 4 GMO Felons

The most common genetically engineered ingredients in processed foods are corn, soy, beet sugar, and vegetable oils that are derived from GMO crops. The natural health crowd refers to them as the "Factory Four." Here's the lowdown on these infiltrators and what to look out for:

Corn. About 90 percent of the corn grown in the United States is genetically engineered. Most of it goes into animal feed and from there makes its way into meat, poultry, and eggs. The rest is converted into corn flour, corn oil, cornmeal, and high-fructose corn syrup—some of the most common ingredients in processed foods.

Soy. This stuff is tinkered with even more so than corn. A full 93 percent of the American soy crop has been genetically altered. Like corn, a lot of it winds up as critter feed, but plenty also goes into your chow in the form of soybean oil, soy milk, soy flour, soy proteins, soy sauce, and soy lecithin.

Beet sugar. More than half of the sugar produced in America comes from sugar beets, a staggering 95 percent of which has been genetically modified. Unless a product label specifically lists "pure cane sugar,"

> ## A Savvy Secret to Sidestepping GMOs
>
> Some makers of nonorganic foods are bypassing GMOs and proudly saying so on their packaging. With most processed foods, though, you need to read labels very carefully because manufacturers use some innocent-sounding words to disguise GMO content. Turn thumbs-down on foods with labels that include any of these tricky terms meant to fool shoppers:
>
> ▶ Aspartame
>
> ▶ Caramel color
>
> ▶ Fructose
>
> ▶ Glucose
>
> ▶ Monosodium glutamate (MSG)
>
> ▶ Tofu
>
> ▶ Xanthan gum

there's a good chance that the stuff has been sweetened with GMO beet sugar.

Vegetable oils. Corn, soybean, canola, and cottonseed oils are all made primarily from GMO varieties. On the other hand, you can rest easy with olive, peanut, grapeseed, coconut, almond, sunflower, and safflower oils because those crops are not genetically engineered—at least not yet!

Labeled for Health

You can make shopping much easier and avoid a whole lot of unhealthy food by looking for one or both of these labels on the packaging:

Certified Organic. By law, any food that sports this label must be produced without genetic engineering and without the use of most synthetic pesticides and fertilizers (including sewer sludge), growth hormones, irradiation, and antibiotics. It also must be certified as meeting those standards by the United States Department of Agriculture (USDA) and/or various state governments. Just about any edible product—whether it's fresh, frozen, dried, or canned—is eligible for the organic designation. That includes fruits and vegetables, grains, meats, dairy products, eggs, coffee and tea, and even processed foods such as ketchup and salad dressings.

Most of the **food** in grocery stores is **factory made**.

Non-GMO Project Verified. This designation by the Non-GMO Project takes organic certification one step further. Not only does it tell you that the food in question contains no GMOs, but it also tests foods to ensure that they have not been contaminated with pollen from nonorganic farms. It only certifies products that have less than 0.9 percent GMO contamination. The organization publishes its list of certified non-GMO products (see "Your Guide to Safe Shopping," above, for details.)

4 Worth Looking For

Three of America's best-loved vegetables and one popular—and normally ultra-healthy—fruit are being genetically modified and sold commercially without any warning labels. Before you plunk down your cash for any of the following quartet, make sure that it's sporting a Certified Organic label.

- Papaya
- Yellow summer squash
- Sweet corn
- Zucchini

Care for a Flame-Resistant Beverage?

No? Well, there's a good chance you're getting it anyway—that is, if you quaff citrus-flavored soda pops or energy drinks. Some of them contain a synthetic chemical called brominated vegetable oil (BVO), which was first marketed as a flame retardant. While this stuff won't kill you, it can make you fat and depressed. That's because it interferes with the function of your thyroid gland, which helps regulate both your mood and your body weight. Imbibing too much BVO can also cause memory loss, nerve disorders, and skin lesions. Water, anyone?

The "Natural" Food Fable

Most of us assume that when we see the word *natural* on a food label, it means that what's inside is wholesome and healthy. The short answer is, naturally, NOT! A "natural" label is simply a designation food companies apply to any product that has received relatively little processing and contains no chemical preservatives. It may or may not be organic, and it may or may not be any different from the regular, unmarked version of the same product. Furthermore, it could easily contain GMOs and a great deal of other stuff that you'd rather not put into your body. (For some ultra-icky examples, see "6 Grossly Gross Ingredients in Processed Foods" on page 102.)

Frightful Phosphates

Your body needs phosphorus. It teams up with calcium and other minerals to build and maintain strong teeth and bones, and it helps transport waste out of your system. But, as with any other mineral, more is not better. The recommended dietary allowance (RDA) of phosphorus is 700 milligrams. Yet, thanks to the potent load of synthetic phosphates in processed foods, most of us are getting

1,500 milligrams or more (sometimes a *lot* more) every day without even knowing it. This overload is being linked to ever-increasing rates of chronic kidney disease, weak bones, and premature death. Your two-part plan for good health:

1. Eat plenty of foods that are naturally rich in *real* phosphorus, such as whole grains; nonprocessed meats, poultry, and fish; eggs; nuts; legumes; and dairy products. This way, an overload is all but impossible because your body absorbs only 40 to 60 percent of the phosphorus content from natural sources.

2. Before you buy any processed food, read the label carefully and pass on anything that contains the letters *phos*. Some of the most common culprits are sodium phosphate, calcium phosphate, and phosphoric acid, but there are 45 different kinds in all. They're used in literally hundreds of packaged foods, from "enhanced meats" (such as self-basting turkey) to frozen dinners and macaroni-and-cheese mixes—and, as unbelievable as it may sound, the FDA does not require food companies to even analyze their products for phosphate levels, much less specify them on their packaging. So it's up to *you* to protect yourself and your family from these deadly demons.

The Harrowing Horrors of Soy

Jaw-Dropping DISCOVERY

For decades, marketing cheerleaders have pitched soy as the ultimate health food. Well, it turns out that this stuff is downright dangerous, both in its natural state and in processed foods—even organic versions. Soy actually contains what scientists call *antinutrients*—substances that literally thousands of studies have linked to cognitive decline, digestive problems, thyroid dysfunction, pancreatic disorders, malnutrition, heart disease, and cancer. And that's only the tip of the soybean. Here are just a few evil examples of these health destroyers:

Goitrogens block your synthesis of thyroid hormones and can lead to thyroid cancer and hypothyroidism.

Hemagglutinin causes your red blood cells to clump abnormally, thereby preventing them from properly absorbing oxygen and distributing the life-giving gas to your tissues.

Phytic acid (a.k.a. phytates) hinders your body's ability to assimilate essential minerals, such as calcium, magnesium, copper, iron, and zinc.

There's a Paint Chemical in Your Salad Dressing

Titanium dioxide is a common ingredient in paint—both house paint and the kind artists use. But the Big Food companies use it on plenty of other "canvases," despite the fact that it is an inorganic chemical with no nutrients whatsoever, rivals diamonds for hardness, and is sometimes described as the equivalent of eating ground glass. And here's the real shocker: The American Cancer Society ranks titanium dioxide among its top five suspected carcinogens. It's also considered a possible trigger for asthma, kidney problems, and Alzheimer's disease. Think about that the next time you're in the supermarket and reach for a bottle of salad dressing. You'll also find it in skim milk, mayonnaise, coffee creamers, ketchup, and icing on cakes and cookies, to name just a handful of horrific examples.

When it comes to processed foods, the FDA can be pretty lenient, to put it mildly. Despite tests to make sure processed foods are safe to eat, those boxes, bags, and cans often harbor disgusting stuff that you really shouldn't put in your body. If these three examples don't send you scurrying to the fresh-food sections of your supermarket, I don't know what will!

▶ An 8-ounce box of macaroni is allowed to contain as many as 225 insect fragments and 4½ rodent hairs.

▶ A 3½-ounce can of mushrooms will pass muster as long as it has no more than 74 mites and 19 maggots.

▶ Maggots can occupy up to 5 percent of the space in any jar of maraschino cherries.

The Deep, Dark Secret of Sprouts

The pitch: Raw-food enthusiasts and other health-conscious folks would have you believe that raw sprouts are nutritional gold mines. In trendy restaurants from coast to coast, they're hailed as an ultra-healthy, crunchy topping for salads and sandwiches.

The truth: While alfalfa, bean, broccoli, and pea sprouts all pack a whopping load of vitamins, minerals, protein, and enzymes, they've been the instigators of at least 40 major outbreaks of food-borne illness over the past 20 years. Even organic versions are often contaminated with *E. coli*, *Listeria*, and *Salmonella* bacteria, and for good reason: These and other dangerous bacteria multiply like mad in the warm, moist conditions that seeds require in order to sprout.

Your best defense: If you favor sprouts for their texture, get the crunch without the risk by shredding cabbage, carrots, or onions onto your sandwiches and salads. On the other hand, if it's the flavor you fancy, cook your sprouts thoroughly before you eat them.

More than **90%** of U.S. **soybeans** are **genetically modified**.

Are Vitamins Killing You?

Like many folks, you probably pop a multivitamin pill into your mouth every day to fill any nutritional gaps in your diet. But unless those supplements are chosen with care, they could be doing you a lot more harm than good. Here are two things to look out for when shopping for vitamin and mineral boosters:

Synthetic vitamins. These are formulated from chemical compounds that do not exist in nature. Some of these substances, such as nicotine and coal tar, are downright toxic. Other synthetic ingredients may not harm you directly, but your body can't absorb them as effectively as it can natural, plant-based vitamins. The fat-soluble vitamins, A, D, E, and K, are especially dangerous in synthetic form. When they build up in your system, they are likely to cause major trouble.

Toxic additives. Just like processed foods, many vitamin/mineral pills contain unnecessary fillers that give them the kind of form, color, flavor, or weight that appeals to shoppers. Be on the lookout for these potentially hazardous chemicals: magnesium stearate or stearic acid, methylcellulose, MSG, silicon dioxide, and titanium dioxide.

Something Fishy Is in Your Fish Oil

Jaw-Dropping DISCOVERY

If you take fish oil supplements to up your intake of ultra-healthy omega-3 fatty acids, be forewarned—some of these products have been found to contain stuff that's anything *but* healthy, such as lead, mercury, cadmium, arsenic, and pesticide residue. While the FDA will crack down on any companies whose potions are found to harbor these poisons, the manufacturers are responsible for ensuring the safety of their products. So don't take any chances. Always choose a brand that displays proof that all individual ingredients as well as the finished product have been tested for safety.

The Tummy-Turning Truth about Eggs

From a nutritional standpoint, eggs are the next best thing to mother's milk. The humble hen fruit has higher-quality protein than any other natural food, plus 39 important vitamins and minerals and every single one of the amino acids that the human body needs. There's just one catch: Depending on where you're getting your eggs, they could be delivering a boatload of junk that you *don't* want in your body. Hens raised on factory farms are nearly always pumped full of antibiotics and arsenic-laden feed to promote growth, and what goes into the chicken goes into the eggs. But wait—it gets worse! According to a study published in the journal *Veterinary Record*, eggs from hens confined in cages (as most of them are these days) are nearly eight times more likely to contain *Salmonella* bacteria than eggs from noncaged birds.

Not Egg-zactly Healthy

A hen's diet isn't the only thing that reduces the nutritional value of commercial eggs (see "The Tummy-Turning Truth about Eggs," at left). Egg cartons nearly always sport pictures of iconic farm scenes because, naturally, egg producers want you to think their hens are scurrying in and out of a cozy red barn, frolicking in the barnyard sun, and foraging for bugs and other goodies. But the real truth is enough to make any animal lover—or egg lover—sick. In most cases, hens spend their entire lives crammed into small cages stacked to the ceiling in a windowless warehouse. On top of that, the chickens are debeaked to keep them from being hurt in such tight quarters, and they undergo forced molting to prolong their egg-laying careers. All this stress, added to the crud in their diets, takes its toll on the nutritional content of their eggs.

Beware of Egg-Carton Labeling Lies

Egg marketers use scads of terms such as *cage-free, free-range, free-roaming,* and *natural* to make you think you're getting hen fruit from the equivalent of Old Mac-Donald's Farm. Well, folks, I'm here to tell you that verbiage is about as meaningless as the word *natural* on other food labels. To get eggs that pack their full nutritional wallop, buy your supply from a local farmer who raises his chickens on grassy pastures. According to studies, eggs from these hens have twice the amount of vitamin E and about two and a half times more omega-3 fatty acids than the kinds less fortunate hens deliver. Your second best option: Look for cartons marked "Animal Welfare Approved," a designation by the Animal Welfare Institute that carries the highest standards of any third-party auditing program.

6 Grossly Gross Ingredients in Processed Foods

When you take a good, hard look at the ingredients listed on processed-food labels, you can find a whole lot of stuff that the FDA deems "generally recognized as safe" (GRAS)—but that might just make you hold your nose and say "Yuck!" Here's a half dozen of the ickiest additives around:

Carmine (a.k.a. Natural Red 4), a food coloring commonly found in ice cream, grapefruit juice, lemonade, and some candies, is made from boiled, crushed cochineal bugs (tiny, scale-like insects that live on cactus plants).

Carnauba wax, which gives a tough-as-nails shine to cars, shoes, floors, surfboards, and other objects that see a lot of heavy wear and tear, is a popular ingredient in gummy candies and chewy fruit snacks.

Castoreum, a flavor enhancer used in candies, puddings, and some frozen dairy desserts, is derived from the castor sac scent glands of beavers, which are located near the critter's anus. You won't see this specific term mentioned on food labels.

Instead, it's generally described as "natural flavorings."

Disodium dihydrogen pyrophosphate, an inorganic chemical, is widely used as a leavening agent in processed baked goods and a color preservative in such edibles as canned seafood and frozen potatoes. It's also highly effective at two other jobs: dispersing the drilling mud used in oil wells and removing iron stains from animal hides during leather processing.

L-cysteine, a dough conditioner that's found in a lot of fast-food desserts and scads of processed baked goods, is made from duck feathers and human hair (frequently imported from China).

Shellac (yes, the old-fashioned furniture finish!) imparts its shiny glow to many sweet treats, such as candy corn, jelly beans, and chocolate mints. You'll see it listed as "confectioner's glaze" or "candy glaze" on the label. Shellac is also used as a coating on aspirin and other "slow-release" tablets. This tasty ingredient is produced by the female *Kerria lacca*, a scale insect that is native to Thailand.

Lethal Bacteria Lurk in Your Meat

The meat and poultry that you buy at the supermarket commonly contain staph bacteria—possibly including the all-but-impossible-to-kill and potentially deadly MRSA strain. The reason: Almost across the board, industrial agribusinesses shoot their livestock full of antibiotics and other veterinary medicines, and this practice fuels the rise of bacteria and other organisms that shrug off all currently available cures. Not scared yet? Then consider these two factoids:

50% of supermarket **meat** may harbor **staph bacteria**.

1. Each year, the MRSA bacteria kill about 19,000 people in the United States (that's more than the number of Americans who die annually from AIDS).

2. A recent study published in the journal *Clinical Infectious Diseases* found that *half* of the meat tested harbored staph bacteria.

Buy Your Milk and Meat from Metallic Cows?

I don't think so. But you're getting plenty of it if you buy common supermarket meats and dairy products. And unfortunately, it's not just beef you need to worry about. Chicken, turkey, pork, and lamb can also be laced with heavy metals, not to mention antibiotics, growth hormones, and pesticide residue. Your best line of defense: Buy all your meat, eggs, milk, and other dairy products from organic farmers whose critters eat good old-fashioned grass—not commercial feeds that are made from genetically engineered grains and filled with other crud, such as animal by-products and metallic compounds.

Don't Get Your Salmon Down on the Farm!

Salmon is one of nature's richest sources of omega-3 fatty acids, which can help to dramatically reduce inflammation throughout your body and cut your risk for heart attack and stroke. There's just one problem: Farmed salmon—the kind you most often find in supermarkets and on restaurant menus—is all but guaranteed to be chock-full of such carcinogenic chemicals as polychlorinated biphenyls (PCBs), pesticides, and antibiotics. To make matters worse, salmon farmers feed their "herds" a mash made from other types of fish that have been ground into fish oil and fish meal. This yucky stuff makes salmon absorb even more toxins into their fat tissue than other kinds of farmed fish do. The simple way to protect yourself: Whether you're shopping or dining out, always insist on wild-caught Alaska salmon. And don't be taken in by a label that says "Atlantic salmon." That's just the fish-farm marketers' way of pulling the wool over your eyes.

Wild and Wicked Fish

Although wild-caught salmon is one of the healthiest delicacies you can put on your plate, the same does not hold true for some other types of fish. In particular, marlin, orange roughy, shark, and swordfish contain extremely high levels of mercury. While the jury is still out on exactly how dangerous this heavy metal is for women beyond their childbearing years, medical pros warn that it's not good for anyone. So play it safe and steer clear of these fish, or at least limit your intake.

2 Shocking Reasons to Shun Shrimp

Americans eat far more shrimp than any other kind of seafood, but before you order up a fried shrimp platter or a shrimp cocktail at your favorite restaurant—or toss any kind of shrimp into your supermarket cart, consider these two gut-wrenching facts:

1. The vast majority of shrimp that's sold in supermarkets and served in restaurants—and virtually everything you get

---

Fiendish Fish Fraud

Jaw-Dropping DISCOVERY

A recent study conducted by the Oceana Foundation revealed that one in three of the seafood samples it examined had been mislabeled. And according to an article in *Food Safety News*, much of that errant verbiage was placed there on purpose so that cheaper fish could be sold at premium prices. Fraudulent labeling is more common in restaurants than it is in grocery stores, but in both places the most likely hoaxes are fillets, nuggets, and other cuts that are much harder to identify by sight.

Be especially wary of imported fish and seafood. By its own admission, the FDA tests less than 3 percent of the stuff that enters our country, which means there's an excellent chance that these foreign arrivals could be mislabeled—or tainted with heaven knows what toxic junk!

at one of the national chains—is imported from places like Thailand. There, the critters are farmed in mangrove swamps that are turned into filthy ponds and loaded with antibiotics and scads of other crud.

2. In the ocean, not only is the supply of shrimp dwindling rapidly, but the methods used to harvest it are destroying astounding quantities of other sea dwellers. For each pound of wild shrimp scraped from the ocean bed, five pounds of so-called bycatch (the other critters caught in the nets) is pulled onto the boat deck and allowed to die—including a lot of endangered sea turtles.

The bottom line: For the sake of your health *and* the survival of the sea's natural balance —not to mention future seafood supplies— forget about eating shrimp. Instead, get your seafood fix from safer and less endangered shellfish sources—clams, mussels, and oysters, for example.

CALL 911

Shellfish allergies can be deadly— and they can come on later in life, sometimes without your knowing it. Symptoms appear within minutes after eating the offending substance. Call 911 immediately if you or a dining companion experiences any of these danger signs:

▸ Dizziness, light-headedness, or loss of consciousness

▸ Rapid pulse

▸ Shock, with a severe drop in blood pressure

▸ Swollen throat or a lump in the throat that makes breathing difficult

Extinction Alert: Fish on the Brink

Don't dodge shark and other kinds of fish just for the sake of your health. Another reason for avoidance is that these creatures are being overfished to the point of extinction, which has serious ramifications for everything that lives in the ocean. Chilean sea bass, rockfish, scallops, shrimp, and bluefin tuna—to name just a handful—are all at high risk. Fortunately, the Monterey Bay Aquarium Seafood Watch® keeps tabs on the ever-growing list. To find out which types of fish are on the brink of vanishing from the sea—and to choose healthy, less endangered alternatives—visit www.seafoodwatch.org. There, you can peruse a searchable database or download a series of regional, printable pocket guides.

1/3 of the **fish sold** in the U.S. is **mislabeled**.

Pest Killers Are Killing You

→ For decades now, we've known that chemical pesticides and herbicides are harmful to human and animal health. Yet, even as more and more studies prove just how deadly these substances are, the chemical industry and giant agribusiness operations bombard us with ever-greater amounts of the poisons. Fortunately, there are ways to protect yourself from the onslaught. As in any battle, the process starts with understanding the enemy.

3 Sickening Facts about Roundup

For decades now, homeowners, golf course groundskeepers, and farmers alike have been reaching for Roundup® to kill pesky weeds. And why not? It's quick, easy, and effective; and the folks who market the stuff pitch its active ingredient, glyphosate, as "biodegradable" and "safe." Well, guess what? The scientific evidence is pouring in, and it's not painting a pretty picture, to put it mildly. Here are three findings that should make you swear off this stuff for good:

Americans use **1.1 billion pounds** of **pesticides** a year.

A French study published in the journal *Chemical Research in Toxicology* found that the levels of glyphosate commonly found in our food—which are far below the amounts permitted in agriculture—can kill human placental, embryonic, and umbilical cells within 24 hours. But that's not all! Roundup has also been linked to spontaneous abortions in farm animals. The bottom line: This stuff is a killer!

It causes cancer. Researchers at the International Agency for Research on Cancer have found that exposure to glyphosate doubles your risk of developing non-Hodgkin's lymphoma, and it's been linked to other malignancies, including breast cancer. But that's not all! More and more research is tying this weed killer to other major health problems, including hormone disruption, obesity, heart problems, and diabetes—and that's just for starters.

It's bombarding us from inside and outside. Every year, nonorganic farmers dump literally millions of pounds of Roundup on their crops. Because it's a systemic chemical, it's absorbed into the plants that we—and farm animals—eat. Scarier yet, the amounts are so excessive that scientists from the U.S. Geological Survey found glyphosate in rain and in the air.

It's gutting your gut. In addition to killing weeds, glyphosate wipes out many pathogenic organisms. (For that reason, it's registered with the U.S. Department of Agriculture as an antimicrobial agent as well as an herbicide.) There's just one freaky problem: Bad bacteria, like *Salmonella*, *E. coli*, and *Clostridium botulinum*, can survive a glyphosate incursion into your digestive tract—but beneficial bacteria, like *Bacillus* and *Lactobacillus*, cannot. In a worst-case scenario, their destruction could lead to "leaky gut," in which your gut lining is so compromised that harmful bacteria and deadly toxins escape into your bloodstream.

A Genetically Engineered Nightmare

In 1996, Monsanto introduced Roundup Ready® Soybeans, which its scientists had genetically altered to resist the company's Roundup herbicide and other products containing glyphosate. They touted GMO technology as a way to reduce the use of chemicals on food crops. Boy, did *that* plan backfire! In the years since then, herbicide use has actually increased by 527 million pounds.

The fact is that engineering seeds so they survive herbicide sprayings that
(continued on page 109)

Herbicide Disaster Alert!

Because Roundup-resistant GMO crops are failing miserably, Monsanto scientists have come up with another, um, brilliant idea: They've engineered seeds that are designed to survive dousing with the old, ugly dicamba herbicide *and* a new Dow AgroSciences product called Enlist™, which combines glyphosate *and* the older, highly toxic 2,4-D weed killer. As of this writing, the Environmental Protection Agency (EPA) is considering whether or not to grant approval. Scientists reckon that if the EPA does give these Frankenseeds the thumbs-up, herbicide use will quadruple. That could spell disaster, given the results of a just-released 30-year study by the International Agency for Research on Cancer. The organization's team found that phenoxy herbicides, which include 2,4-D and dicamba, are clearly associated with three types of non-Hodgkin's lymphoma. These chemicals have also been linked to other cancers, as well as hypothyroidism, Parkinson's disease, and suppressed immune function. (As a side note, you Vietnam vets will recall that 2,4-D was an active ingredient in the infamous Agent Orange.)

Killer Convenience Foods

It's not only fresh fruits and vegetables that retain dangerous pesticide and herbicide residue. Many of the packaged foods you eat are loaded with those deadly chemicals. According to tests conducted regularly by the FDA, this is the unhealthiest handful:

Bread. Grains of all kinds are routinely sprayed with insecticides. In its most recent analysis, the FDA detected malathion residue on most samples of bread (rye, white, *and* whole wheat), as well as on flour tortillas and crackers.

Breakfast cereals. Wheat-based cereals harbor the same bug-killer residue that bread does. Beyond that, most popular breakfast foods are made from corn, soy, and/or sugar derived from sugar beets—three crops that are genetically engineered to withstand massive doses of pesticides.

Ketchup, spaghetti sauce, and salsa. Commercial farmers spray the heck out of tomatoes in the field, so these three and other tomato-based foods retain significant pesticide residue. The most common is 2-chloroethyl linoleate, which has been linked to nerve and liver damage.

Canned chili. Like other canned foods, chili gets a thumbs-down because of the toxic bisphenol A (BPA) used to line the cans (more on that score coming up). Tomatoes and beans—two key ingredients in most types of chili—are heavily doused with pesticides.

Frozen dinners. It's no secret that these convenience foods are laced with heaps of sodium, artificial flavorings, and other nasty junk. But some of them—particularly frozen lasagna and burritos—have been found to contain organophosphate pesticides in the same class as DDT.

Snack foods. Pretzels and crackers—especially butter crackers, graham crackers, and saltines—contain high levels of organophosphate pesticide residue. And potato chips are notorious for their supply of a nerve- and liver-damaging pesticide called chlorpropham. It's widely used on safflower and soybeans, the source of the oils in which many chips are fried.

The takeaway? If you're going to use these time-savers at all, fork over a little more money for the organic versions!

would normally kill them is a losing battle. Just as the overuse of antibiotics has led to resistant supergerms, this onslaught of weed killers has fueled the emergence of weeds that stand up and shout "Boo!" to glyphosate. (The first one appeared in 1996, the same year Roundup Ready Soybeans hit the market. Now there are more than two dozen species of these superweeds.)

NOTE: *Superbugs are also on the rise in GMO farm fields across the country, causing farmers to ramp up their use of pesticides, big-time.*

2,4-D + Dicamba = Travelin' Trouble on the Double

Make that *big* trouble! When nonorganic farmers spray the ultra-toxic 2,4-D or dicamba on their fields, the disgusting stuff doesn't just stay there, as Roundup does. Instead, it quickly morphs into a gas that floats off in the air. This aerial bombardment can hurt you and your loved ones in four horrifying ways:

YIKES! Even at current levels, 2,4-D is responsible for more drift-related crop destruction than any other herbicide. Just one horrendous example: In 2012, migrating 2,4-D killed off nearly 15,000 acres of cotton and an entire pomegranate orchard in California.

It destroys your garden. The new GMO crops will allow growers to spray their fields with this killer combo later in the season, just at the time when your tomatoes, peppers, and squash are leafing out and are most susceptible to the noxious gas.

13 different **pesticides** are used on **nonorganic strawberries**.

It stabs organic farmers in the back. Even when these chemical gases don't kill plants outright, they often cause severe twisting and other deformities that render the harvest unsaleable. Researchers at Ohio State University estimate that drift from corn and soy fields treated with 2,4-D or dicamba will cause anywhere from a 17 to 77 percent reduction in marketable produce for nearby organic farmers. And, of course, whatever fruits and veggies do survive the attack will cost you a lot more at your local supermarket or farm stand.

It decimates your pest-control squad. In your yard and in natural field border areas, drifts of dicamba and 2,4-D kill off plants that harbor bees, butterflies, and birds that are essential for pollinating a great many crops—along with literally millions of predatory insects and other good guys, like bats and toads, that control destructive pests in organic farms and gardens.

It can kill your pets. Studies at Purdue University and the National Cancer Institute have found that dogs who are exposed to 2,4-D have increased risk for both malignant lymphoma and bladder cancer. In fact, even accidental exposure to the heinous chemicals can also cause lethargy, weakness, vomiting, convulsions—and consequently death—in all domestic and wild animals.

Astonishing Ways to Eat Safer for Less

➡ Contrary to what a lot of folks think—and food marketers *want* you to think—eating a healthier diet does not have to mean dropping a lot more dough on food. In fact, armed with a few simple strategies, you can up the quality of your edibles while actually reducing your grocery budget—not to mention saving buckets of bucks on health-care costs.

2 Bonus Benefits of Organic Food

Avoiding pesticides, herbicides, and other dangerous substances is a mighty powerful reason to opt for organic foods whenever you possibly can. But crud-free chow has a couple of other feathers in its cap that you should know about:

It tastes better. Consumer studies show that organic foods have richer flavor than their counterparts that are grown with synthetic fertilizers and sprayed with chemical pesticides.

It's better for you. Synthetic fertilizers kill off beneficial microorganisms in the soil that supply fruits and vegetables with their most important life-giving nutrients. In fact, a recent survey examining more than 40 years' worth of scientific studies found that organic produce has much higher levels of vitamin C, iron, magnesium, and phosphorus than conventionally grown versions.

The Weird Truth about Organic Food Prices

True or false? Organic food is a gigantic rip-off.

SOMETIMES TRUE, BUT MORE OFTEN FALSE. While some unscrupulous supermarkets and specialty stores do jack up prices to target dedicated organic-food shoppers, in most cases there is a valid reason behind those bigger numbers. The fact is that growing organic produce or raising organic-grade livestock on a commercial scale involves considerably more than just saying "No!" to synthetic chemicals, GMOs, and antibiotics. It demands systematic, long-term planning, detailed record keeping to meet government certification standards, and a major investment in equipment and supplies—which all add up to the higher price of most organically grown food.

Of course, there are exceptions. Even in supermarkets, organic foods don't always cost more than their conventional counterparts. For example, in my local store, the price of a box of cherry tomatoes is the same for both the organic and conventionally grown varieties. The same is true for pasta. Also, just like everything else, organic foods go on sale frequently. When that happens, the cost often drops below that of conventional brands. So keep your eyes open—a healthier diet could cost a lot less than you think!

The Dirty Dozen and the Clean 15

Each year, the Environmental Working Group (EWG) releases two lists that make it a great deal easier to eat healthier

Make a Farmer Your Friend

One of the best ways to cut the high cost of organic food—and have a lot of fun at the same time—is to buy your fruits, vegetables, eggs, meats, and dairy products direct from the source. Chances are, a short drive from home will take you to organic farms with roadside stands or, better yet, pick-your-own fields, where you'll find excellent edibles at a fraction of the cost your local supermarket probably charges. If there's no room in your schedule for a country jaunt, visit a nearby farmers' market that includes organic growers. Besides fresh-picked produce, you're likely to find cut flowers, homemade jams and jellies, yummy baked goods, and even free entertainment. To locate organic farms and markets in your area, check out www.localharvest.org, or search online for "organic farmers' markets."

without the time and expense it can take to go whole-hog organic. One roster presents the 12 conventionally grown fruits and vegetables that EWG's scientists have analyzed and found to retain the largest amounts of pesticide residue. The clean slate identifies the 15 least pesticide-laden types of produce that you're likely to find in your local supermarket. Here are the good, the bad, and the ugly for 2014:

The Dirty Dozen (from most to least pesticide-laden)

1. Apples
2. Strawberries
3. Grapes
4. Celery
5. Peaches
6. Spinach
7. Sweet bell peppers
8. Nectarines (imported)
9. Cucumbers
10. Cherry tomatoes
11. Snap peas (imported)
12. Potatoes

There are **more pesticides** in **apples** than any other fruit.

Dishonorable mention goes to kale, collard greens, and hot peppers because, while their levels of retained pesticide don't qualify them for the top 12, the insecticides that they are generally sprayed with pose major risks to human health.

The Clean 15 (from least to most pesticide-laden)

1. Avocados
2. Sweet corn
3. Pineapples
4. Cabbage
5. Sweet peas (frozen)
6. Onions
7. Asparagus
8. Mangoes
9. Papayas
10. Kiwi
11. Eggplant
12. Grapefruit
13. Cantaloupe
14. Cauliflower
15. Sweet potatoes

Don't Be Fooled by Food Expiration Dates

If you're confused by all of the expiration dates printed on food packages, you're not alone. Whether it's a deliberate move by food companies to make you toss out perfectly good edibles before their time is debatable, but here's the lowdown on what that label lingo really means:

"Sell by" means that the store should move the product off its shelves by that date, but you still have ample time to consume it before the quality goes downhill. Take milk, for example. If the carton says, "Sell by July 25," you have a good week or so beyond that date to drink up before it will be unsafe (or at least highly unpalatable) to drink.

"Best if used by" is a form of quality assurance. It's provided by the manufacturer to suggest how long the product will be at its peak of flavor and freshness. Usually, a package label will say something like "Best if used by July 25." Again, this is only a guideline. It doesn't mean that (for instance) your bag of walnuts will suddenly become inedible at midnight of that day. They will simply begin to slowly decline in flavor and texture.

"Use by" or "Expires on" is a whole other kettle of fish. In this case, if you don't use the product by the date listed, you are likely to see a marked deterioration in both product quality and safety.

Sink or Swim

If you refrigerate eggs outside of their original carton, you won't have a sell-buy date to guide you. So how do you know whether to keep the eggs or pitch them? It's simple: Set one of them into a bowl of cold, salty water. If it sinks, hang on to the eggs (but use them as soon as you can). If the "guinea pig" rises to the surface, toss 'em all out.

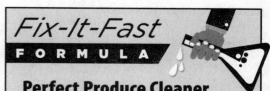

Fix-It-Fast FORMULA

Perfect Produce Cleaner

When you buy conventionally grown fruits or vegetables—even if they're not on the Dirty Dozen list (at left)—it's all but guaranteed that they contain some chemical residue. In the case of organic produce, it may have been sprayed with a botanical pesticide such as rotenone or pyrethrum, or with something that you'd simply rather not eat, like garlic oil. This powerful potion will get rid of all unwanted additives (including garden-variety dirt).

1 cup of white vinegar
1 tbsp. of baking soda
Juice of ½ lemon
1 cup of water

Combine all of the ingredients in a spray bottle, and shake it well. Then, before you eat any fresh produce, or use it in a recipe, give each piece a good spritzing, and let it sit for five minutes. Rinse thoroughly, and you're good to go.

Deflect Dietary Danger

Even if your local supermarket doesn't offer a big supply of organic foods, or you just need to keep an eagle eye on your food budget, you

Nix the #1 Chemical Source

Studies show that meat, milk, and other dairy products retain much more pesticide residue than vegetables and fruits do—in addition to harboring antibiotics and other toxic crap that is routinely pumped into conventionally raised livestock. So do yourself a favor and buy organic versions of any animal-derived foods, even if that means trimming your overall intake of those menu items or pinching pennies elsewhere in your budget.

can still reduce your chemical intake considerably. Here are two simple ways to enjoy a healthier diet without going whole-hog organic:

Consider what you consume. Aside from bypassing the fruits and vegetables on the Dirty Dozen list (see page 112), remember that when pesticides are sprayed onto produce such as leafy greens, tomatoes, broccoli, berries, and grapes, the chemical goes directly onto (and often into) the edible plant parts. For that reason, these foods belong at the top of your buy-organic list. On the other hand, root vegetables like carrots, beets, and onions, as well as thick-skinned fruits like melons, have more natural protection, so less of the sprayed substance will reach the parts you eat. That means you can rest a little easier with conventionally grown versions of these foods.

Consider your eating habits. Most likely, there are certain foods that you and your family consume in quantity nearly every day—maybe milk, bananas, or tomatoes, or processed foods such as cereals and ketchup—and others that you eat less often. Simply by seeking out organic versions of your steady favorites, you'll cut your potential chemical intake dramatically.

Avocados are the **safest nonorganic** food choice.

Sensational Storage Strategies

When you go to the trouble and expense of seeking out organic produce, you sure don't want it to go belly-up before its time. These guidelines will help you keep your produce at the peak of its flavor and nutrition for as long as possible.

Apples. Store them, unwashed and uncovered, in the refrigerator, away from onions and any other odor-producing foods. They'll stay fresh for up to two weeks.

Leaf lettuce. Put the entire bunch into a jar full of water, just as you'd do with a cut flower. Then put a big plastic bag over the whole thing and set it in the fridge.

Mushrooms. Remove them from the plastic packaging they came in, and keep them in a paper bag in your refrigerator. They'll stay fresh twice as long.

Peaches. Pop them into the fridge, unwashed and uncovered. They'll retain their juicy-fresh flavor for a week or so.

Peppers. Stash them, unwashed and uncovered, in the refrigerator crisper for up to two weeks.

> ## The Best-Kept Secret for Keeping Food Fresh
>
> Food goes downhill fast when it's not kept cool enough. So check the temperature in both the refrigerator and freezer compartments. In order to slow the growth of mold and bacteria, the fridge should stay below 40°F, and the freezer should be chillin' along at a frosty 0°F.

Strawberries. You should eat them right away, but if that's not possible, tuck 'em, unwashed, in the coolest part of the fridge, where they'll keep for up to three days.

Zucchini and summer squash. Store in a plastic bag in the refrigerator for up to a week.

Precise Potato Pointers

Whether you opt for ever-popular bakers or more colorful, nutrient-rich varieties, never store your potatoes in the refrigerator, or anyplace else where the temperature gets below 40°F. If you do, they'll develop a sweet taste and turn brown when you cook them. Instead, store your spuds in a cool (45° to 50°F), humid (not wet), dark place with good ventilation. Whatever you do, avoid storing taters in warm places, such as under the sink or in a cupboard that's close to a sunny window. In those spots they will likely sprout and shrivel up and could attract bugs and rodents. And if potatoes are exposed to light during storage, they'll turn green and produce a bitter, toxic substance called solanine. Throw away any that are mostly green, but if there are just a few colorful patches, slice them off, making sure to get all of the green parts out, and then you can safely use the rest of the spud.

3 Timely Tomato-Storage Tips

The tomato may be the crown jewel of the garden, but when it comes to storage, it's a temperamental little bugger. This handful of hints will help you give it the TLC it needs:

A Fine Freezer Fruit

Although tomatoes don't fare too well in the refrigerator (see "3 Timely Tomato-Storage Tips," at right), they do just fine in the freezer. What's more, they don't need any fancy treatment before you freeze them. Just wash them, cut out any bad spots, put them on baking sheets, and slide the sheets into the freezer. Once the tomatoes have frozen, store them in freezer containers. (The skins will crack during the freezing process, making the fruits easier to peel when they've thawed out.)

Hint #1. Tomatoes retain the most flavor when you keep them at room temperature (55°F or above). If they're fully ripe and fresh from the garden (or farm stand), they'll keep for a day or two. But keep them away from direct sunlight. They'll overheat and ripen unevenly, or spoil more quickly.

Hint #2. To bring unripe tomatoes to the eating stage faster, tuck them into a brown paper bag with an apple or a banana. Both fruits give off ethylene gas that speeds the ripening process. But never refrigerate a tomato that's not fully ripe. The cold will destroy the flavor and stop the ripening process in its tracks!

Hint #3. If you have to store your tomatoes for more than two days, you'll need to do the unthinkable and put them in the fridge. For best results, put them in the butter compartment—it's the warmest place—and use them as soon as you can.

Store Your Onions Outside the Box

Outside the icebox, that is. These pungent bulbs (and garlic, too) should never be stored in the fridge. Instead, keep them in a cool, dry place using this method: Drop a bulb into a panty hose leg, tie a knot, drop in another one, and so on. Then hang the bulging pouch from a wall hook in your pantry—or from the ceiling, if it's low enough. When you want to use one of the bulbs, cut just below the knot above it.

Put Your Herbs on Ice

When you put fresh herbs in the fridge, they can turn into a wilted mess right before your eyes. On the other hand, when you freeze them, they retain their fresh-picked flavor, aroma, and nutrient content for months. So wash 'em up, wrap the bunches (one kind per bunch) in aluminum foil, and stash them in the freezer. Another option: Chop the herbs, and freeze them in glass containers; or puree chopped herbs with water, butter, or olive oil. Then pour the mixture into ice cube trays. When the cubes are frozen, pop them out of the trays, and store them in containers or freezer bags.

It's What's Outside That Counts

➡ **If you think that the gunk added to processed foods and the pesticides and herbicides used on farmers' crops are the only dietary hazards you need to be concerned about, think again. The pans that you cook with, the containers you stash your leftovers in, and even the food wraps that you've used for years may be destroying your health.**

The Nauseating Truth about Nonstick Pans

Some folks like to use nonstick cookware because it requires less fats and oils than regular pots and pans do. Other people simply enjoy the fact that these slick surfaces make for easier cleanup. Unfortunately, when these kitchenware coatings start to crack, chemicals called perfluorooctanoic acids leach into your food. These nasty nellies have been linked to a number of health problems, including high cholesterol and ADHD, in adults as well as children. So do yourself a favor: Ditch the nonstick stuff and cook with safe materials. Glass, cast iron, stoneware, and untreated stainless steel are all good choices.

Nonstick pans can be **deadly**.

The Potent Perils of Popcorn

Who would ever think that one of America's favorite, and potentially healthiest, snacks could actually be harming you—that is, if you opt

Old-Fashioned Movie Theater Popcorn

Remember all those Saturday afternoons when you and your pals sat in your hometown movie theater, cheering for the good guys in the white cowboy hats and munching the world's greatest popcorn? Well, guess what? You can re-create that old-time, healthy taste treat right in your own kitchen. This recipe makes two theater-size servings.

3 tbsp. of coconut oil*

⅓ cup of organic popcorn kernels

2 tbsp. of melted butter (or more to taste)

Salt and pepper (optional)

Heat the oil in a 3-quart saucepan over medium heat. Put three or four popcorn kernels into the pan, and cover it. When the kernels pop, add the remainder so they form an even layer on the bottom of the pan. Replace the cover, remove from the heat, and wait 30 seconds. Return the pan to the heat, keeping the lid slightly ajar (this way, steam can escape, keeping the popcorn drier and crisper). As soon as the kernels start popping, move the pan back and forth over the burner until several seconds elapse between pops. Then remove the lid, and dump the popcorn into a wide bowl. Toss it with the melted butter and the seasonings, if desired. Then fire up the DVD player, and dig in.

* Or substitute another oil that has a high smoke point, such as peanut or grapeseed oil.

for the microwavable stuff in the snack-food section of your local supermarket. Not only is the bag lined with weird nonstick chemicals that have been linked to thyroid disease and other ills, but the corn itself contains artificial colorings, flavorings, chemically altered oils, and other gunk that can lead to obesity, diabetes, and (yes) even cancer. So eat popcorn in its healthy state by popping it up using the recipe at left.

The Monstrous Menace of Plastic

Unless you've recently arrived from Mars, you know that bisphenol A (BPA), a type of plastic commonly found in things like canned-food linings, travel cups, and water bottles, has been linked to rising rates of heart disease, breast cancer, prostate cancer, and assorted other serious ills. Well, scads of new studies are showing that other kinds of plastic may be just as toxic, especially when they're heated in a microwave oven or filled with hot foods or beverages. Health and nutrition experts advise getting the following two plastics out of your kitchen and the rest of your house—now!

Polyvinyl chloride (PVC). The dangerous elements here are phthalates, which are highly toxic and migrate freely from PVC to anything that touches it—for example, food, drink, or your mouth. Even small doses can cause or contribute to heart disease, cancer, and reproductive problems. You'll most often find PVC in plastic bags and wraps as well as in plastic squeezable bottles, where it's indicated by #3 inside the recycling triangle on the product.

Polystyrene. One of its key ingredients is styrene (a.k.a. vinyl benzene), which the EPA describes as "a suspected carcinogen" and "a suspected toxin to the gastrointestinal, kidney, and respiratory systems, among others." It comes in two forms. The foam kind is commonly used in disposable coffee cups, take-out food containers, egg cartons, and meat packaging. In solid form, you'll find it in disposable cutlery, yogurt cups, food-storage containers, and the dishes used in microwavable meals. Its presence is indicated by #6 in the recycling triangle on the bottom of product containers.

A Creepy Reason to Can Cans

A recent study by the Centers for Disease Control and Prevention (CDC) estimated that a whopping 92.6 percent of Americans aged six and above have measurable amounts of BPA in their systems. The number one source of this potentially deadly chemical: canned foods. Granted, it's difficult to avoid tins altogether, but whenever possible, opt for soup, chili, tomatoes, beets, and similar foods that come in glass jars or Tetra Pak® boxes rather than cans. Your body will thank you!

Throw *All* the Plastic Bums Out!

REMARKABLE REMEDY

Of course, I realize that's not really possible in this day and age. But studies galore are beginning to show that quite likely no form of plastic is truly safe—at least not over the long term and not in the horrendous quantities used in our homes and offices. While none of us can swear off plastic altogether, there are simple ways to cut back enough to greatly reduce our safety risk. For starters, begin replacing your plastic food-storage containers with glass versions. Ditch your plastic water bottle or traveling coffee cup in favor of a stainless steel model. Instead of relying so much on microwavable meals, start cooking more. (Besides lessening your exposure to toxins and eating healthier, you'll save a whole lot of money!)

Grow Your Own

➡ The surest way to cut back on the pesticides and other toxins in your food is to grow your own fruits and vegetables. Don't get me wrong! I'm not suggesting that you try to grow all your own produce. That would be a full-time job and then some! But even tending a few pots of mini vegetables on your deck or herbs on a sunny kitchen windowsill can go a long way toward reducing your intake of health-destroying poisons.

3 Surprising Secrets to Successful Gardening

Vegetables, fruits, and herbs thrive on the same kind of chemical-free TLC that ornamental plants do. (You'll find the whole lowdown on that in "Poison-Packin' Posies," starting on page 321. So if you're setting out to plant your first food garden, before you buy a single seed, ponder these simple guidelines for happy—and successful—growing:

The **lumber** in **raised beds** can **poison** your crop.

Keep it small. When you're new to growing vegetables, follow my golden rule for happy gardening: Decide on a size that you can handle cheerfully and comfortably, then reduce it by a third.

Keep it near your house. Or as close as your yard's layout will allow. This way, you'll be better able to spot tiny weeds before they grow into big ones. You'll notice insect pests while there's still time to pick them off by hand or send them fleeing with a spray from the garden hose. Plus, you'll know just when your new vegetables are ready for picking, and you won't miss a minute of their sweet, fresh flavor!

Keep it within reach of your hose. Otherwise, you'll spend a lot of time toting a watering can back and forth because vegetables are a thirsty bunch. Most of them require at least an inch of water every week, and some need more than that.

The Bountiful Benefits of Raised Beds

Besides saving space in your yard, growing crops in raised beds is also the best way to ensure both good drainage *and* better moisture retention. But those aren't the only reasons to use these elevated marvels. Just consider the following advantages:

A broader plant palette. An enclosed, raised bed is a big, bottomless container, so you can fill it with any type of soil that suits the requirements of any kind of plant.

Earlier planting. The soil in raised beds warms up earlier in the spring because more of it is exposed to sunlight. That means you can get such heat lovers as tomatoes and peppers off and running that much sooner.

Easier maintenance. You don't have to reach so far to pull weeds and harvest crops. In fact, because the beds can be placed as high as you want, it's possible to garden comfortably even if you use a wheelchair or have trouble bending over.

Good looks. Since the walls can be made of just about any material that holds soil, raised beds are often an attractive addition to your yard.

Problem prevention. The walls hold the soil (and plants) inside, even in heavy rain, and they help deter weeds and many pests to boot.

2 Need-to-Know Facts about Raised Beds

While it *is* true that you can build a raised bed from just about any material under the sun, there are a couple of points you must keep in mind to ensure the health-giving goodness of your food—or even the survival of your crops.

Don't Grow Frankenfood!

You may think that if you intend to grow your crops using organic methods, it doesn't matter what kind of seeds or transplants you start with. Well, think again, friend! It's crucial that you use only organic seeds and seedlings for two reasons:

▶ Conventional seed producers use literally tons of pesticides and fungicides on their seed crops. And those noxious chemicals will stay in the plants that you grow. What's more, if your planting list includes sweet corn, yellow squash, or zucchini, nonorganic versions of those seeds could well be genetically modified.

▶ Organic seeds, produced without the use of synthetic chemicals, are better adapted to organic growing conditions. Therefore, they'll perform better in your garden.

If your local garden center doesn't carry organic versions of the seeds you want, search online for (you guessed it) "organic seeds." You'll find scads of reliable mail-order sources.

Fact #1. Don't use pressure-treated lumber for your raised beds. It contains toxic chemicals that can leach into the soil, and possibly into the plants you'll soon be eating.

Fact #2. If you live in a hot climate, build your beds from light-colored material that reflects the sun's rays—for example, stone, or wood painted with white water-based paint. If the sides are dark, the intense heat they absorb could cook your plants' roots.

Make a Super-Simple Soil Sandwich

The best and easiest way to make a planting bed in any kind of soil—or even on a hard surface like a patio or driveway—is to whip up one of these "sandwiches." Here's the simple four-step process:

Color It Happy

Believe it or not, the color of your pots can play a crucial role in the success or failure of your garden. This is particularly crucial with black containers, which capture and hold heat. That can be a big advantage in a cool climate, especially if you're growing heat-loving vegetables like tomatoes. But during a hot summer, the sun's rays will turn that pot into an oven that will bake your plants' roots before you know it. So if you live where the weather gets steamy, stick with white or pale tones.

Step 1. Build the framework for your raised bed. If it's on your lawn and you have clay soil or (worse) hardpan, puncture the ground in a few places, using a garden fork or even a hammer and metal rod. This will enable earthworms to penetrate the nasty stuff and eventually help soften it.

Step 2. Lay a 1- to 2-inch-thick layer of newspaper over the bed, overlapping the edges as you go and trampling down any tall weeds. Then soak the paper thoroughly with water.

Step 3. Spread 1 to 2 inches of compost over the paper. Then cover the compost with 4 to 6 inches of organic matter. Leaves, pine needles, dried grass clippings, shredded paper, and seaweed will all work like a charm.

Add alternate layers of compost and organic matter until the stack reaches about 12 to 20 inches high.

Step 4. Top the stack off with 4 to 6 inches of a half-and-half mixture of compost and good-quality topsoil. Then water it well, wait two weeks, and plant to your heart's content.

PART 2

Are You on a Fast Track
to an Early Grave?

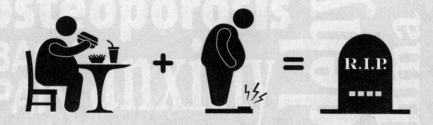

In the days before vaccines, antibiotics, and miraculous surgical techniques, most afflictions that caused folks to die at young ages were not preventable—for example, scarlet fever, smallpox, infected wounds, or complications of childbirth. Today, thanks to modern medical science, those kinds of tragedies are all but unheard of. Instead, each year, millions of people kick the bucket, or become disabled, in the prime of life from conditions that they would never have gotten if they had simply taken better care of themselves. So consider what follows a wake-up call to make sure you don't join that unfortunate crowd.

The Fatal Fat Factor

Despite constant warnings about the dangers of packing on too many pounds, the rate of obesity continues to soar. Granted, in a time when we're constantly surrounded by unhealthy food and bombarded by ads urging us to eat more of it—not to mention spending more time in our cars or parked at our desks—it's not easy to get (or stay) slim and trim. But it's worth every bit of time and effort it takes because shedding your excess pounds is the single most important thing you can do to improve your health and lengthen your life.

Fat Kills!

➡ And not just every now and then. Obesity is second only to smoking as the leading cause of preventable death in the United States. Plus (are you listening, ladies?), it's the number one risk factor for postmenopausal breast cancer. So get with the program, and start slimming down and shaping up pronto!

8 More Reasons to Drop the Pounds

Obesity and lesser degrees of being overweight are renowned for their role in causing diabetes, cardiovascular disease, cancer, and stroke. But when your weight exceeds what's normal for the size of your frame, you're also begging for these eight less-heralded health hazards:

1. Bladder problems

2. Carpal tunnel syndrome

3. Gallbladder disease and gallstones

4. Gout

5. Liver and kidney disease

6. Menstrual irregularities

7. Osteoarthritis

8. Sleep apnea

Are You Just Pleasingly Plump?

How do you know when you've crossed the line from "chubby" to full-blown obesity? Medical pros base that determination on your body mass index (BMI), a number arrived at by dividing your weight by your height. You can find out exactly where you rank by checking the Body Mass Index Table on the website of the National Heart, Lung, and Blood Institute (www.nhlbi.nih.gov/guidelines/obesity/bmi_tbl.htm). But here are the guidelines for adults of statistically average height (5 feet 4 inches for women; 5 feet 10 inches for men):

Normal. BMI 24.9 or below. In terms of weight, that translates into 144 pounds or less for a woman and 173 pounds or less for a man.

Overweight. BMI 25 to 29.9. A woman in this category tips the scales at 145 to 173 pounds. A man weighs 174 to 208 pounds.

Obese. BMI 30 to 39.9. The female weight range here is 174 to 231 pounds. For an obese male, it's 209 to 277 pounds.

Extremely obese. BMI 40 or higher. This dangerous designation goes to a woman who weighs 232 pounds or more and a man who registers 278 pounds or above.

The Sinister Skinny on Belly Fat

The most ominous kind of fat is the type that collects at your abdomen. That's because most of it is what scientists call visceral, or deep, fat. We all need some visceral fat to cushion our organs. But if you gain too much weight, your body runs out of safe places to store visceral fat, so it's forced to stash the excess inside your organs, including your liver, and in too-thick layers around your heart. A spare tire around your belly is a red flag that you've reached the danger zone—and you're a walking invitation for

 If there's any doubt in your mind about how dire the obesity epidemic is, take a gander at these two fiendishly frightening—and foreboding—facts:

1. According to the Johns Hopkins University School of Public Health, the rate of being overweight and obese is nearly four times what it was 40 years ago, and if current trends continue, by 2030 a whopping 86 percent of American adults will be overweight or obese!

2. Estimates place obesity-related health-care costs in the United States at $190 billion a year, and if waistlines continue to expand at their current rate, by 2030 the yearly total will be at least $50 billion higher than that. And that's not counting the extra health-care costs incurred by overweight folks who don't quite meet the definition of obese (see "Are You Just Pleasingly Plump?," at left).

all the ugly by-products of obesity, including high blood pressure, breast cancer, and colon cancer. If you're a woman and your waist size is 35 inches or more, or if you're a man with a 40-inch waist or larger, you're on a fast track to big trouble, so start losing weight now!

2 out of 3
Americans are
overweight.

Fat Fries Your Brain

Study after study has fingered depression as a major contributor to obesity and its unavoidable offshoot, diabetes. Well, guess what? The sinister sword cuts both ways. These two physical conditions also wreak havoc on your mental health. Consider the findings:

- Obese people and those with related conditions, such as diabetes and cardiovascular disease, perform worse on cognitive tests than folks who are leaner and healthier.

- Thanks to new imaging techniques, scientists know that as obese people age, their brains literally shrink, especially in the areas that control clear thinking and positive emotions. So the more overweight you are, the more likely you'll develop dementia and depression.

- These reveal-all pictures also show that the brains of obese patients appear to be 16 years older than those of normal-weight folks of the same age.

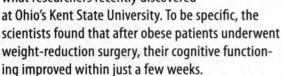

Losing Pounds Leads to Clearer Thinking

The mere fact of being fat fouls up the wiring in your brain that enables you to think clearly. At least, that's what researchers recently discovered at Ohio's Kent State University. To be specific, the scientists found that after obese patients underwent weight-reduction surgery, their cognitive functioning improved within just a few weeks.

Jaw-Dropping DISCOVERY

NOTE: *This is not to suggest that you should even consider going under the knife unless your doctor strongly advises it. There are plenty of safer (albeit slower) ways to drop your brain-fogging fat!*

Scary Secrets of Weight-Loss Surgery

Weight-loss (a.k.a. bariatric) surgery has become a booming industry—to the tune of $3.6 billion a year, with an estimated 400 Americans going under the pound-peeling knife *every day*. For extremely obese folks whose health is declining rapidly, this quick fix can be truly lifesaving. But that doesn't mean it's the right choice for you. Before you opt for an operation, have a serious heart-to-heart with your doctor, and consider these risks:

Post-op complications. A "fat-ectomy" carries the same risks as any other abdominal surgery, including a host of aftereffects. Some, like nausea, vomiting, and diarrhea, are merely bothersome. Others, like wound infections and abdominal hernias, are painful and may require additional surgery.

Fatal consequences. Some bariatric patients suffer fatal heart attacks, bleeding ulcers, blood clots to the lungs (a.k.a. pulmonary embolism), and leaks in the new surgical gut connections. And people over age 60 are at higher risk for all of these lethal problems.

More surgery. Even after a highly successful weight-reduction operation, patients frequently require body-contouring surgery to tighten up sagging skin. Many folks develop gallstones that require gallbladder removal. And vitamin deficiencies and malnutrition are common afflictions because the surgery hinders your body's ability to absorb nutrients efficiently.

Surgery Is Just the Start

If you've struggled for years to lose weight and nothing has worked, bariatric surgery may seem like the miracle cure you've been praying for. But don't count on it. Besides carrying all the risks of any other invasive surgery (see "Scary Secrets of Weight-Loss Surgery," at left), it's not a slam-dunk solution to your problem. That's because it does nothing to address the psychological and emotional reasons that made you obese in the first place. Unless you adopt healthier eating habits, a more active lifestyle, and a different attitude toward food, you could gain back a good bit of the fat the surgeon's knife shaved away. So before you put your life in the hands of the OR staff, ask yourself whether you can, and will, accept the procedure for what it really is—just the first step toward your slimmer, fitter future.

Beware of Cellulite Cures

True or false? Cellulite is simply an annoying cosmetic issue, and spa treatments will help get rid of it.

FALSE! Those pockets of fat that give your skin an unattractive "cottage cheese" or "orange peel" appearance are indications that your liver and

Lively Liver Tonic

Your liver performs more than 200 crucial functions in your body, including eliminating toxic substances from your blood, and producing bile, which is essential for digestion. Simply making fresh parsley a regular part of your diet will help keep that vital organ running smoothly. But every once in a while, give it an extra boost with this tasty cocktail.

½ cup of fresh parsley leaves, finely chopped

½ cup of organic beet juice

½ cup of organic carrot juice

Put all of the ingredients in a blender, and pulse until they're thoroughly combined.

your lymphatic system may not be functioning at their peak—and that lackadaisical performance could have dangerous implications for your whole body. That's because this dynamic duo's purpose is to rid your system of toxins and pathogens of all kinds, as well as your body's waste products and other debris. Plus, a weakened liver causes your other organs to become overactive and stressed out. And sluggish lymphatic flow can throw your body's immune system out of whack. So take this as a wake-up call, and clean up your act. Specifically, revamp your diet, and for heaven's sake, get up off the couch! Regular, moderate exercise is an absolute must for improving your liver function and re-energizing your lymphatic system. And while a spa massage can be relaxing and stress-reducing, it won't cure your cellulite!

You Are What You Eat

➜ Every time you turn around, you see another hustler claiming that your unwanted pounds will slide right off if you just pop this pill, drink that miraculous shake, or eat only certain foods. Well, if you believe such a promise, I can give you a good price on a bridge in Brooklyn. The fact is the only way to lose weight, and stay trim and healthy, is to eat a sensible, wholesome diet and get regular exercise.

3 Daffy Diet Delusions

With so many folks overweight, it's understandable that a lot of them are desperately seeking a slick trick that will make their excess baggage melt away like an ice cube dropped on a hot sidewalk. Well, friends, there is no magic bullet for weight loss. In particular, don't be taken in by this trio of rampant misconceptions:

Wheat is wicked and gluten is ghastly. A lot of folks—including the authors of some highly successful diet books—would have you believe that the instant you eat a slice of bread or a forkful of spaghetti, your belly will blow up like a hot-air balloon. Nonsense! Of course, eating too much wheat will make you gain weight—just the same as an excess of any other food will. On the other hand, eaten in moderation, whole wheat is a valuable part of a healthy diet. As for the gluten that wheat contains, unless you have celiac disease, it's perfectly harmless (see "The Great Gluten Rip-Off" on page 69).

Going organic will make you lose weight. The notion has sprung up in certain circles that chemicals in food make you fat, and if you simply switch to an all-organic diet, your poundage will plummet. Hogwash! While it is true that eating organically grown food will help you avoid a lot of harmful toxins, shoveling down (for instance) a pint of double-chocolate fudge ice cream will have the same effect on your waistline regardless of whether the originating cows ate pesticide-free grass or genetically modified grain.

Diet food makes you drop pounds. Baloney! All those "miraculous" weight-loss cookies, bars, and other pseudo-foods that you see in stores and on the Internet are the solid equivalent of diet soda (see "The Shocking Truth about Diet Soda" on page 66). They're highly processed products made from artificial

Fork Up Forbidden Food

REMARKABLE REMEDY

The surest route to a failed diet is to go cold turkey on any particular kinds of food or drink. That's because forbidding yourself to ever eat (let's say) a few French fries or a slice of cake inevitably leads to cravings for the "no-no" treat. More often than not, such avoidance results in binges that cause you to gain weight rather than lose it—and sends your stress level soaring when you bash yourself for falling off the wagon. Despite what promoters of certain diets may tell you, there are no "good" or "bad" foods. There are just good and bad eating habits. The only way to lose weight and keep it off permanently is to change how you think about food so that you can alter your eating habits for the better.

sweeteners, artificial flavorings, and worthless fillers that trick your brain into thinking that you're eating real food. For a short time, you do feel full, but because your body isn't getting the nutrients and calories that should coincide with a satisfied tummy, your hunger returns with a vengeance. So you eat more. And more . . .

The Great Weight-Loss Plan Rip-Off

We've all seen the big, bright ads with dramatic before-and-after pictures and glowing promises: "Mary Smith lost 50 pounds on the XYZ program, and you can too!" Or the celebrities who crow in TV commercials about dropping the pounds effortlessly on the ABC diet plan.

95% of dieters **regain** their **lost pounds**.

Then at the bottom of the page or screen, they lay out the triple-digit prices you can expect to pay for a supply of their packaged dinners, desserts, shakes, and what have you—along with the tiny-print disclaimer that these results are not "representative of all participants on the program."

You're darn tootin' they're not "representative"! Although these regimens have helped many dieters lose weight, follow-up studies show that all but a tiny percentage of those gullible folks gained it completely back—and then some. The cold, hard fact is that losing weight and keeping it off require a lifetime shift in behavior and the role food plays in your life, and these product-targeted programs offer no guidance at all in that regard. So once you get tired of eating (and paying for!) the branded products and venture into "normal" edibles, the pounds pile right back on.

CALL 911

Diets that greatly restrict your caloric intake or confine you to only one or two types of food can cause major health damage. If you're on any kind of quick weight-loss plan, and you experience any dizziness, severe headaches, vomiting, or diarrhea—head for the ER. You may be seriously dehydrated, or worse.

Red Flags on Fad Diets

It's all but impossible to resist a plan that promises to produce quick weight loss and an instant boost to your health. Unfortunately, these easy-way-out slenderizing schemes rarely, if ever, help you achieve your optimum weight and stay there. What's more, they can hand you more health problems than you had to begin with. In particular, turn two thumbs down on diets that meet any of these descriptions:

They confine the menu largely to one food or type of food. Prime examples of these are the Atkins Diet and similar low-carb, high-protein diets. They are not nutritionally sound, have little scientific evidence to back them up, and can even lead to serious problems, such as loss of muscle density, enlarged kidneys, and renal failure.

They promise fast weight loss. On plans guaranteeing you'll lose 2 pounds a week or more, you probably will lose weight quickly in the beginning, but most of it will be in the form of water, not fat. After the initial week or so, the pounds will drop more slowly. Plus, as soon as you stray from the diet, you'll rapidly return to your original weight. Worse, though, if you stay on the regimen for any length of time, you could deprive your body of enough vital nutrients to cause severe damage to your health.

They rely on "chemical reactions." Or perhaps they refer to "scientific proof" but have no evidence to back up their claims. One infamous example is the diet that has you begin each meal with half a grapefruit on the premise that it contains fat-burning enzymes. (It doesn't.)

Fad diets have been around since the days of ancient Rome, when folks confined the menu to figs and water when they wanted to drop a toga size or two. But pound-shedding ploys don't come any nuttier than this trio, which has made just about every list of the Most Dangerous Diets of 2014. Steer clear of these:

The alcorexia diet has you severely restrict your intake of solid food so you can "bank" as many as 1,500 calories per week for alcoholic beverages. That's equivalent to approximately 15 glasses of red wine or about 15 shots of hard liquor.

The corset diet works on the premise that wearing this tight undergarment will compress your stomach, so you'll eat less. It also compresses your other internal organs, including your liver and kidneys, restricts the flow of oxygen through your whole body, and slows down your metabolism.

The cotton ball diet has you soak cotton balls in fruit juice and swallow them—thereby guaranteeing malnutrition and begging for intestinal blockages. On top of that, most cotton balls are not pure (much less organic) cotton, but also contain polyester fibers and heaven knows what noxious chemicals.

Detox Debunked

Proponents of detox (a.k.a. cleansing) plans pitch them as a way to clear dangerous toxins from your body, but many folks use them to slim down quickly for a big event such as a wedding or a body-baring beach vacation. Well, don't you do it! While you *will* lose weight rapidly, most of it will be water, just as it is with other crash diets. When you resume your normal eating patterns, the number on the scale will shoot right back up again. But that's not the worst of it.

Fasting and other aggressive cleansing methods used in these routines often deliver the unpleasant side effects of constipation, aches, pains, fatigue, flu symptoms, brain fog, and even colon damage. Plus, some plans incorporate herbs and other supplements that can produce serious drug interactions.

Detox diets are especially dangerous for people with underlying health conditions such as diabetes or high blood pressure. The bottom line: The time to start losing weight for a special occasion is months, not weeks, before the big day!

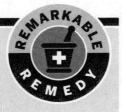

12 Steps to a Slimmer, Healthier You

For some people, overeating is far more than a bad habit—it's a genuine addiction, akin to alcoholism or drug abuse (see "Addiction Advisory: 7 Signs That You May Be Hooked" on page 6). If you recognize your behavior patterns in that rundown, do yourself a favor and give Overeaters Anonymous a try. To find a chapter near you, visit www.oa.org. The organization's 12-step process may not be your cup of tea, but if you do click with the program, you could find, as legions of failed dieters have, that for the first time in your life, *you're* the one calling the shots—not the slave-driving food that's constantly at the forefront of your mind.

The Astonishing Danger of Distracted Eating

We all know that a huge percentage of auto accidents are caused by misguided multitaskers who think they can safely control their cars while (for instance) talking on their cell phones, guzzling their morning coffee, or even applying makeup. Well, guess what? Eating when your mind is focused elsewhere can also produce highly unhealthy results. Of course (unless you're behind the wheel of a car), it won't kill you or harm innocent bystanders, but it can make you fat—or at least put a major crimp in your weight-loss efforts. According to a recent study published in *The American Journal of Clinical Nutrition*, distracted eaters are likely to consume up to 50 percent more calories than folks who devote their full attention to the matter at hand. In fact, they also eat more at the next meal or snack because their minds never fully registered what they consumed on the previous occasion.

Here's the good news: If you routinely gobble lunch at your desk or eat dinner parked in front of the TV, you can cut your calorie consumption in a big way simply by kicking that habit. At home, turn off the television, computer, cell phone, and any other electronic devices. At work, flee your cubicle for the quietest space you can find. Then sit down, and concentrate on enjoying your food. Take small bites, chew slowly, and savor the flavor of every mouthful. That way, both your body and your brain will be satisfied—with a lot less intake than you probably thought possible.

To Shrink Your Belly, Shrink Your Plate

Jaw-Dropping DISCOVERY

Waistlines aren't the only things that have expanded over the past 40 years. Since the 1970s, the typical dinner plate has grown in size from 10 inches in diameter to 12 inches or more (in some cases, a *lot* more). And that gives you an absolutely effortless way to drop your unwanted pounds. Simply by trading in your oversize plates for versions that are 2 inches smaller, you'll serve yourself 22 percent fewer calories per meal. That act alone can make you lose 2 pounds in 30 days—and, most likely, you won't even notice the decrease in the amount of food on your plate.

Quit the Clean Plate Club

There are scads of reasons why so many people in our country are overweight, but one of the most common lies in three little words: "Clean your plate." If you grew up hearing that command around the family dinner table, it's a good bet your subconscious mind still hears it loud and clear every time you sit down to eat. The solution: Trick your inner eight-year-old into pleasing Mom *and* eating sensibly with these simple strategies:

- When you place your order in a restaurant, ask the waiter to put half of your serving in a doggie bag *before* he brings it to your table.

- Whenever possible, shun buffets (including salad bars). The enticing array of goodies makes it all but impossible to resist putting one of everything on your plate until you've got a mound the size of Mount McKinley.

- At must-attend business or social events that serve food buffet-style, choose the smallest plate offered. Then plant your attention firmly on your fellow attendees and the action at hand, so you'll be less tempted to go back for seconds.

3 Ways Fiber Helps You Win at Losing

It's ironic that many trendy diets severely restrict one of the most powerful weight-loss aids of all: fiber. If you're fighting a never-ending battle of the bulge, consider this amazing fact: Simply by eating more whole grains, nuts, fruits, and vegetables (including root veggies with their skins), you could lose a couple of pounds a month without cutting a single calorie. That's because fiber pulls off a trio of fabulous fat-fighting feats:

1. It tricks your tummy. Many calories in fiber-rich foods can't be digested, but they do fill you up. So you feel full with fewer calories than you would normally eat.

2. It puts an end to hunger pangs. Water-soluble fiber absorbs water in your stomach and swells up to form a thick gel. This, in turn, alerts your brain that you're full. It also slows down the flow of food out of your stomach, which keeps you satisfied longer and releases a steady, prolonged supply of energy. So you can go about your business without the constant need to nibble.

3. It empowers your slimming hormones. The fiber in fruits and vegetables raises the levels of GLP-1, a hormone in your gastrointestinal tract that—like the tummy gel—slows down digestion, makes you feel full longer, and helps you lose weight.

NOTE: *Increase your fiber intake gradually. Although a sudden surge of it won't hurt you, it can trigger uncomfortable gas and bloating.*

Strange but True: Fat Burns Fat

That is, if you choose the right kinds. Studies show that a couple of dynamic dietary fats increase your body's ability to burn fat and also fend off food cravings. These two superstars can light a fat-shredding fire in your inner furnace:

Conjugated linoleic acid (CLA). The most powerful pyrotechnic performers are beef, full-fat dairy products, and egg yolks—ideally produced by grass-fed critters. When beef cattle, dairy cows, and chickens are fed genetically modified (GMO) grain or other processed feed, their CLA output plummets. There is also one potent vegetarian source of this ferocious fuel: white button mushrooms such as the ones you'll find in your local supermarket.

Monounsaturated fat. Avocados, flaxseed oil, nuts, and olive oil are all high in this ultra-healthy weight-loss helper.

A Berry Weird Way to Lose Weight

We all know that our sense of smell is the one most closely tied to our memories. But scents do much more than just carry our minds back to bygone days. They also stimulate all sorts of mental and physical functions. For instance, studies show that smelling strawberries prior to exercise causes you to burn more calories. So before you head off on your next power walk, hit the

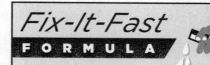

Fix-It-Fast FORMULA

Fabulous Fat-Burning Smoothie

You couldn't ask for a more delicious way to burn fat—and give a big-time boost to your health—than this slimming superstar. This recipe makes two servings.

2 green-tea bags

¾ cup of boiling water

2 cups of blueberries*

12 oz. of whole-milk vanilla yogurt

3 ice cubes

2 tbsp. of ground flaxseed

2 tbsp. of unsalted almonds

Steep the tea bags in the water for five minutes. Remove them, and while the tea cools, whirl the remaining ingredients in a blender until smooth. Add the tea, and blend for a few more seconds. Then pour the potion into a tall glass, and drink to your good looks and good health!

* Or substitute other berries of your choice, either fresh or frozen.

treadmill at the gym—or even get ready to mow the lawn—pull some berries out of the fridge, and take a good long whiff!

But strawberry isn't the only aroma that can help you slim down. In a study by the Smell & Taste Treatment and Research Foundation, 3,193 volunteers who frequently sniffed the scents of peppermint, green apples, or bananas throughout the day lost an average of 30 pounds in six months!

The Legend of Negative Calories

Some folks claim that your excess pounds will slide right off if you confine the bulk of your intake to negative-calorie (a.k.a. catabolic) foods that contain fewer calories than your body uses to digest them. Are they right? Yes and no. While it is true that a few edibles, such as celery, do require more energy to metabolize compared with the number of calories they provide, no scientific study has demonstrated the catabolic prowess of any particular food!

That being said, nutritional scientists tell us that, in general, your body uses about 10 calories for every 100 calories it breaks down—which means there are a lot of ultra-nutritious metabolic champs that can help you slim down while keeping (or getting) your health in tip-top shape. Consider these, for instance:

Diet foods make you eat **more calories**.

- Apples
- Asparagus
- Berries
- Broccoli
- Citrus fruits
- Eggplant
- Lettuce
- Melons
- Pears
- Peppers
- Pineapple
- Plums
- Sweet potatoes
- Zucchini

Wacky Ways to Pack on Pounds

➜ You say you're putting on weight, even though you don't think you're eating any more than usual? I'm not surprised. A whole lot of factors, from the decor in your kitchen to the pals you hang around with, can make you shovel in more food without even realizing it. And a few physical conditions cause pounds to pile up, regardless of how many calories you are (or aren't) taking in. The good news is that once you know the nature of the problem, it's easy to get your fat-burning engine back on track.

. . . .

Your Kitchen Is Porking You Up

If your house is like most, the kitchen is action central—which may be partly to blame for your weight problem. If that statement sounds way-out wacko, consider this fact: Kitchens are typically 50 percent larger than they were 35 years ago, and in most households they've become the location of choice for paying bills, watching television, and cruising the Web—all activities that provide snacking opportunities galore. Studies show that people who routinely eat while doing something else consume more food and eat more frequently—devouring, on average, the equivalent of an entire extra meal per day. Your pound-dropping mission: Move the computer and TV out of the kitchen. Shift bill-paying and other paperwork chores to the den or family room. And when you talk on the phone, do it where there's no food in sight!

Lighting Invites Overeating

As bizarre as it may sound, the lighting in your kitchen and dining room may be hampering your weight-loss labors. It works in two ways: Bright lights raise your stress

Countertop Clutter Wallops Your Willpower

In most households, the kitchen counters attract all kinds of stuff, from baseball caps to supermarket receipts and week-old newspapers. If you think those littered surfaces are merely an aesthetic issue, think again. Not only does clutter lead to appetite-boosting stress, but it also makes it harder to maintain healthy eating habits. That's because it's a whole lot easier to grab a fattening frozen dinner from the freezer or order a pizza than it is to dig through the mess to clear a cooking surface. So get that stuff outta there *now*! Toss out the obvious junk (like last week's papers). Then gather up everything that you don't routinely use in the kitchen, and take it elsewhere. Finally, round up the things that do belong in the kitchen—for example, culinary magazines and cooking gadgets that have migrated to the countertops—and tuck them away in designated drawers or cabinets.

level, which in turn stimulates your appetite and causes you to eat more than usual. On the flip side, low lighting lowers your inhibitions—unsurprisingly making you eat more. The simple solution: When you're preparing meals or setting the table, crank up the wattage as high as you'd like, but when it's time to eat, dim the scene to about 240 total watts in incandescent bulbs or 75 to 100 watts for compact fluorescents. And between meals, keep all kitchen lights off. That sends a clear message to your subconscious mind that the "restaurant" is closed!

Bright lights will make **you eat** more.

The Deadly TV Diet

Numerous studies have shown that adults whose TV viewing exceeds three hours a day are more prone to weight gain than less-devoted viewers are, and they're nearly twice as likely to be obese. If that glowing screen has become an ever-present fixture in your life, use these tricks to trim your waistline:

Banish TV from the bedroom. Watching TV in bed is a proven cause of weight gain and an invitation to chronic insomnia to boot.

Schedule your viewing time. At the beginning of each week, make a list of the shows that you'd like to watch, and add up the time they'd keep you in front of the tube each day. If any day's programming totals more than three hours, either forget it or record any must-see footage, and watch it on a day when the lineup is less enticing.

Don't eat in front of the screen. If you have a snack in hand every time you turn on the tube, it becomes a habit, not unlike how some folks reach for a cigarette as soon as they have a drink in hand. Plus, it is mindless eating that packs on pounds (see "Your Kitchen Is Porking You Up," on page 137, for the details). So if you almost always munch while channel surfing, make a concerted effort to stop.

Fewer TV Hours = More Pounds Lost

According to a recent study at the University of Vermont, simply trimming the amount of time you spend watching television can make you lose weight—with no effort whatsoever.

The details: Researchers installed monitoring devices on the television sets of 36 overweight and obese adults, who were then divided into two groups for the three-week study. One team had monitors that turned their sets off after three hours of "on" time, while the other bunch continued their normal viewing routine. All the volunteers wore armbands that measured calorie expenditure, and all were interviewed each week about their eating habits.

The results: Although there was no significant difference in how much any of the participants ate, those whose viewing time was limited to three hours burned an average of 119 more calories a day, and lost an average of 1½ pounds—without engaging in any kind of exercise program or cutting their food intake. On the other hand, the "guinea pigs" who put in their usual amount of boob-tube time lost nary an ounce.

The takeaway: Limit your TV time to three hours a day or less. The more screen time you shave from your schedule, the more pounds you're likely to shed—regardless of what you do during those "found" hours.

Warm, Cozy Homes Fuel the Fat

According to a recent study published in the journal *Obesity Reviews*, the increasingly warm temperatures in our homes, offices, and cars could be, in part, what's making us chubby. That's because, as

Obesity Is Contagious

Jaw-Dropping DISCOVERY

No, that doesn't mean that fat "germs" fly through the air in the same way cold and flu viruses do. Rather, obesity tends to get passed along because people within social networks share (often unconsciously) many of the same behavioral traits—including their eating and other lifestyle habits. For example, one study found that your likelihood of being obese is 57 percent greater if one or more close friends are obese, 40 percent greater if a sibling is obese, and 37 percent greater if your spouse is obese.

Don't get me wrong—I'm not suggesting that you should drop your nearest and dearest like hot potatoes! Instead, try these two ploys:

▶ Have heart-to-heart discussions with friends or family members whom you think might like to join you in adopting healthier behaviors.

▶ Join a weight-loss support group, a fitness center, or an activity-oriented group such as a hiking, biking, or skating club. That way, you'll be much more likely to meet folks who share your desire to be healthy and active.

numerous studies have shown, when you're cold—even mildly chilly—your body activates your supply of brown fat as a way to generate heat, burning calories in the process. Conversely, the warmer your environment is, the fewer calories you burn. Even if you're not overweight now, kicking your brown fat into action can help keep you from picking up unwanted pounds in the future. And the R_x couldn't be simpler: Just turn down your thermostat, open a window while you're driving, or nix a sweater when you might otherwise reach for one. Anything that'll cool you down by a few degrees will do the trick.

By 2030 a whopping **86%** of American adults will be **overweight or obese**.

Cool Down to Slim Down

In a study published in *The Journal of Clinical Investigation*, researchers exposed a group of men to 66°F temperatures for two hours a day for six weeks. Meanwhile, a control group went about life as usual in their normal living temperatures. The results: PET scans showed that the guys exposed to the lower temps had increased levels of brown-fat activity, and they burned 200 extra calories per day. They also had 5 percent less body fat mass. On the other hand, fat levels and calorie-burning action of the comfortably warm bunch remained unchanged.

2 Household Allies Are Stabbing You in the Back

You say that you're eating less and exercising more, but the pounds still aren't dropping off as they should? Well, if your home is like most, it's filled with a couple of hormone-disrupting "miracle" substances that have been strongly linked to obesity. These are the treacherous twins that you want to dodge as much as possible:

Slick-surface treatments. Nonstick cookware, greaseproof food wrappers, and microwavable popcorn bags, as well as stain-proof and waterproof fabrics, all get their super shedding power from a chemical called perfluorooctanoic acid (PFOA). As long as your nonstick kitchenware is in good shape, it's safe to use, but once the surfaces become scratched, cracked, or chipped, replace your gear with cast iron or untreated stainless steel versions.

Vinyl products. The trouble-causing chemicals in polyvinyl chloride (PVC) are organotins and phthalates. And the worst part is that over time PVC breaks down into tiny particles, so most likely the dust in your home is full of the stuff. Your best defense: Vacuum and clean thoroughly, and when it's time to replace vinyl flooring, look for friendlier options (see "Menacing Materials" on page 263).

8 Signs That Your Bulging Beltline Is Not Your Fault

If you've gained a lot of extra weight lately, even though your eating habits and activity level haven't changed, there's a good chance you can pin the blame on your underachieving thyroid gland. Have your doctor test you for hypothyroidism if your sudden weight gain is accompanied by any of these other symptoms:

1. Achy muscles and joints, for no apparent reason
2. Almost constant tiredness and trouble falling asleep
3. Anxiety and depression
4. Chronic constipation
5. Cold feet
6. Extremely dry hair and skin
7. Forgetfulness and an inability to concentrate
8. Vanished sex drive

The Fattening Fungus among Us

The *Candida albicans* fungus is best known for causing agonizingly itchy genital infections, but according to natural health pros, an overgrowth of this yeast in your gut can also cause fluid retention and weight gain or the inability to lose weight. This fungus is always present in your digestive tract, but two common elements of modern life—overuse of antibiotics and a diet

Sleep More, Weigh Less . . .

Jaw-Dropping DISCOVERY

Or maybe more. Scads of scientific studies have shown that spending either too little *or* too much quality time between the sheets can make you gain weight. For most adults, the optimum is seven to nine hours of shut-eye a night. If you're heftier than you should be, and you routinely sleep longer than that, see your doctor to rule out any underlying health conditions or drug-related causes. On the other hand, if you're neglecting snooze time in favor of more "productive" endeavors, set your priorities straight right now. (For the whole skinny on slumber, see "Good Health—Sleep on It!" on page 17.)

that's too high in sugar—can kick it into serious overdrive. *Candida* symptoms vary widely from one person to another and may or may not include the classic itch, as well as all the signs of hypothyroidism (see "8 Signs That Your Bulging Beltline Is Not Your Fault" on page 141). But two sure indicators that you should see your doctor for a diagnosis and treatment are oral thrush (a white film on your tongue or in your mouth) and a constant craving for sweet treats.

Move It!

⮕ We all know (I hope!) that to lose weight, you have to burn more calories than you take in. Recently, though, scientists have discovered that even slender folks can build up dangerous amounts of internal fat if they don't get regular exercise. But don't worry! There are plenty of ways you can incorporate health-giving movement into your day without taking up running, hiring a personal trainer, or spending hours a week at the gym.

Don't Let Exercise Undermine Your Diet

While it is true that the only way to lose weight is to burn more calories than you take in, trying *too hard* to keep the "fire" going could sabotage your efforts. That's because when a lot of folks embark on an intensive exercise program, they start eating more than they did before. In some cases, they think they're burning more calories than they really are, so it's okay to toss back (for instance) an after-workout candy bar or two. But most people don't even realize that they're upping their food intake. Whichever of those categories you fall into, these three tricks will help you stay on track:

Eat sooner. Studies have shown that eating meals within 15 to 30 minutes after exercising makes you less likely to eat back the "fuel" you've just burned than you would be if you wait longer.

Guzzle water. It's often easy to mistake thirst for hunger. So when you find yourself eating more than you should on workout days, try drinking more water than you normally do. That could solve the problem lickety-split.

Give yourself a treat that you can't eat. If you think you deserve a prize for your physical labor, by all means go for it. Just make sure it's something inedible.

NOTE: *It's a good bet that your bad habit of thinking of food as a reward for good behavior is a big part of what got you to an overweight state in the first place!*

Ditch the Workout and Drop the Weight

If your chosen form of exercise—whether it's running, swimming, or working out at the gym—leaves you too hungry to eat sensibly, give up the activity. Instead, find ways to move your body more without actually exercising. Puttering in your garden, walking the dog, sweeping the floor, and washing your car all burn calories galore, but because your mind doesn't count these and other everyday activities as "real exercise," it's highly unlikely that they'll set off your starvation alarm bells (see "Don't Let Exercise Undermine Your Diet," at left).

A Colossal Collateral Benefit

Although you reap enormous health dividends each time you leave your car behind and walk somewhere, *(continued on page 145)*

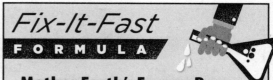

Fix-It-Fast
F O R M U L A

Mother Earth's Energy Bars

Whether you're walking, cycling, or trotting across a shopping-mall parking lot, you can suddenly find yourself craving an energy boost. So keep a few of these tasty and nutritious treats tucked in your pocket, purse, or saddle pack, and reach for one whenever you need a power fix.

Butter or vegetable oil

1 egg

½ cup of brown sugar

I tsp. of vanilla extract

I cup of granola

½ cup of chopped, dried fruit*

½ cup of chopped nuts*

3 tbsp. of dark chocolate chips (preferably organic)

Generously rub the butter or vegetable oil onto an 8-by-8-inch square baking pan. Crack the egg into a medium-size bowl. Add the brown sugar and vanilla, and mix thoroughly. Stir in the granola, dried fruit, nuts, and chocolate chips, and mix until combined. Scrape the mixture into the baking pan, pressing it firmly with your hand, making sure that the surface is covered evenly. Bake for 25 minutes at 350°F. Cool, cut into bars (whatever size you like), and wrap each one in wax paper or aluminum foil.

* Use your favorite kinds!

Walking Whittles Your Waistline and Lengthens Your Life

Throughout this book, I've been telling you that simply walking for 30 minutes a day can not only help you lose weight but also lower your stress level, reduce your risk for lethal diseases, and even make you happier. Well, one of the simplest ways to reach that target is to get out of your car for 30 minutes a day and spend that time walking instead of driving.

Of course, you don't have to limit your daily walk-don't-drive time to half an hour. Nor do you need to rack up the time in one fell swoop, or to hit the full 30-minute mark each and every day. The bottom line is that the more minutes you devote to this transportation trade-off throughout the day, the more rewards you'll reap! Consider these six easy ways you can replace horsepower with foot power:

1. Walk to and from work, church, errands, and social gatherings whenever you can. When that's not possible, drive to within 15 minutes or so of your destination, park the car, and hoof it the rest of the way.

2. If you and your coworkers routinely drive to and from lunch, walk instead. The "from" portion of the jaunt is especially effective from a weight-loss standpoint because walking within 30 minutes after eating increases calorie burning by as much as 30 percent. So when you only have time for a one-way walk, snag a ride to the restaurant and return to the office on foot.

3. When you drive downtown or out to the mall, don't circle the block or the parking lot until you find the spot closest to the door. Instead, do just the opposite: Ease into a space that's far removed from the building entrance, and stroll on in from there.

4. Nix drive-up windows at banks, coffee shops, the post office, and other places. Instead, park the car and amble inside.

5. Whenever you take public transportation, get off a stop or two early, and then walk to your destination.

6. At work, use restrooms, copy machines, and so on that are farther away from your office.

your body isn't the only beneficiary of this deal. It's also a boon to your bank account. For starters, less driving results in less money spent on gasoline and all the other liquids that your gas guzzler consumes, including motor oil; antifreeze; and brake, transmission, and windshield-wiper fluids. What's more, you'll reduce wear and tear on the vehicle, and that will translate into lower maintenance costs and, ultimately, a longer life for old Betsy. Most likely, you'll also save money on parking fees (and tickets, too!).

Depending on how often the car is left behind, you could even qualify for a low-mileage discount on your auto insurance policy. That's because insurance underwriters know that the less time you spend behind the wheel, the less likely you are to be involved in an accident. (Chalk up yet another health benefit of walking rather than driving!)

Trade Foot Power for Pedal Power

If you'd rather cycle than stroll, I have even better news for you: Replacing a 30-minute drive with a half-hour bike ride will help you shed even more weight than walking does for the same amount of time. That's because you'll be moving your legs faster and traveling a lot farther. To be specific, walking for 30 minutes at the rate of 3 miles per hour will burn a little over 128 calories. Riding a bicycle for the same length of time at 12.4 miles per hour will burn roughly 274 calories, so get rolling!

3 Terrific Tips for Happy Hoofing

You can **lose 25 pounds** in a year just by **walking** for 1 hour a day.

Unlike most athletic pursuits and exercise routines, walking requires absolutely no special clothing or equipment. But to maximize your comfort level (and, therefore, the likelihood that you'll stick with the program), keep these tips in mind:

Baby your feet. Wear the most comfortable shoes you can find. For longer distances (say, when you're doing 15 minutes or more at a single stretch), shoes that are specially made for running or power walking are your best bet. For short strolls or occasions that call for something a little dressier than sneakers, simply wear whatever footgear feels best to you and goes well with your outfit. Whatever you do, though, steer clear of high, spiky heels because, with every step you take, they subject the balls of your feet to as much as (are you ready for this?) 2,000 pounds of pressure! And that takes an enormous toll on your knee and hip joints.

Accessorize your outfit. Consider buying an inexpensive pedometer that you can clip to your belt, waistband, or coat. Counting the steps you take each day is a lot like watching the dollars add up in a savings account: The more the numbers increase, the more motivated you are to nudge them upward even further. Aim for 10,000 steps a day. Studies show that the average American takes 3,000 to 5,000 steps per day, but to stay healthy and fend off chronic diseases, you need to double the amount. So step lively!

Lose the luggage. Granted, there may be times (when you're hoofing it to work, for instance) when you have to tote a purse, a briefcase, or both. But whenever possible, leave those carrying cases at home. Instead, wear clothes that have enough pockets to hold such essential take-alongs as your wallet, reading glasses, and/or shopping list. It's a fact: The less stuff you have to lug along, the more enjoyable your trek will be.

The Incredible Calorie-Burning Power of Housekeeping

Lots of folks love the camaraderie of working out at a gym, where they're surrounded and encouraged by their fellow weight-loss warriors. But if you're not that social by nature, you don't care for formal workout routines—or you simply don't have the time or money to squander on a health club member-

Push Excess Pounds Away

If you'd like to give a down-home boost to your weight-loss labors—and you have a small, fairly flat lawn—here's a "reel" sweet idea: Exchange your powered lawn mower for a manual reel mower. Using it to mow your lawn will burn about 400 calories an hour, compared with 250 for a powered push mower and 175 for the riding version. Plus, it'll tone your muscles and rev up your heart rate far beyond what you'd achieve with any powered machine. By the way, if the only reel mower you've ever known was the one you muscled around your parents' lawn on Saturday mornings, don't worry—that old dinosaur has been reborn, with a much lighter body and smoother-working parts. So do your body a favor, and take one for a test drive, er, test push.

ship—don't fret: Just by performing routine chores around the old homestead, you can easily roast enough calories to fuel your pound-shedding process and tone up your muscles to boot. Here's a handful of examples:

Digging in your yard burns about 630 calories per hour, in addition to toning the muscles in your calves, thighs, arms, and shoulders. Plus, if you go at it vigorously for 20 minutes or more, you can increase your heart rate and strengthen your cardiovascular system at the same time.

Raking leaves for an hour can burn 450 calories, and the resistance offered by the leaves helps tone all the major muscle groups in your body.

Scrubbing the bathroom burns 400 calories an hour and tones your arm and shoulder muscles.

> You can **burn** up to **450 calories** an hour **raking leaves**.

Sweeping and mopping a floor burns about 240 calories an hour and gives you a great upper- and lower-body workout.

Washing the car burns 286 calories an hour and helps tone your arms and abdominal muscles.

The exact number of calories a person burns during any activity varies greatly, depending on gender, age, weight, and individual metabolism. An Internet search for "calorie burn calculator" will bring up scads of sites where you can type in your vital stats and learn how many calories you'll expend on common chores, ranging from loading your dishwasher to washing your dog, as well as more athletic endeavors such as swimming, dancing, and hitting the rowing machine at the health club.

Diabolical Diseases

6

Throughout this book, I've been telling you about all the ways that our modern American lifestyle is wrecking our health. In this chapter, we're going to zero in on some of the most dreaded diseases that may befall you if you tread that path of sloppy habits and overexposure to noxious chemicals. The good news is that if you mend your ways, it's possible for you to avoid many, if not all, of these demons—or at least greatly lessen the likelihood that they'll send you to meet your Maker before your time.

Savvy Cancer Survival Strategies

Few, if any, diseases strike more dread in our hearts than cancer. For that reason, it's all too easy to panic when yet another study pops up in the news claiming that some nearly unavoidable chemical, food, or activity causes cancer. It's enough to make you want to crawl into a cave and stay there. Well, don't do that, folks. Instead, just use your common sense and do the best you can to get your body into tip-top shape and keep it there.

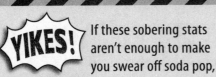

YIKES! If these sobering stats aren't enough to make you swear off soda pop, I don't know what is!

▶ Men who drink a single sugar-sweetened soda per day increase their risk for aggressive prostate cancer by 40 percent.

▶ Postmenopausal women who quaff nondiet soda on a regular basis up their likelihood of developing uterine cancer by 78 percent.

▶ Folks of either sex who toss back two or more regular *or* diet sodas a day raise their risk for pancreatic cancer by a whopping 87 percent.

2 Malignant Myths Busted

Malignant myth #1: Eating sugar causes cancer to grow faster.
FACT: All the cells in your body depend on glucose (a.k.a. blood sugar) for energy. Research has shown that cancer cells do consume more glucose than normal cells, but eating sugar does *not* make them grow bigger or spread faster. And quitting sugar cold turkey will not make your cancer any better—unless a high-sugar diet is contributing

to excess poundage. Being overweight or obese can hinder cancer recovery and raise your risk of a relapse.

Malignant myth #2: Underarm deodorants and antiperspirants can cause breast cancer.

FACT: According to both the American Cancer Society and the National Cancer Institute, there is no conclusive evidence to support this notion. But given the number of strong chemicals in many of these products, it can't hurt to go with a safer organic, or at least all-natural, brand.

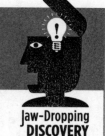

Chalk Up Another Win for Exercise

Jaw-Dropping DISCOVERY

More and more scientific studies are showing that regular exercise can help prevent cancer, ease the side effects of radiation and chemotherapy, and lessen the chance that cancer recurs. And here's the *big* news: If you have cancer of any kind, exercising on a routine basis can cut your risk of dying from it by 53 percent. So get a move on—*yesterday*!

A Hair-Raising Risk

For years, we've heard speculation that hair dye causes cancer. Is it true? Nobody knows for sure. Some studies have linked hair-dye ingredients to certain types of cancer. Other research has found no such connection. So what's a health-conscious hair colorer to do? Make your to-dye or not-to-dye decision with these considerations in mind:

1. Hair dye comes in three basic types: temporary, semipermanent, and permanent. As you might expect, the chemical load increases with the level of staying power.

2. Generally, the darker a dye is, the more potentially dangerous coloring compounds it contains.

3. As with any known or suspected carcinogen, the extent of risk depends in large part on your degree of exposure. Hairstylists, who work with dyes and other chemical-laden beauty products day in and day out, are far more vulnerable than, let's say, a woman who has her gray strands covered every six weeks or so.

4. Your chances of acquiring a malignancy from hair dye or anything else are greater if you already have other strikes against you, such as obesity, smoking, poor nutrition, or an inactive lifestyle, or if you routinely use many other products that contain harsh chemicals.

The Backyard Barbecue: Festive Summer Pastime—or Deadly Health Risk?

Summer wouldn't be summer without the smoke, sizzle, and tantalizing aroma of backyard barbecues. But the notion has spread that these get-togethers are giving us cancer. Is cooking meat on a charcoal grill really dangerous? According to experts, including those at the American Institute for Cancer Research, the answer is, probably not.

However, it *is* true that cooking meat at overly high temperatures, or charring it over direct flames, causes the formation of two problematic substances, heterocyclic amines (HCAs) and polycyclic aromatic hydrocarbons (PAHs). Both have been linked to cancer in laboratory animals, but the jury is still out on the risk they pose for humans. Consuming large quantities of red meat, no matter how it's cooked, is bad for you. But enjoying grilled foods in moderation is just fine.

Grilled meat in moderation **won't hurt** you.

4 Great Guidelines for Safer Grilling

Health experts offer these four simple pointers for making your grilling safer and healthier for all concerned:

1. Trim away excess fat to prevent it from dripping, flaring up, and burning the meat.

2. Brush coals to the periphery, and grill your meat above the center to reduce flare-ups. If necessary, use a drip pan.

3. On a gas grill, set the temperature at medium-high, and flip the meat frequently as it cooks to prevent charring.

4. Marinate your meat for at least 60 minutes in a vinegar- or lemon-based marinade that includes herbs—for example, basil, marjoram, mint, oregano, rosemary, sage, savory, and thyme. These antioxidants will reduce HCA and PAH production by 99 to 100 percent.

Chocolate Fights Cancer

As we explained earlier (see "Clobber Cancer with Chocolate" on page 87), this delicious confection contains compounds called polyphenols that help slow the growth of cancer cells. But we're not talking about chowing down on chocolate cake, chocolate pudding, or the cheap chocolates you get by the bagful. It's *dark* chocolate—not the lighter, sweeter milk chocolate—that's the champ when it comes to battling the Big C. So be sure to choose chocolate that consists of more than 70 percent cocoa.

The Top 10 Cancer-Trouncing Foods

One key to staying in the pink of health is to eat a wide variety of wholesome foods. But when it comes to preventing or slowing the growth of cancer cells, nutritionists tout these 10 all-stars:

- Apples (preferably organic)
- Berries of all kinds
- Cruciferous vegetables, such as broccoli, Brussels sprouts, cabbage, and cauliflower
- Dark green or red leafy veggies, such as romaine lettuce, Swiss chard, kale, and collard greens
- Flaxseed
- Garlic
- Grapes, especially red and purple varieties
- Legumes, including beans, peas, lentils, and peanuts
- Tomatoes*
- Whole grains, including barley, bulgur, whole-wheat flour, oatmeal, and brown rice

Tomatoes deliver more lycopene when they're cooked or processed into such foods as juice, sauce, and ketchup. Look for the organic kinds, and limit your purchases of canned tomato products to avoid the toxic BPA used in can linings (see "A Creepy Reason to Can Cans" on page 119.)

Colonoscopy Prep Made Easy

REMARKABLE REMEDY

Make that *easier*. Prepping for a colonoscopy is far more unpleasant than the procedure itself. It entails a 24-hour process of cleaning out your colon by only drinking clear fluids and a foul-tasting "beverage," and the routine can make your rear end as sore as the dickens. Fortunately, there are simple ways to solve both of those problems.

The ingoing process. Just add a teaspoon of vanilla extract to the drink. It'll go down a lot more smoothly!

The outgoing process. The evening before you start prepping, mix a few drops of lavender essential oil per ounce of witch hazel. Dip a dozen or so cotton pads in the solution, and then stash them in the freezer. The next day, use them as often as needed to bring powerful relief to your sitting area. **NOTE:** *If you have any of the frozen pads left over, save them for soothing future cuts, scratches, or insect bites.*

Diabetes—How Sweet It Ain't!

➥ Hand in glove with the obesity epidemic, diabetes rates have skyrocketed in recent decades. But, while being over your fighting weight makes you a prime candidate for what old-timers called "sugar," there are plenty of other risk factors that may be painting a big D target on your back. Some of these conditions you bring on yourself; others are passed down through your genes. But none of them guarantees that you *will* get diabetes. If you make some major lifestyle changes—fast—you may be able to dodge a bullet.

Diabetes Demystified . . .

And remystified. "Huh?" I hear you saying. Here's the deal: Historically, there have been two main types of this dastardly disease:

Type 1, a.k.a. juvenile or insulin-dependent diabetes, is a classic example of an autoimmune disease in which the body mistakenly identifies normal cell tissue (in this case, insulin-generating cells produced by the pancreas) as outside invaders and attacks them. Type 1 most commonly strikes during childhood or adolescence, and its victims can survive only with the help of frequent insulin injections. About 5 percent of diabetics fall into this category (see "Juvenile Diabetes: It's Not Kid Stuff Anymore" on page 157).

2 out of 3 diabetics **die** from **heart disease** or **stroke**.

Type 2, a.k.a. adult diabetes, is a metabolic condition in which the pancreas either stops producing insulin or loses the ability to use it effectively enough to control blood sugar levels. It accounts for about 95 percent of cases. While some folks in this classification may need insulin injections, very often the disease can be controlled with oral medications, or simply by weight loss, exercise, and healthier eating habits. **NOTE:** *A variant of type 2, called gestational diabetes, sometimes occurs in pregnant women, and then it vanishes after the baby is born.*

Here's the fly in the ointment. In recent years, doctors have been diagnosing more and more adults who have type 1 diabetes or a latent form of it, sometimes referred to as type 1.5. These people test positive for the antibodies that attack the pancreatic cells, but they may or may not develop the full-blown autoimmune disease. The medical community has no idea why this "cross-pollination" is occurring, but researchers at the country's top medical schools are hard at work looking for answers.

Diabetes Is a Stealthy Stalker

One of the most frightening facts about type 2 diabetes is that you can have it for years before any symptoms appear. Plus, when they first show up, they may be so mild that you don't even notice them—or simply fail to recognize them as signs of serious trouble. If you experience any of the danger signals listed below, hightail it to your doctor for a blood glucose test.

- Areas of darkened, often velvety, skin on your neck, armpits, or joints

- Blurred vision

- Constant fatigue

- Increased hunger accompanied by weight loss

- Increased thirst and frequent urination

- Numbness or tingling in your hands or feet

- Slow-healing wounds or frequent infections

- Unexplained itching

Are You on a Collision Course with Diabetes?

No one knows exactly why some people develop type 2 diabetes while others

Previews of Coming Atrocities

Health-care statisticians tell us that one out of every three Americans has prediabetes, which means that their blood sugar levels are higher than normal, but not quite high enough to qualify as type 2 diabetes. But here's the really scary part:

▶ Unless it's diagnosed and dealt with, prediabetes will most likely morph into the genuine article in 10 years or less.

▶ If you have prediabetes, the long-term havoc wreaked by the disease itself—especially damage to your heart and circulatory system—may already be under way.

▶ While prediabetes may produce classic type 2 symptoms, in many cases, you won't have a clue that anything's gone awry.

Now for the good news: If you clean up your act—that is, start eating better, work more physical activity into your daily routine, and maintain a healthy weight—you may be able to bring your blood sugar level down to normal before major trouble sets in.

don't, but certain factors have been proven to put you at greater risk. If one or more of the items in the list below hits home, get a blood glucose screening to rule out either active or prediabetes.

What You're Stuck With

Your genes. If a parent or sibling has type 2 diabetes, your chance of getting it escalates.

Your race. For reasons unknown, diabetes is far more prevalent among African Americans, American Indians, Asian Americans, Hispanics, and Pacific Islanders than it is among Caucasians of European descent.

Your bout of gestational diabetes. If you had it during a pregnancy, you are more likely to get type 2 later in life.

Scented candles may ignite diabetes, but these aromatic mood setters aren't the only fragrant felons lurking in homes from coast to coast. Studies show that exposure to phthalates—chemicals used in synthetic fragrances, as well as in many plastics—can actually double your risk for contracting diabetes. Scientists reckon that phthalates disrupt your hormones in a way that hinders your body's ability to metabolize and regulate fat. Even at low levels, these substances promote weight gain, thereby making you a prime candidate for diabetes.

What You Can Change

Your inertia. The less you move your body, the more you up the odds that you'll get the Big D. And this danger applies even if you're pencil thin.

Your weight. Both obesity and lesser degrees of overweight pose major risks. But belly fat is particularly apt to send your glucose into the stratosphere because the bigger your spare tire is, the more resistant your cells become to insulin.

Your overall health. High blood pressure, high levels of triglycerides in your blood, and low levels of HDL (good) cholesterol all contribute to insulin resistance. And when you combine those conditions with the two factors mentioned above, you're begging for big-time trouble.

4 Steps to Stop Diabetes

Chemicals called phthalates are used in synthetic fragrances (see how scented candles may deliver diabetes in the Yikes! box, above).

Having these floating around in your household air may not directly cause diabetes, but they dramatically increase the chance that you and your family will get the disease. So, especially if you have risk factors that can't be eliminated, or if you've been diagnosed with prediabetes, strengthen your defenses with these four simple measures:

1. Send scented candles packin'—and air fresheners, too, including sprays, gels, and plug-ins. Instead, burn beeswax candles that produce air-cleaning negative ions. If you like pleasant aromas drifting through the air, bring in fragrant fresh flowers, or make herbal potpourris (for the simple formula, see Healthy Herbal Potpourri, at right).

2. When you buy cosmetics or personal-care products of any kind, read the labels carefully, and turn thumbs down on anything that has the word *parfum* or *fragrance* in the ingredient list. To find safe, natural alternatives, check the Environmental Working Group's Skin Deep® Cosmetics Database at www.ewg.org.

3. Choose unscented versions of laundry and household cleaning products. You'll find them in your local supermarket right next to the odiferous kinds.

4. As much as possible, shun products that are made of flexible plastic and vinyl. Phthalates are used in the manufacture of household staples ranging from shower curtains, wallpaper, and vinyl mini-blinds to food packaging and plastic wrap, as well as pet toys and beds. (And, yes, in case you're wondering, these hormone-disrupting demons are just as dangerous for Fido and Fluffy as they are for you.)

Healthy Herbal Potpourri

REMARKABLE REMEDY

To scent the air in your home without the dangerous chemicals found in commercial products, whip up your own aromatic blend. Simply combine 13 cups of your favorite dried herbs and/or flowers with 1 ounce each of orrisroot and sweet flag powder (all available in health-food stores, herbal-supply stores, and online). Then fill bowls or baskets with the mixture, and set them out wherever you like. Pour any leftover blend into glass jars with tight-fitting lids, and store the containers in a cool, dark place.

1 in 3 American adults has **prediabetes**; **89%** of them **don't know** it.

Sleep Deprivation = Diabetes Risk

If you're among the legions of folks who don't get enough quality sleep—whether the reason is clinical insomnia or the desire to pack more action into your day—here's a tidbit you need to know: After just one night of poor sleep, your body can show signs of insulin resistance, which is a major risk factor for diabetes. Routinely spending less than six hours asleep makes the danger skyrocket. If you already have diabetes, sleep deprivation can undermine efforts to control blood sugar. For tips on how to get a good night's sleep, see "Good Health—Sleep on It!" on page 17.

Fix-It-Fast
FORMULA

Banana-Walnut Smoothie

In addition to providing your daily dose of disease-fighting cinnamon, this delicious drink serves up a major load of vitamins, minerals, and protein. Whip it up and take it along as an on-the-go breakfast, or enjoy it as a healthful snack.

1 banana, peeled and sliced

1½ cups of milk

¼ cup of chopped walnuts

2 tbsp. of honey

½ tsp. of cinnamon

Put all of the ingredients in a blender, puree until smooth, and drink up.

A Sweet Trick for Dodging Diabetes

Numerous studies show that adding ½ to 1 teaspoon of cinnamon to your diet every day could be enough to help control blood sugar levels and avoid this dreaded disease. That's because it can improve the ability of your body's cells to recognize and respond to insulin—a process that goes haywire in diabetics. But if you already have either type 1 or type 2 diabetes, consult your doctor before you start dosing yourself with cinnamon—or anything else!

And that's not the only good news about this tasty spice! Research shows that consuming just ½ to 1 teaspoon of cinnamon each day can also lower your LDL (bad) cholesterol, lessen your risk for chronic diseases of all kinds, and may reduce the growth of leukemia and lymphoma cancer cells. Wondering how to get your daily dose of cinnamon? It's a snap—just

Inactivity raises your **risk** for **diabetes**.

sprinkle it on cereal, toast, or English muffins; add it to your coffee or tea, stir it into a dish of yogurt, or blend it into a healthful drink, such as the delicious Banana-Walnut Smoothie (at left).

The Nose Knows

In people with diabetes, blood sugar can plummet to dangerous levels, resulting in a state called ketoacidosis. When this happens, a diabetic can feel nauseous and confused and can even pass out. But many people are unaware of any change in their system. What does change, though, is the odor of their breath. No human on earth can detect the subtle difference in aroma, but dogs can. That's because, depending on the breed, a pooch's sense of smell is anywhere from 1,000 to (yes, you're reading this right) 100 million times more sensitive than ours. For that reason, a number of nonprofit organizations around the country now train and supply these lifesaving companion canines to diabetics. Here are four of the finest outfits:

- Dogs Assisting Diabetics (www.dogsassistingdiabetics.com)

- Dogs 4 Diabetics (www.dogs4diabetics.com)

- Early Alert Canines (www.earlyalertcanines.org)

- National Institute for Diabetic Alert Dogs (www.nidad.com)

Juvenile Diabetes: It's Not Kid Stuff Anymore

This nightmarish childhood disease is now more often called by the problem it leads to: insulin-dependent diabetes. That's because more and more adults are being diagnosed with the type 1 form. Why? No one knows with any certainty, but scientists are working around the clock to find the reasons, and they're constantly developing more effective ways to treat the condition and its many side effects.

If there is any consolation, unlike with type 2 diabetes, which can perform its dastardly deeds in your body for years before being diagnosed, the symptoms of type 1 strike quickly, developing over just weeks or months. And, unlike type 2 indicators, the clues are not subtle. These are the signs that you need to see your doctor—*fast*:

▶ Constant hunger, accompanied by weight loss

▶ Extreme thirst and dehydration and the need to urinate—often

▶ Heavy, labored breathing

▶ Stupor or unconsciousness

▶ Weakness and loss of muscle power

Give Heart Disease the Heave-Ho

➡ We all know that heart disease (a.k.a. cardiovascular disease, or CVD) is the number one killer in the United States. But here's a factoid that you may not know: A full 99 percent of heart disease is preventable. So get with the program—*now*!

Being Skinny Won't Save Your Heart

While it is true that overweight and obese folks are most likely to get ticker trouble, even those who are as slim as fashion models die of heart attacks every day. That's because a predisposition to the plaque that clogs coronary arteries can be passed along in your genes, and it carries no warning signs. So do yourself a favor: Make sure you know the levels of your dangerous (LDL) and good (HDL) cholesterol, as well as your triglycerides, and do everything you can to keep them where they should be (see "High Cholesterol—Stop That Block!" on page 166). And for God's sake, if you smoke, stop it *right now*! Smoking—regardless of your weight or any other risk factor—puts you on an ultra-fast track to a heart attack.

CALL 911

If you even think you or someone you're with might be having a heart attack, dial 911 and (unless you're the victim) begin CPR *immediately*! Your clue will be one or more of these signs:

▶ Cold, sweaty skin

▶ Light-headedness, dizziness, fainting, or shortness of breath

▶ Pain, pressure, or a feeling of fullness in the chest

▶ Pain radiating from the chest to the arms, shoulders, neck, or back

▶ Weakness, anxiety, or shortness of breath

In addition to, or instead of, those symptoms, women often experience jaw pain, a feeling of breathing in ice-cold air, and/or overwhelming exhaustion or fatigue.

The Myth of the Lifesaving Cough

True or false? When you're having a heart attack and you've called 911, you can ensure your survival by coughing repeatedly and very vigorously until the EMT crew arrives.

ABSOLUTELY FALSE! Although this logical-sounding advice

regularly circulates in e-mail chains, it will do nothing to keep you among the living. But these three steps might:

1. At your first inkling of a heart attack, chew—don't swallow—an aspirin (any strength you have on hand will do).

2. Unlock your door so the paramedics can get in quickly.

3. Until help arrives, repeatedly squeeze the end of the little finger on your left hand as hard as you can. As wacky as it sounds, this acupressure technique has been reported to do what the coughing gambit won't—namely, save your life.

A Doggone Purrfect Secret to a Healthy Heart

Over the years, a huge body of scientific research has shown that, by and large, pet owners are happier and healthier than folks who do not share their homes with furry companions. And now, after examining scads of studies, the American Heart Association has issued a statement saying that owning a pet can reduce your danger of cardiovascular disease and improve your odds of surviving a heart attack. There are four reasons:

Owning a **pet** may **protect** you from **heart disease**.

1. Increased movement. Dog owners who walk and play with their pets are 54 percent more likely to get the level of physical activity recommended for good heart health. But having a cat in the household also demands that you get up off the couch and move your body around—and every step helps.

2. Lowered key numbers. Owning a pet, whether canine or feline, has been directly linked to lower blood pressure and LDL (bad) cholesterol levels and a lower likelihood of obesity—thereby mitigating three major risk factors for heart disease.

3. Reduced stress. Research shows that simply looking at a beloved pet calms you down in two ways: Your body releases a powerful feel-good chemical called oxytocin and, at the same time, decreases its output of the stress hormone cortisol.

4. Social interaction. This is an especially important factor if you live alone because study after study has found that interacting with animals (just as with people) leads to better health—including a

Cats Are Medical Miracle Workers

Believe it or not, cat owners have been found to have (depending on which studies you read) a 30 to 60 percent lower risk of heart attacks than folks who do not have a feline in the household. Apparently, the secret lies in kitty's purr, which medical pros have termed a "natural healing mechanism" because it emits low-frequency vibrations that, in addition to making you less prone to cardiovascular problems, may help strengthen and repair bones, relieve pain, and heal wounds—not to mention how relaxing it can be just to pet a purring cat that's curled up on your lap.

stronger heart—and a longer life. Plus, when you have a dog, in addition to benefiting from his companionship at home, you get daily opportunities to boost your social time by taking Fido out to mix and mingle with human neighbors and passersby.

Give Blood, Save Yourself

Studies show that donating blood on a regular basis can lower your risk of heart disease—and possibly cancer and Alzheimer's disease to boot! This generous gesture is especially helpful if, like many folks, you eat too much red meat, thereby consuming an overload of iron, which can help trigger the formation of dangerous free radicals. But when your blood flows out of your body and into the hanging bag, it reduces the amount of troublemaking iron in your system. Don't count on blood-drive dates alone, though, to keep your iron supply at a healthy level. Also go easy on beef and other red meats. Health-care experts generally recommend eating no more than a few deck-of-card-size servings per week—and the less, the better.

Say "Cheers!" to a Healthy Heart

For years, health gurus have told us that drinking red wine in moderation can help keep our hearts in good working order. Well, sipping a bit of bubbly every day may be even more helpful for our tickers. A study at the University of Reading in England found that drinking two glasses of champagne (or other sparkling wine) a day improves the functioning of blood vessels, thereby reducing the risk of heart disease and stroke. In another study, published in the *Journal of*

(continued on page 162)

Your Pills Can Kill You

Whether you're battling heart disease, high blood pressure, or any other condition that includes a daily dose of meds, you need to be aware that each year 106,000 people die in U.S. hospitals from "adverse drug reactions." But the actual number of victims is higher, because many hospital deaths attributed to various diseases are actually caused by the meds patients were taking to treat the condition. The estimate also fails to include two huge categories:

1. Drug-related deaths that occur at home and are not reported as having any such connection.

2. Deaths and near deaths caused by such over-the-counter (OTC) products as nonsteroidal anti-inflammatory drugs (NSAIDs). For example, each year, bleeding ulcers triggered by aspirin and related drugs kill more than 16,000 people and send another 200,000 to the hospital.

Ugly Unintended Consequences

Overdosing ranks high on the list of reasons for death by medication. Other culprits are allergic reactions and the interaction of various drugs with each other, or with natural remedies. But even used as directed, a great many drugs, both R_x and OTC, deliver dire consequences, ranging from liver damage to nerve disorders, diabetes, kidney disease, and stroke.

Your Lifesaving Action Plan

I'm not telling you to fire your doctor and start dosing yourself with concoctions that you find on the Internet! Modern drugs can, and do, save lives. But it pays to take precautions:

• Find an MD who can help you reduce your need for certain drugs, or decrease their side effects, by making lifestyle changes and using natural remedies.

• Whenever you see a doctor, bring a detailed list of everything you're taking, including prescription and OTC drugs, as well as herbal remedies, nutritional supplements, and vitamins.

• Ask the doc about possible food interactions with the drug(s) you're about to get.

Agricultural and Food Chemistry, researchers found that the same pleasant Rx also protects the brain from injuries occurring during a stroke and in people with Alzheimer's disease, Parkinson's disease, and other illnesses.

According to the scientists, the secret lies in the vivacious vino's high concentration of particular kinds of polyphenols (powerful antioxidants), which are lacking in nonsparkling wines. These potent substances help regulate cells' response to injury and clear out dangerous chemicals from your body. What's more, these astounding compounds can cross your body's blood-brain barrier and confer their good deeds on your entire central nervous system.

Every **74 seconds** **2** Americans **die** of **heart disease**.

YIKES! A recent study found that adults who watched television for more than four hours a day were a whopping 80 percent more likely to die from cardiovascular disease than their counterparts who spent fewer than two hours in front of the boob tube. If that isn't enough to make you tuck your TV into a back room—or even boot it out the door—I don't know what is!

Avocados Deliver Double-Barreled Heart Protection

Believe it or not, these creamy green treats contain larger supplies of two powerful heart-guarding compounds than you'll find in any other commonly eaten fruit—in some cases, up to seven times as much! These are the big guns:

Beta-sitosterol inhibits the absorption of cholesterol from your intestines into your bloodstream, thereby reducing your risk of heart disease. Research has also shown that beta-sitosterol reduces inflammation, boosts the immune system, and may hinder the growth of cancerous tumors.

Glutathione is a powerful antioxidant that not only helps prevent heart disease, but also boosts the immune system, encourages a healthy nervous system, slows the aging process, and may help fend off cancers of the mouth and pharynx. The bottom line: If you're not already a fan, it's time you learn to love avocados!

Get Soaring Blood Pressure Numbers Down

➡ **While high blood pressure itself is not a disease, the condition puts you at a greatly elevated risk for every heart problem under the sun. What's even more sobering, though, is that your blood pressure can be sky high without your even knowing it.**

Don't Let Your Doc Raise Your Numbers

A do-it-yourself blood pressure monitoring kit gives you a dandy way to keep tabs on your vital stats between doctor's appointments. But it can give you even more peace of mind *after* your visit with the doc. How so? Because of an ultra-common condition known as white-coat hypertension. It's caused when a doctor or nurse walks into the examining room (wearing a white lab coat or not), and your anxiety level automatically leaps skyward—accompanied by your blood pressure. If going to the doctor makes you anxious, there is nothing you can do to lower your reading while you're in the office, but chances are your blood pressure will begin returning to normal once you get outta Dodge and head for home. When you arrive and settle in, you can confirm the good news by using your blood pressure monitor and checking the numbers for yourself. You'll rest a whole lot easier afterward.

Pets Can Make Blood Pressure Plummet

Jaw-Dropping DISCOVERY

When scientists at the State University of New York at Buffalo wanted to research the connection between pet ownership and blood pressure, they went to some of the most highly stressed folks on the planet: New York City stockbrokers. All 48 volunteers (24 men and 24 women) had high blood pressure, all were on potent medications to control it during stressful situations, all had lived alone for at least five years, and all were willing to adopt pets. Half of the bunch, selected at random, were directed to acquire a cat or dog of their choice, while the other 24 subjects remained critter-free. By the end of the six-month study, every single one of the pet "parents" had significantly more stable blood pressure readings than the non-adopters had. As you might expect, when the brokers in the control group learned the results of the study, a whole lot of them dashed out and enlisted furry roommates of their own!

Triumphant Disease-Trumping Tonic

Worldwide studies show that a mixture made of apple cider vinegar, garlic, and honey can cure or help prevent almost every ailment under the sun, including high blood pressure, asthma, and cancer, as well as Alzheimer's disease, arthritis, obesity, ulcers, muscle aches—and even the common cold. Here's the simple formula:

1 cup of raw organic honey

1 cup of unfiltered apple cider vinegar

8 peeled garlic cloves

Water or fruit juice

Mix the first three ingredients in a blender on high speed for 60 seconds. Pour the mixture into a glass jar that has a tight-fitting lid, and let it sit in the refrigerator for five days. Then every day (ideally before breakfast), take 2 teaspoons of the blend stirred into a glass of water or fruit juice. Researchers especially recommend using fresh orange or 100 percent grape juice.

Celery Can Lower Your Blood Pressure?!

Yep. This highly underrated vegetable contains an oil that can be one of your strongest allies in sending your numbers downward. It works its magic by allowing the muscles that regulate your blood flow to dilate, thereby taking the pressure off those life-giving, fluid-carrying "canals." So far, researchers have not come up with any particular intake of celery that's required to perform this prodigious feat, so just incorporate this crispy, crunchy (and ultra-low-calorie) champ into your diet as much as you can.

Scallions Satisfy Salt Cravings

If you're on a sodium-restricted diet to control your blood pressure, and you really miss being able to let the salt flow freely, here's good news: Eating a scallion or two with each meal can be just the ticket to satisfy your appetite for salty foods. So trim and wash a bunch of scallions (a.k.a. green onions), wrap them in a damp paper towel, and stash them in the fridge, where they'll keep for up to a week. Change the moist wrapping every other day to maintain maximum freshness.

More Mg + K = Lower BP

Adequate intake of both magnesium (Mg) and potassium (K) is essential for maintaining proper blood pressure. If you need to get

1/2 of all **women** over 45 have **high blood pressure**.

your numbers down, or simply want to stay on an even keel, pack plenty of these health workers into your daily diet:

Magnesium. The RDA is 350 mg for men; 280 mg for women. Good sources include baked potatoes, bananas, broccoli, dairy products, nuts, pumpkin seeds, spinach, and wheat germ.

Potassium. Men and women both need at least 2,000 mg per day. You'll find it in avocados, baked potatoes, bananas, cantaloupe, dried fruits, milk, mushrooms, tomatoes, and yogurt.

3 Fabulous Folk Remedies Foil High Blood Pressure

While it is true that our unhealthy 21st-century lifestyle has contributed to the soaring rates of high blood pressure, the condition itself has been plaguing mankind since the dawn of time. That's why, long before the arrival of sophisticated medicines—or even nutritional supplements—ordinary folks had their own highly effective ways of solving the problem. Here's a trio of the best:

1. Scrub and peel five medium-size potatoes, then simmer the skins in 2 cups of water for 20 minutes. Drink 1 cup of the strained brew twice a day.

2. Three times a day (with each meal), drink a potion made from ½ teaspoon of cream of tartar mixed with ½ teaspoon of lemon juice in

The Stunning Secret of Onion Skins

REMARKABLE REMEDY

Like many other vegetables and fruits, onions hold health-giving treasure in their skins. Specifically, onion skins contain massive amounts of quercetin, a compound that has almost miraculous power to lower blood pressure and LDL (bad) cholesterol, reduce inflammation, fight allergies, relieve depression, treat some forms of cancer. . . . The list goes on and on. There are two simple ways you can tap into this medicinal gold mine anytime you make soup, stew, or rice:

▶ Toss a whole, unpeeled onion or two into the pot, and fish the bulb out before you serve the dish.

▶ Whenever you peel onions, save the skins in a paper bag. Then stuff a handful of the peels into a cheesecloth pouch, and put it into the cooking pot. At serving time, discard the skins. Wash and save the pouch for next time.

8 ounces of water. For the sake of convenience, you can multiply the recipe and store it in the refrigerator for up to 48 hours.

3. Steep 6 tablespoons of dried raspberry leaves* in 4 cups of just-boiled water for 40 minutes, then strain. Either drink the tea hot, put it in the fridge to chill (it will keep well overnight), or pour it into ice-pop molds and freeze them.

Available in health-food stores, herbal-supply stores, and online. You can also harvest wild or cultivated raspberry leaves in spring or midsummer (when the healthful compounds are most potent). Dry them indoors, away from light, to prepare them for use.

High Cholesterol—Stop That Block!

➔ It's an almost universally known fact that high cholesterol puts you on the high road to heart trouble. But a number of myths could be preventing you from achieving a healthy level. Fortunately, some surprising new findings and age-old tricks can help speed up your quest for lower numbers.

The Other Heart-Hurtful Stuff That's in Your Blood

Although cholesterol gets most of the attention when the topic turns to heart health, a fat called triglycerides can also cause serious problems if the level in your blood rises to 150 mg/dl or above. Fortunately, you can send your numbers downward simply by losing weight, getting more exercise, and cutting back on sugars and processed foods.

A Monstrous Misconception about Cholesterol

Common assumption: Cholesterol is cholesterol, and it's all bad.

THE TRUTH: The total amount of cholesterol in your system does matter—less than 200 milligrams per deciliter of blood (mg/dl) is considered healthy; any more than that indicates you could be headed for heart trouble. But there are two types of cholesterol, and how your blood stacks up in regard to them determines how close you are to major trouble. Low-density (LDL) cholesterol is the villain that causes plaque to build up in your arteries, and you want to keep it to a minimum. High-density

(HDL) cholesterol appears to actually help prevent arteriosclerosis, and the more of it you have, the merrier your heart will be. Here's an easy way to remember which is which: LDL cholesterol is Lousy; HDL cholesterol is Happy.

The Fiendish Facts about Statins

If you're taking statins, which are commonly prescribed to lower cholesterol, here's a need-to-know tidbit for you: These powerful drugs can nearly triple your risk of impaired kidney function and increase your likelihood of hemorrhagic stroke by 66 percent. And that's in addition to a truckload of other common side effects, ranging from muscle pain and fatigue to memory loss, insomnia, irritability, sexual dysfunction, and peripheral neuropathy (a painful nerve disorder that affects arms, hands, legs, or feet).

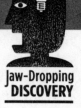

Hen Fruit Is Your Friend

Jaw-Dropping DISCOVERY

We all know that eating eggs will make your blood cholesterol skyrocket, right? Wrong! Medical pros now tell us that, contrary to the old wives' tale, you can eat eggs till the hens come home, and they won't send your cholesterol levels out of whack. In fact, a recent study found that eating eggs on a regular basis (presuming your diet is not overly high in other kinds of fat) can actually raise HDL (good) cholesterol and decrease your level of the bad LDL version.

On top of all that, while statins do make cholesterol levels drop in almost everybody, studies have shown that they are effective at preventing fatal heart attacks and strokes *only* in people who have a history of cardiovascular disease. When these meds are used as preemptive measures for folks with no existing heart problems, they reduce the risk of death from ticker-related causes by less than 2 percent. (To put that figure in perspective, see "Cats Are Medical Miracle Workers" on page 160.) So do yourself a favor: If you've had even a mild side effect from statins, talk to your doctor about either lowering your dose or switching to safer natural remedies. And do it ASAP because the longer you live with the collateral condition, the more damage it can do to your health, and the longer it may take you to get rid of it.

Statin drugs **increase** your **risk** of **stroke**.

Fix-It-Fast FORMULA

Artichoke Cholesterol-Control Tonic

The globe artichoke contains a fierce cholesterol-fighting compound called cynarin. Unfortunately, the highest concentrations of it are found not in the tasty artichoke heart, but in the bitter, stringy leaves. So how do you extract their heart-healthy goodness? Why, with this fabulous formula, of course!

5 ¼ cups of artichoke leaves

2 pints of unflavored vodka or gin

Crush the leaves slightly, and put them in a large glass jar with the liquor. Screw the lid on, and place the container in a cool, dark place for 10 days. Then strain the liquid into a clean jar or bottle that has a tight-fitting lid. Take 1 tablespoon of the tonic twice a day between meals.

The Inside Scoop on Unfiltered Coffee

You've probably heard the rumor that unfiltered coffee, such as espresso, latte, and the kind made in those fancy French press gadgets, can raise your LDL cholesterol. And you might be assuming that it's just a bunch of hooey invented by folks who market coffee filters, right? Not so fast. It turns out that filtering coffee actually does remove a compound called cafestol that can, indeed, increase your levels of the dreaded artery clogger. There is one catch, though: You need to use a paper filter. The reusable gold type doesn't cut the mustard for this job, so be sure to stock up on the paper versions when they're on sale.

A Freaky Cause of Cholesterol Catastrophes

Everybody talks about the effect of diet on cholesterol—both good and bad kinds. But more and more studies are showing how big a role stress plays in the DL drama. To be specific, stress raises your levels of villainous LDL cholesterol and lowers the amount of its good-guy counterpart, HDL. However, when you cope with stressful, emotionally straining situations in a positive way, you actually increase the HDL cast. This lets them carry on one of their most important missions: mopping up all of that excess LDL in your blood. For the full lowdown on stress and how to control it, see "All Stressed Out" on page 41.

1/2 of all **women over** age **50 die** of heart disease.

Strike Back at Stroke!

➔ It's probably safe to say that for most of us, the prospect of a stroke—either our own or one befalling someone we love—ranks right up there with cancer and Alzheimer's disease as a horrifying nightmare. But here are two comforting thoughts to keep in mind as you face down your fears: The vast majority of strokes can be prevented, and scientists are learning more and more about how to do just that.

Stroke Strikes in 2 Ways

This devastating blow to the brain comes in two forms:

Ischemic stroke is the most common type. It occurs when blood can't get to the brain, most often because a clot or fatty deposit is blocking a blood vessel. High blood pressure, high cholesterol levels, smoking, sleep apnea, and a family history of stroke all put you at high risk for this demon.

Hemorrhagic stroke is directly tied to high blood pressure. It occurs when a blood vessel bursts in your brain. So start getting those numbers down *now*!

Words to the Wise: Clogged Arteries Cause Ministrokes

A ministroke, known in medical circles as a transient ischemic attack (TIA), is often a wake-up call that a full-blown ischemic stroke is on the way. A TIA happens when

> **CALL 911**
>
> If you think that you or a companion is having a stroke, don't hesitate for a second—make a mad dash to the ER. The docs can sometimes stop an ischemic stroke in its tracks with an enzyme called tissue plasminogen activator (tPA), but it *must* be administered within three hours of the onset of symptoms—and the sooner the better. These are the stroke danger signals:
>
> ▶ Weakness or numbness in the face, arm, or leg on one side of the body
>
> ▶ Difficulty speaking or understanding others
>
> ▶ Dimness or impaired vision in one eye
>
> ▶ An unexplained dizzy spell
>
> ▶ A severe headache with no apparent cause
>
> Even if the symptoms pass quickly, get immediate help because you may have had a TIA, which means the real deal could be barreling down the pike.

blood flow to the brain is blocked for only a few moments before it's resumed, and you're back to normal again—at least for a while. Most often, it's the direct result of arteriosclerosis (a.k.a. clogged arteries), but high blood pressure, diabetes, and smoking can also trigger a TIA.

Every 40 seconds, someone in the U.S. has a **stroke**.

Killer Coasters

If you think that the worst trouble you can get from one of those super-colossal roller coasters is a queasy stomach (or tossed cookies), think again. In some cases, those twists, turns, and bone-jarring plunges can cause bleeding in your brain that could trigger a stroke. So do yourself a favor: If you suffer from frequent headaches, you have high blood pressure, arteriosclerosis, or cardiovascular problems of any kind, or you're on blood-thinning meds, stay off those big mamas! Even if you aren't among the high-risk crowd (at least not to your knowledge), be alert for the major danger signal—a postride headache—and if one occurs, see a doctor immediately.

Send Artery Plaque Packin'

REMARKABLE REMEDY

Arteriosclerosis, a.k.a. clogging of the arteries, is caused by plaque, a combination of LDL cholesterol, calcium, fatty food substances, and other matter. It builds up over many years as a result of smoking, lack of exercise, and poor diet. If that description fits your lifestyle (but you haven't been diagnosed with the condition), keep clogs—and strokes—at bay with this simple remedy: Once a day, finely mince two peeled garlic cloves, mix them in half a glass of orange juice or water, and drink it down. Don't worry that you'll walk around with dragon breath. As long as you don't chew the garlic bits, you won't suffer any aromatic side effects.

An Alarming Reason to Turn Down the Volume

For years, research has suggested that noise can raise your stress level and blood pressure to highly unhealthy levels. Well, a growing body of evidence is now showing a direct correlation between noise and stroke. For example, one recent study in Denmark exposed 51,000 people to road traffic sounds ranging from 40 to 82 decibels (dB). The results: For every 10-dB increase in volume, the risk of stroke increased by 14 percent in subjects 65 and younger, and it rose 27 percent in folks over age 65. Just to put those numbers in perspective, here are average ratings for some common sounds:

- Quiet room: 40 dB
- Normal conversation: 65 dB
- Vacuum cleaner: 70 dB
- City street: 85 dB
- Power mower: 107 dB
- Amplified music or chain saw: 110 dB
- Gunshot: 140 dB
- Jet aircraft at takeoff: 180 dB

NOTE: *For every 10-dB increase in volume, your perception of the loudness doubles.*

The Astonishing Stroke-Preventing Power of Tea

Black tea—the regular stuff sold in your supermarket—has been linked to a reduced risk of stroke and heart disease. A study published in the *Archives of Internal Medicine* found that 800 elderly men who drank 4 or more cups of tea a day had a 69 percent lower risk of stroke than those who downed fewer than 2.6 cups. Scientists reckon it works because the antioxidants in tea maintain the health of the circulatory system and reduce the likelihood of blood clots.

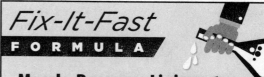

Fix-It-Fast
FORMULA

Muscle-Recovery Liniment

If you've suffered a stroke and are working your way back to health, this warming potion can help boost blood circulation to any paralyzed muscles. (But only use it, or any remedy in this book, with your doctor's or therapist's blessing.)

2 oz. of powdered rosemary*
1 oz. of powdered English lavender flowers*
½ oz. of powdered cayenne pepper
1 qt. of rubbing alcohol

Combine all of the ingredients in a glass jar that has a tight-fitting lid (a clamp-lidded canning jar is perfect). Let the mixture stand at room temperature for seven days, shaking it well each day. Then strain the contents into a clean bottle. Once or twice a day, rub the liniment onto your afflicted body parts.

* Available in health-food stores, herbal-supply stores, and online.

Breaking: Broccoli Boosts Your Stroke Defenses

After analyzing the diets of more than 100,000 people for 14 years, researchers at Harvard came to a maybe not-so-surprising conclusion:

The more fruits and vegetables the volunteers ate, the less likely they were to suffer a stroke. But here's the surprising part: According to this and many other studies, the most effective foods for fending off (or recovering from) strokes—and heart attacks, too— are cruciferous vegetables, which include broccoli, Brussels sprouts, cabbage, cauliflower, and kale. And, for the real kicker: The American Heart Association tells us that when it comes to protecting yourself from a stroke, crunching your crucifers on a routine basis ranks right up there with controlling your blood pressure and engaging in regular physical activity. Put that trio together, and you've got a genuine dream team!

Asthma—Breathe Easy!

➡ Breathing is something that most of us take for granted. But for folks with asthma, the simple act of inhaling is a constant struggle. And the ranks of those who wage this battle are on the rise—over the past 25 years, asthma rates have quadrupled and the number of deaths from asthma attacks has doubled. Whether you're included in those staggering statistics, or simply want to avoid making the list, the tips, tricks, and tonics here can help.

Being Ladylike Is Lethal

Studies show that after age 20, women are more likely than men to develop asthma, and the risk increases with age. But the sobering news doesn't stop there. Women are also more likely to be hospitalized for asthma and to die of an attack. To top it all off, those who take estrogen supplements for 10 years or longer significantly raise their risk for acquiring this atrocious ailment. The bottom line: Don't panic—but *do* make every effort to clean up your act and eliminate as many other asthma risk factors as possible.

4 Shocking Causes of Asthma

About three-fifths of all asthma cases are hereditary. And while no one knows for sure what triggers attacks in folks whose genes do not predispose them to the condition, natural health practitioners point their fingers at these four factors:

1. The modern American diet (MAD) and its two ugly offspring: chronic inflammation, which causes your airways to swell up and become clogged with mucus, and nutritional deficiencies, which make you more prone to diseases of all kinds, including asthma. (You can read all about MAD in Chapter 3.)

2. An overload of chemicals in our food, water, and air—indoors and out—that both weaken your immune system and throw your hormones out of balance.

3. Increasing levels of allergens, such as mold, mildew, and toxin-bearing dust mites in homes and offices.

4. A tidal wave of tension, anxiety, and stress, all of which contribute to or worsen every health problem under the sun.

Another Pressing Peril of Plumpness

Harvard researchers have found that women who are 30 percent over their normal weight for their height are more than twice as likely to develop adult asthma than ladies who are not packing extra pounds. So if you're bearing a bulge, and you want to keep—or start—breathing freely, your mission is clear: Strive to lose weight at a sustainable rate of about a pound a week through regular exercise and healthful eating (*not* a crazy quack diet!). Within four months or so, you should drop enough weight to greatly lessen the chance that your bronchial tubes will betray you. If you already have asthma, your inhaler should begin to see a lot less action.

HRT Can Take Your Breath Away

For years, the media has made much of studies showing that hormone-replacement therapy (HRT) increases a woman's risk for heart

Deliver Fast First Aid

When you're near someone who suffers a severe asthma attack, proceed as follows:

1. Have the victim sit down with his back straight and head up.

2. Put both hands on the person's lower stomach, and apply upward pressure.

3. If you have no other remedy on hand, administer a cup of strong, cold black coffee to help restore normal breathing.

attack, stroke, and breast cancer. But here's a stunner that hasn't gotten as much airplay: Thanks to its load of supplemental estrogen, HRT can double your risk of developing asthma. Especially if this bronchial nightmare runs in your family, ask your doctor about a lung-friendlier, OTC alternative called Promensil®. Its key ingredient, red clover, delivers herbal estrogen that helps reduce hot flashes and other menopausal discomforts without the dangers of the heavy hitters in traditional HRT meds.

Alleviating Asthma Is a Laughing Matter

No, I'm not suggesting that asthma, or any other lung problem, is something to be taken lightly! Rather, I'm passing along the good, scientifically proven news that laughing is a guaranteed way to help you breathe easier. That's because it improves the exchange of air in your lungs, thereby revving up oxygen circulation and clearing out accumulated mucus. So do your breathing apparatus a favor: Increase your exposure to whatever tickles your funny bone, whether that entails signing up for daily e-mail joke delivery, listening to comedians via CDs or radio on the way to work, or making movie and TV comedies—new or old—a bigger part of your viewing time.

50% of **asthma** sufferers have **allergen-triggered** attacks.

2 Astounding Asthma-Bashing Beverages

A couple of common—and ultra-healthy—drinks can often stop asthmatic episodes cold turkey, or at least lessen their severity.

• **Cranberry juice.** Take 2 tablespoons of pure, unsweetened cranberry juice 30 minutes before each meal and at the onset of an attack. Just be sure to use 100 percent cranberry juice (not juice combos), with no sugar or preservatives added.

- **Garlic milk.** As soon as you feel an attack coming on, peel and chop 10 garlic cloves, and add them to ¼ cup of milk. Heat the moo juice to boiling, then strain out the garlic. Let the milky "tea" cool to a comfortable temperature, and drink it down.

That Old Cliché about Apples . . .

Is worth taking to heart if you've got asthma. A recent study at the University of Nottingham in England found that asthmatics who ate more than five apples a week really did keep the doctor away. The volunteer subjects had less wheeziness and other symptoms, as well as improved overall lung function. But wait—there's more! The nutrients, enzymes, and biochemical compounds in Adam's favorite fruit have also been proven to help lower high blood pressure and LDL (bad) cholesterol; prevent or dissolve gallstones; keep blood sugar under control; and fend off or relieve scads of other potentially deadly conditions, including colon cancer, cardiovascular disease, stroke, and coronary heart disease.

And here's more good news: Apples pack the same healthy wallop whether you eat them fresh, dried, frozen, or cooked—or drink them in the form of 100 percent apple juice or cider. Just stick to organic apples in all their forms to ensure you're not exposing yourself to dangerous pesticides. (For more about the unnatural chemicals on and in our food, see Chapter 4.)

The Hidden Healing Secrets of Citrus Peels

REMARKABLE REMEDY

Studies have found that a chemical called limonene, which is found in the rinds of all citrus fruits, can provide potent protection against obstructions in your bronchial tubes. But that's not all! In addition to easing your wheezing woes, limonene may help prevent breast, colon, and prostate cancers. You can put this a-peeling healer to work in three ways:

1. Sniff it. Fold a piece of peel between your fingers, and squeeze it. Then slowly inhale the refreshing aroma.

2. Eat it. Add freshly grated lemon, lime, orange, grapefruit, or tangerine peels to stir-fries, salad dressings, baked goods, and rice. Or top your toast, bagels, and muffins with marmalade.

3. Bathe in it. Stuff cheesecloth bags or panty hose feet with crushed citrus peels, and toss them into your bathwater. Whatever you do, though, never put loose rinds—or any other solid material—in the tub, or your cleared-up wind pipes will come at the expense of clogged-up drain pipes!

Crippling Chronic Pain

Although pain, like that caused by arthritis, back problems, migraines, and other agonizing ailments, won't kill you outright, it can strongly hinder your ability to function physically and can also lead to intense depression. Furthermore, untreated chronic pain can damage your immune system, making you susceptible to a whole passel of fatal diseases.

Arthritis—Get Your Joints Jumpin'!

➡ **As with many other ills, arthritis is on a fast upward track across our land, and for two major reasons. One is our ever-growing girth (obesity is the leading cause of arthritis). The other is our aging population. It's a basic law of physics that the older we get, the more wear and tear we put on our joints—even if we're in tip-top shape.**

Obesity is renowned for its role in our explosive diabetes epidemic, but according to the Centers for Disease Control and Prevention (CDC), obesity is also the single leading cause of osteoarthritis (OA). And the more you weigh, the sooner OA is likely to set in, and the more severe your symptoms will be. That's because as our bodies grow older, our cartilage slowly starts to wear out, and the fluid between the joints begins to dry up. When you put a bigger load on those joints than they were designed to handle, the wearing-out and drying-up processes happen a whole lot faster.

2 Tall Tales about Arthritis

With so many people suffering from arthritis, it's no wonder that there is a mountain of misinformation floating around about what causes arthritis and how to cope with it. These are the two most prevalent misconceptions:

Tall tale #1: All joint pain is arthritis.
FACT: Tendinitis, bursitis, and soft-tissue injuries can also cause joint pain. So before you try any do-it-yourself remedies, get a diagnosis from a rheumatologist.

Tall tale #2: Arthritis is arthritis—period.
FACT: There are more than 100 forms of arthritis. They operate in slightly different ways, and some are more

debilitating than others. Again, a rheumatologist can tell you which kind (if any) you've got and the best ways to treat it.

A Trio of Joint-Jolting Terrors

Out of all types of arthritis, these are the three most common varieties:

Osteoarthritis. This is the most prevalent type, and it results from either injury or wear and tear on your joints. If your hips or knees ache when you climb out of bed in the morning, and you were a jock or a dancer in high school or college, it's all but guaranteed that OA is the culprit.

Rheumatoid arthritis (RA). This is an autoimmune disease that occurs when the immune system malfunctions and attacks your body. Over time, the resulting inflammation can cause severe joint damage and deformities. This very serious condition demands top-notch medical care, but many of the same pain-relieving and mobility-enhancing tricks that work for OA can also work wonders for RA sufferers.

Gout. Contrary to folklore, gout is not limited to old men who eat too much rich food. Rather, it can strike anyone whose body cannot eliminate uric acid effectively. The excess acid settles in your joints, where it forms needle-like crystals, which in turn cause swelling and severe pain. (You'll find more grist on gout beginning on page 201.)

Psoriatic Arthritis: A Despicable Double Whammy

All by itself psoriasis is a nightmare come true. But up to 30 percent of folks who suffer from it are slammed with an added woe: an associated inflammation of the joints called psoriatic arthritis. And there's no telling how it might manifest. It can affect multiple joints or only one. It can attack the spine or cause fingers and toes to swell up like sausages. Lesions may develop on finger- and/or toenails. Eyes often become red and sore. Psoriatic arthritis usually strikes people between the ages of 30 and 50, but it can also start in childhood. In extreme cases, surgery may be necessary. When symptoms are less severe, your doctor's R_X will probably be a combo of arthritis and psoriasis remedies.

The Whole Nine Yards about Knuckle Cracking

If you're a lifelong knuckle cracker, you've no doubt been told over and over again that it's putting you on a fast track to arthritis. Well, guess what? According to numerous studies, as well as the orthopedic experts at Harvard Medical School, it's doing no such thing. But there are plenty of other reasons to kick the habit. Aside from annoying the daylights out of people around you, repeatedly cracking your knuckles can spur the development of skin pads or calluses over your joints, weaken your grip, cause your hands to swell up, and even damage the ligaments in your fingers. So stop it already!

4 Deadly Nightshades

If you suffer from arthritis, *and* you love spuds and tomatoes, this news will not be music to your ears, but it could be a sweet lullaby for your aching joints: Vegetables in the tomato (a.k.a. nightshade or *Solanaceae*) family can intensify arthritic pain. To find out whether you're sensitive to these foods, either get an allergy test or—simpler and a whole lot cheaper—go cold turkey on the entire clan for a month or so, and see if you feel any relief. These are the suspects in question:

1/3 of **arthritis** sufferers **get no exercise**.

- Eggplant
- Peppers (sweet or hot)
- Potatoes (sweet potatoes are okay)
- Tomatoes

2 Hidden Hazards of Topical Pain Creams

Folks who use pain-relieving ointments and creams to soothe their achy joints and muscles know they work every bit as well as aspirin does. And there's a good reason: Many of them contain salicylates, the main ingredient in aspirin. That could translate into big trouble in two ways:

1. Salicylates interact with many kinds of drugs, so if you're on meds of any kind—either prescription or OTC—check with your doctor before using a topical rub.

2. People who are allergic to aspirin can have a reaction when the medicine is absorbed into their body. If you know that you're allergic to aspirin, read the package labels carefully and (of course!) bypass any product that contains the offending substance.

Are You Asking for Osteoarthritis?

You don't have to be a gung-ho athlete to put yourself at high risk for developing OA. There could be potent dangers lurking in your everyday routine. Like these, for instance:

The shoes you wear. If you opt for high heels day in and day out—whether they're pencil-thin stilettos or chunkier versions— you're all but begging for OA in your knees. Plus, high-heeled shoes (or boots) that are pointy or tight can also lead to arthritis of the toes. Wearing dress-up pumps on special occasions isn't likely to cause damage, but for daily wear, choose footgear with ample toe room and sturdy heels that are no more than 1 to 2 inches high.

The loads you tote. Walking with heavy bags (or any other weighty objects) in your hands, with your arms stretched downward, puts an undue strain on shoulders, elbows, wrists, and fingers. So when your shopping haul weighs any more than a couple of pounds, cradle the bag in both arms, or use one or two long-handled canvas sacks slung over your shoulder(s). If you routinely carry a heavy briefcase to work or school, consider trading it for a wheeled model or one with a shoulder strap.

The pounds you pack. Obesity is the leading cause of osteoarthritis because excess weight puts enormous stress on your knees and hips. Need more incentive to trim the fat? Then consider this fact: By shedding just 10 pounds, you'll reduce the stress on each knee by a full 40 pounds!

The moves you don't make. Couch potatoes are prime targets for OA. Conversely, in the words of the Arthritis Foundation's recent awareness campaign theme, "Moving is the best medicine." Even if you're not overweight, regular physical activity is a must for strengthening the muscles that support your joints—and keeping the joints themselves flexible. But there is one caveat: Running, especially on hard pavement, is murder on your knees. So opt for more easygoing activities, such as walking, yoga, or even bowling. Better yet, sign up for an aquatic exercise class, like the ones conducted by the Arthritis Foundation. To find a location near you, visit www.arthritis.org.

Your Painkillers Could Be Killing You

Jaw-Dropping DISCOVERY

Nonsteroidal anti-inflammatory drugs (NSAIDs) are renowned for their ability to ease the discomfort of arthritis and myriad other aches and pains. But more and more research is fingering these miracle meds as a prime cause of leaky gut syndrome, a breakdown of the intestinal lining that keeps harmful substances from passing out of your gut and flowing through your body. Not only can that motley array of toxins intensify the joint pain you're trying to erase, but—depending on the number and nature of the roving pathogens—they may trigger or contribute to far more serious conditions, including diabetes, asthma, and autism, as well as immune system disorders such as celiac disease, Crohn's disease, and (yes) rheumatoid arthritis.

Popping an aspirin or ibuprofen every now and then isn't likely to hurt you, but chronic use of these meds just might, especially if they're potent doctor-prescribed versions. In fact, studies in Great Britain have found that 70 to 80 percent of people who take prescription-strength NSAIDs for just two weeks will get leaky gut syndrome.

3 Super-Safe Supplements That Soothe Sore Joints

While aspirin and other NSAIDs may deliver dangerous side effects (see "Your Painkillers Could Be Killing You," at left), a trio of supplements can help ease your pain and, according to natural health pros, may actually heal leaky gut syndrome. You can find these winners at health-food stores and online at sites that carry natural health and nutrition products:

- Colostrum
- Deglycerinated licorice (DGL)
- L-glutamine

NOTE: *If you're on prescription meds for arthritis or any other condition, check with your doctor before you start taking these or any other supplements.*

An Un-bee-lievable Arthritis Remedy

As outrageous as this may sound, many physicians are using bee venom to treat arthritis patients who do not respond well to conventional medications. The practice is called apitherapy. The results have been impressive in both OA and RA sufferers, and there are no serious side effects. The secret to success lies in two ingredients: melittin, an anti-inflammatory agent that is said to be about 100 times stronger than cortisone, and adolapin, which also fights inflammation and pain. But arthritis isn't the only condition that apitherapy can relieve. It's also being used across the country to treat lower-back and shoulder pain, asthma, high blood pressure, multiple sclerosis, hearing loss, and even premenstrual syndrome.

Apitherapy ABCs

Bee venom therapy is nothing new. The ancient Egyptians wrote about it in their medical texts, and Hippocrates, the Father of Medicine, routinely used it to treat joint pain and swelling in the fifth century B.C. But before you rush out for a dose of bee juice, keep these particulars in mind:

- Relief is not a slam dunk. Although the docs who use apitherapy report excellent results, some patients—and some conditions—respond better than others.

- The injections or bee stings (which some doctors use) can be painful, and you may need more than a dozen of them before your condition improves.

- This goes without saying (I hope!), but if you're allergic to bee stings, this cure could kill you.

Eat to Treat RA Pain

For years, medical pros have been singing the praises of the Mediterranean diet for its ability to prevent or treat conditions ranging from heart disease, diabetes, and stroke to poor vision, osteoporosis, and excess weight—as well as to simply increase

For OA Relief, Count to TENS

REMARKABLE REMEDY

If you have osteoarthritis, you could join the legions of sufferers who have opted for acupuncture. It's been proven to relieve pain and improve mobility for weeks after treatment. You say you don't fancy having needles stuck in your knees or elbows? Not to worry! Transcutaneous electrical nerve stimulation (TENS) can work just as well with no poking required. A TENS unit is a battery-powered device, smaller than a deck of cards, that you attach to your belt or waistband. It delivers electrical impulses (painlessly!) through your skin, thereby increasing endorphins—naturally occurring narcotics in your body—that inhibit pain impulses arising from the spinal cord. Although TENS won't cure your arthritis, it may greatly ease the aches in your joints. Ask your doctor if TENS is tops for you!

your life span. Now, it turns out that it can also reduce inflammation caused by rheumatoid arthritis and help stop painful flare-ups in their tracks. For the full scoop on this medical marvel, see "The Big Diet Lie" (below).

Fix-It-Fast FORMULA

Hot Healing Liniment

This dandy DIY potion will bring warm relief to your aching joints—and sore muscles, too.

1 cup of grated fresh ginger

1 tsp. of cayenne pepper

1 tsp. of vegetable glycerin*

2½ cups of unflavored vodka

Combine the first three ingredients in a large jar that has a tight-fitting lid (a 1-quart clamp-lidded canning jar is perfect). Pour in the vodka, and shake vigorously for 30 seconds or so to blend the contents. Stash the container in a cool, dark place for four weeks, shaking it for 15 to 20 seconds every day. When time's up, pour the potion through a strainer lined with a paper coffee filter, making sure that you press all of the fluid out of the grated ginger. Funnel the liniment into a clean bottle, cap it tightly, and store it in a dark, room-temperature cabinet, where it should keep for about two years. Then, whenever your joints need relief, massage the potion into the ailing areas and say, "Ahhh . . . that feels better!"

* Available in most drugstores.

The Big Diet Lie

Don't let anyone fool you: The Mediterranean diet is not one of those regimens that force you to count calories and swear off all the foods you love most. Rather, it's a way of life that emphasizes healthy foods and minimizes (but does not make you give up) not-so-good dietary choices. Here's a quick overview of the life-extending guidelines:

- Heaping helpings of fruits, vegetables, whole grains, nuts, seeds, and herbs.

- A variety of foods—fresh, in-season, locally grown, and organic, whenever possible. This helps to ensure the maximum delivery of health-giving micronutrients and antioxidants.

- Plenty of extra virgin olive oil.

- Moderate amounts of cheese, milk, yogurt, fish, poultry, and eggs.

- Minimal amounts of sugar, saturated fat, and red meat.

- Moderate consumption of red wine (optional).

- Regular physical activity to promote healthy weight, muscle tone, and overall well-being.

Chipping Away at Joint Health

Potato chips—and scads of other processed foods—are commonly made with vegetable oils that are high in omega-6 fatty acids. These fats increase inflammation in your body, thereby intensifying arthritis pain (or any other kind). Your best feel-better policy: Whenever you're shopping for processed foods, especially snacks or baked goods, read the labels carefully, and steer clear of anything that contains more than trace amounts of corn, safflower, soybean, or sunflower oil. And for cooking purposes, go with olive oil or nut oils such as almond, coconut, peanut, or walnut. They're all rich in unsaturated fats, which, aside from *not* worsening your misery, actually enhance the health of your joints.

Obesity is the **leading cause** of **arthritis.**

Save Your Spine from Back and Neck Pain!

➡ Just about every adult on the planet has had a backache at one time or other. But if there is any doubt in your mind about how widespread the problem is, consider this fact: Back pain is the second-leading cause of lost work time (the common cold is first). Here's another shocker: Chronic back and neck pain is the number one reason that people undergo a surgical procedure.

2 Dangerous Myths about Back Pain

At least 8 out of every 10 people experience disabling back pain at some point in their lives. So no wonder multitudes of misconceptions have sprung up about its origins and treatment. Here are two that could cause you a whole lot of misery.

Myth #1: Back pain sufferers should stay in bed.
FACT: For the first day or two after an injury, staying in bed, or at least taking it easy, will help calm your pain and avoid any further damage to the tissues. But loafing any longer than that can actually hinder the healing process. Instead, you should see a physical therapist, who can develop an exercise program that's tailored to your specific diagnosis and pain level.

Myth #2: Pain is a fact of life—so get used to it!

FACT: Chronic pain of any kind is very debilitating and must be treated; otherwise, it can affect your immune system and lead to additional serious conditions. If an aching back is interfering with your daily activities, see a doctor now, before the problem gets worse.

CALL 911

While it is true that in most cases a backache is a straightforward problem, it can be a warning sign of a potentially life-threatening condition. If any of the situations below apply to you, get medical help immediately.

▶ Your back pain is accompanied by either bowel or bladder incontinence or progressive weakness in your legs.

▶ You have a fever.

▶ You've experienced unexplained weight loss.

▶ The pain occurs after a fall, car accident, or other physical mishap.

▶ You suffer from osteoporosis or multiple myeloma (a.k.a. Kahler's disease).

▶ You have a history of breast, lung, or prostate cancer, which can spread to the spine.

3 Cunning Coconspirators

Although all backaches have physical origins, a trio of other factors can play a considerable role in how severe the pain is and how long it lasts. Here's the terrible triad:

1. Depression or anxiety. Either one—or worse, a combination of the two—greatly intensifies your discomfort.

2. Insomnia. Getting too little shut-eye, for whatever reason, can contribute mightily to back pain.

3. Stress. It causes your muscles to tense up, thereby increasing your misery.

Pack On Pounds at Your Peril

Besides putting you at high risk for such life-threatening conditions as heart disease, diabetes, and stroke, being overweight makes you prone to spinal problems of all kinds. In particular, carrying excess fat around your belly makes you a prime target for lower-back pain. Doctors prescribe health-related weight loss for women whose waists measure more than 35 inches and men with waist measurements of more than 40 inches. Overall, to relieve any current back pain and prevent future trouble, you should drop to within 10 pounds of your ideal weight.

The Mind-Boggling Truth about MRIs

Common assumption: In order to accurately pinpoint the source of your back or neck pain, an MRI or a CT scan is necessary.

FACT: In all but a tiny percentage of cases, a health-care pro can successfully diagnose and treat your problem based on a complete medical history and a thorough physical exam. What's more, these expensive tests often reveal common abnormalities, such as a degenerated disk, that cause no trouble at all and probably never will. Yet they can fail to show any problems in a person with great pain. The bottom line: Unless you're prepping for surgery, ask your doc if you can skip the scans.

When Money Hurts

Hey, guys! Do you experience back or hip pain whenever you sit for a while, but you can't figure out the source? It could be in your pants. If you habitually carry a thick wallet (or your cell phone) in your back pocket, there's a good chance it's putting pressure on your sciatic nerve. So move the offender to a jacket pocket. You just might enjoy a miraculous recovery!

Jaw-Dropping DISCOVERY

Smoking triples your **risk** of **spinal degeneration**.

Another Diabolical Danger of Smoking

Some folks who suffer from chronic pain—in their backs or anyplace else in their bodies—find that a quick smoke gives them blessed, albeit temporary, relief. Well, if you're in that unfortunate crowd, I have news for you: Smoking will actually make your pain worse in the long run (that is, if you don't puff your way into a disease that kills you first). In addition to its other vile deeds, puffing the wicked weed slows healing, hinders blood circulation, and increases your risk for degenerated disks. So quit the sticks now!

The Worst Hazard on the Golf Course

If you're thinking of taking up golf, or you're new to the game, here's a dirty little secret you should know: This seemingly benign pastime can be murder on your spine. Nearly all golfers develop backaches or suffer from injuries ranging from twisted muscles to pinched nerves, ruptured disks, spinal stenosis, and sciatica. But you don't have to join the crowd. Just take this handful of simple precautions to stay safe on the links:

- Make sure your clubs fit you perfectly. If the shafts are either too long or too short, you're asking for trouble from the get-go.

- Start slow. If you're a beginner, or you haven't played for a while, spend some quality time on the driving range before tackling the full course.

- Condition your body. Focus on exercises that incorporate rotation, as well as strengthen the muscles in your back, abdomen, pelvis, and buttocks.

- Stretch before, during, and after each round.

- Rest between games. Swinging a golf club is not a natural human movement, and playing day after day puts more strain on your body than it is designed to handle.

Just Say, "Om"

Yoga can be one of the most effective treatments of all for chronic back pain—but only if you keep these two pointers in mind:

1. Opt for Hatha yoga, which features gentle stretching, deep breathing,

---

Fix-It-Fast FORMULA

Extreme-Relief Muscle Massage Oil

When a round of golf—or any other strenuous work or play—leaves you so stiff and sore that you can hardly move, a massage with this ultra-potent blend is just what the doctor ordered. (It's also highly effective for relaxing tight, painful neck muscles.)

10 drops of rosemary oil*

5 drops of lavender oil

5 drops of lemon oil

5 drops of peppermint oil

5 drops of Roman chamomile oil

1 oz. of sweet almond oil

Drip the first five essential oils into a glass bottle that has a tight-fitting lid. Add the sweet almond oil, screw on the top, and shake thoroughly. Then massage the blend into all the strained, painful areas for deep-down relief—or have your spouse do the honors. For an even deeper, more effective treatment, book an appointment with a professional massage therapist, and take the potion with you.

* All the oils are available in health-food stores, herbal-supply stores, and online at sites that specialize in essential oils.

and relaxing poses. Avoid the trendy, action-packed styles that could actually cause more trouble than you've already got.

2. Find a highly skilled instructor who has extensive experience working with back pain sufferers and who promotes a noncompetitive, stress-free atmosphere in class.

Bottoms-Up Back Relief

Believe it or not, soaking your feet in a lavender bath can pulverize muscle pain in your back, or anywhere else in your body. Just fill a basin with hot, but not scalding, water, and for every quart of H_2O, stir in 5 to 10 drops of lavender oil. Settle into a comfy chair, put your tootsies in the potion, and relax for at least 10 minutes. The fluid will get the blood flowing all through your system, just like an internal hot compress—and that's exactly what your muscles need for quick healing.

Sensational Sciatica Solution

REMARKABLE REMEDY

The sciatic nerve is your body's biggest nerve, and it can also produce one of its biggest pains. But—as unlikely as it may seem when that "fire" is shooting down your leg—you *can* relieve the discomfort. Just mix equal parts of castor oil, arnica oil, and St. John's wort oil, and gently massage the mixture onto the nerve track. Begin at your buttocks, and go down the back of your leg. If you have a disk problem, massage the oil into that area, too. Repeat as needed for soothing relief.

NOTE: *You can buy arnica oil and St. John's wort oil in health-food and herbal-supply stores, as well as online.*

Sneaky Spinal Self-Deception

Optimism is a wonderful trait—but not when it morphs into denial about a potentially dangerous condition. Here are a couple of fibs your subconscious mind may be using to convince you that, barring unforeseen injuries, you're safe from back problems.

Americans spend **$50 billion** a year to treat **lower-back pain**.

Fib #1: Only folks who are out of shape get back trouble, and I'm active and as fit as a fiddle.
THE TRUTH: Yes, physical exercise can go a long way toward preventing back injury. But if you focus on one activity that uses a particular set of muscles—say, bowling, tennis, or dancing—you're

actually increasing the likelihood of developing back pain. Because you build up tension in one area, weakness tends to occur in other places. The key to fending off trouble is to develop an exercise program that strengthens and stretches all of your muscle groups.

Fib #2: I know that fat people are prone to backaches, but I'm skinny, so I don't have to worry.

THE TRUTH: Although being overweight is a major cause of back problems, the reality is that they can strike anyone. Furthermore, if you're too thin—whether the cause is a naturally tiny appetite or full-blown anorexia—you're a prime candidate for bone loss, which could easily result in fractured or crushed vertebrae. The bottom line: Strive to maintain the optimum weight for your height and bone structure.

Your Job Can Be a Real Pain in the Neck

That's because the vast majority of neck pain is caused by muscle tension. Leaning over a work surface, hunching in front of a computer screen, or slouching at the wheel of your car all make neck muscles tighten up. So can emotional stress generated by constant deadlines, testy meetings, and clogged highways. Then the vicious circle begins: When your muscles tense up, the blood flow to them decreases, thereby triggering pain, which, in turn, increases your tension. The good news is that this cause-and-effect scenario makes neck trouble a prime candidate for successful DIY treatment.

50% of people with **neck pain** don't seek **treatment**.

1. Eliminate as much emotional stress as possible, and learn to deal with the rest in a healthy manner (see "All Stressed Out," beginning on page 41).

2. Resolve the ergonomic issues—that is, the physical positions in which you work, sit, and sleep (more on that score in "3 Slick Tricks for Pulverizing Neck Pain," below, and "Sleep Better, Hurt Less" on page 190).

3. Get—and stay—in shape. The stronger and more flexible you are, the less likely you'll be to suffer from neck pain. In particular, well-toned stomach muscles are a must for keeping your whole spine in good working order.

3 Slick Tricks for Pulverizing Neck Pain

This trio of simple actions will put you on the fast track to freedom from distress:

Practice the complete breath. This yoga exercise opens up airways and is a sure-fire way to relax and soothe the sore muscles in your neck. Visit www.americanyogaassociation.org for the how-to.

Keep your work at eye level. Looking down or reaching up for long periods of time is guaranteed to give you a sore neck. Adjust the height of your desk, chair, or computer monitor so that you're looking straight at the screen. If you do a lot of reaching up—for instance, to pull supplies from shelves—use a stool, stepladder, or elevated platform to bring you even with your targets.

CALL 911

While it is true that most neck pain is the direct result of stress and muscle tension, it can be a sign of far more serious trouble. Make a mad dash to the ER in any of these instances:

▶ The problem was caused by a fall or other accident.

▶ The pain radiates down your arms and legs.

▶ Your neck discomfort is accompanied by a headache, numbness, tingling, or weakness.

▶ Your vision is disturbed in any way.

Change your habits. Poor posture puts a huge strain on neck muscles. So do seemingly innocent activities, such as washing your hair in the sink, cradling a phone receiver between your ear and shoulder, or falling asleep in a chair and winding up with your head at an awkward angle. Identify and change behavior patterns that keep your neck in unnatural positions for any length of time. And for Pete's sake, do what your mother (or your drill sergeant) always told you: Stand—and sit—up straight!

Sleep Better, Hurt Less

For years, experts on spinal health have advised us that sleeping in the wrong position and using the wrong bedding can cause chronic neck pain. (The R_X for trouble avoidance: Sleep on your back or side on a firm mattress, using a pillow that is neither too high nor too stiff.) Well, now it appears that sleep itself plays a major role in neck pain. In a study at the Harvard Medical School, researchers compared musculoskeletal pain in more than 4,000 healthy volunteers with and without sleeping problems, including difficulty falling asleep, trouble staying asleep, waking prematurely in the morning, and nonrestorative sleep. The result: People who reported moderate to severe difficulty in at least three of those four categories were significantly more likely to develop chronic pain during the yearlong study than those who reported little or no trouble in the snooze department.

Head Chronic Headaches Off at the Pass!

➡ Anything from a skipped meal or a stressful day at work to a sudden change in the weather can make your head hurt. But if the same trigger starts the nasty throbbing time and time again, it's all but guaranteed that the problem is in your genes. According to headache specialists, about 90 percent of people who get chronic cluster headaches have a family history of them. Fortunately, although you can't do anything to change that, there is plenty you can do to ease your torment.

1 in 6
Americans **suffers** from **chronic headaches**.

6 Typical Headache Triggers

The vast majority of headaches—both chronic and occasional—are brought on by stress or nervous tension. So before you start popping pain relievers or searching for crazy remedies, try to pinpoint the reason your head hurts. That should help you find the most effective solution. Ponder the past 24 hours, and ask yourself these questions:

1. Did I get a good night's sleep?

2. Have I eaten well?

3. Have I had a bowel movement?

4. Am I facing a pressing work deadline?

5. Have there been changes or unusual events (for better or worse) at home or work?

6. Is there something I'm dreading (like dental work or a job interview)?

90% of **chronic headache** cases are **genetic** in origin.

The Crazy Coffee Connection

An overload of caffeine can cause a headache—but so can abruptly swearing off the stuff. For those of you who routinely drink four to six cups of coffee a day, and then suddenly stop, it's all but guaranteed that your head will hurt like the dickens. So if you want to break the coffee habit, reduce your intake gradually over a month or so.

3 Common Headache Beliefs Busted

Belief #1: Pollen allergies cause headaches.
FACT: Not so. Your allergy may clog your sinuses, leading to head pain, but the pollen itself is not the culprit. Therefore, any allergy medication you're taking will not relieve the ache in your head. You need to treat the two conditions separately.

Belief #2: Food sensitivities cause chronic headaches.
FACT: Sometimes yes, but more often not. According to specialists in the field, food affects only one in three chronic-headache sufferers. Very often, people mistake a food allergy for a highly common pain trigger: low blood sugar. To solve that problem, eat at least three meals a day, every day, to keep your blood glucose levels stable.

Belief #3: If you have a chronic headache, there's a good chance that you have a brain tumor.

CALL 911

If a severe headache comes on suddenly—especially if you're over age 50—or if you also lose consciousness, your speech becomes slurred, or you experience partial paralysis, nausea, vomiting, and/or a fever, get help *immediately*! You may have a suffered a stroke or have a potentially deadly aneurysm or brain tumor.

(continued on page 193)

10 Zany Ways to Cure a Headache

Over the years, folks have come up with more headache remedies than you can shake an aspirin bottle at. Here's an assortment of the weirdest—and, surprisingly, most effective:

1. Soak for 20 to 30 minutes in a steamy hot (but not burning!) bath while holding an ice pack on your head. The combination of heat and cold will ease the pain by drawing blood away from your head and narrowing the blood vessels in your scalp.

2. Tape a fresh mint leaf on the part of your head that hurts the most, and keep it there until you feel relief.

3. Stick your tongue out about ½ inch, and bite down on it as hard as possible without hurting yourself. Hold the position for 10 minutes—no less and no more.

4. Soak a large white cloth in vinegar, wring it out, and tie it tightly around your head. Keep it in place until the pain is gone.

5. Slice a fresh lime in half, and slowly but firmly rub a cut side on the site of the ache. The pain should vanish pronto.

6. Stand up straight with your arms hanging loosely at your sides. Then swing your arms back and forth in unison (not staggered). The motion will direct blood flow away from your aching head to your hands, thus easing the pain.

7. Quickly drink two glasses of Gatorade® or a similar sports drink, one after the other. You'll put your electrolytes back in balance and stop the throbbing in its tracks.

8. Stuff two tennis balls into a sock. Then lie on your back and wedge the sock behind your neck with one ball on each side. They'll relax your neck muscles and chase away the pain-causing tension.

9. Hold a pencil in your mouth sideways, without biting down. Your jaw muscles will automatically relax, thereby relieving one of the most common causes of tension headaches: strain on the muscles that connect your jaw to your temples.

10. Guzzle a glass or two of water. Dehydration is a leading cause of headaches. If that's what triggered your pain, it should vanish in a flash. Then be sure to stay hydrated throughout the day, to avoid a relapse.

FACT: Not by a long shot. Only very rarely does a headache—no matter how agonizing or long-lived—signify a brain tumor. That being said, your pulsing pain could indicate any number of other serious conditions, so play it safe and see your doctor.

A Simple Solution for High-Tech Headaches

It should come as no surprise that one of the most common causes of headaches is staring at a computer for hours on end. The easy good-riddance routine: Leave your desk every half hour or so, or at least shift your eyes away from the screen and focus them on a point as far away as possible. That should nix your noggin pain for good!

Move On from Migraine

If you're among the millions of Americans who suffer from migraines, you know the upheaval and turmoil these often days-long episodes can cause in your life. But before we move on to some helpful hints on how to conquer, or at least coexist, with the enemy in your brain, you might take some comfort in this piece of historical trivia: Lewis Carroll, Charles Darwin, Thomas Jefferson, Robert E. Lee, and Vincent van Gogh (to name just a handful of famous folks) battled severe migraines throughout their lives, but they still managed to accomplish a thing or two along the way.

Misleading Migraine Lore

More than 37 million Americans suffer from migraines. But as common as the condition is, it remains a mystery to a lot of folks—

Painkillers Can Bite Back

Jaw-Dropping DISCOVERY

If you routinely take either OTC or prescription medications of any kind to treat chronic headaches, don't be surprised if your pain returns with a vengeance. Scientists don't know exactly why these so-called rebound headaches occur, but most likely it's because repeated use of the drugs changes the way certain pain pathways and receptors work in your brain. Anything from simple aspirin, Tylenol®, and Excedrin® to potent narcotics can cause problems. Taken in the prescribed amounts every now and then, the meds are generally safe and effective, but if you reach for them too often, or exceed the normal dosage, you could find yourself with a low-grade headache that just won't say uncle.

including many doctors. Here are a few of the misconceptions floating around out there:

Misunderstanding #1: A migraine is just a bad headache.

THE TRUTH: Migraine is a neurological disease characterized by flare-ups that may not even include a headache. In fact, for an accurate diagnosis of a migraine attack, there must be symptoms other than headache.

Misunderstanding #2: Only women get migraines.

THE TRUTH: The disease is most prevalent in women, but it can attack anyone of any age.

Misunderstanding #3: Migraines are not life-threatening, just annoying.

THE TRUTH: Although the attack itself may not be life-threatening, associated complications and risk factors can be. For instance, studies have shown a link between migraine and cardiovascular diseases, including stroke. Other research has confirmed a strong connection between migraine and suicide, even when major depression is not present.

More than **37 million** Americans **suffer** from **migraines**.

YIKES! Believe it or not, there is no specific medical test for migraine. To ensure an accurate diagnosis, you must track your own symptoms and confer with a doctor who is an expert in migraine treatment (see "3 Keys to Coexisting with Migraines," at right). What's more, several migraine symptoms mimic those of other illnesses. So if you experience a pain or an odd sensation that you've never felt before, hightail it to the ER!

6 Sinister Signs of Migraine

Unlike your garden-variety headache, a migraine attack presents an agonizing assortment of symptoms. They may include any or all of these:

1. Throbbing, pulsating pain on one side of the head

2. Light sensitivity

3. Sound sensitivity

4. Nausea

5. Vomiting

6. Blurred vision

The Awful Aura

More than a third of migraine attacks begin with an *aura*. No, not the kind where you can predict the future or see into other realms. This aura could be a show of lights or spots dancing before your eyes, or suddenly feeling cold, even when you're in a warm room. These are some other common opening acts:

- Abrupt, unexplained mood change
- Food craving
- Frequent yawning
- Sudden burst of energy
- Tingling sensation in your body

3 Keys to Coexisting with Migraines

There is no cure for migraine, but you can take charge of your treatment. Here's how:

1. Write all about it. Record all the circumstances surrounding each attack, including your sleeping patterns, activities, mood, and everything you've eaten.

2. Team up with the right doctor. Not all neurologists are migraine specialists. And not all migraine specialists are neurologists. Find a doc who understands the condition and will work with you to formulate one or more treatments that work best for you.

3. Speak up. Tell the doctor everything about your symptoms and how they affect your activities. That way, the two of you can come up with a plan to keep your life on a steady course.

Don't Drink to Your Migraine Misery

If you're a fan of draft beer, I have some sorry news for you: Hoisting a pint of your favorite brew might be giving you a monstrous migraine. That's because, like many types of food, beer on tap contains tons of tyramine. So do unpasteurized beers and ales. You wine lovers need to exercise caution, too, because both red and white versions can cause trouble. The tyramine content of vino varies greatly, though, so check with your doctor or fellow migraine sufferers to pinpoint the safest kinds.

To Halt Migraines, Toss the Tyramine

Tyramine is an amino acid that occurs naturally in your body and helps to regulate blood pressure. It's also found in a great many foods.

For most people, that poses no problem, but for many migraine sufferers, it brings on major episodes. To find out whether tyramine is triggering your torment, try eliminating these prime sources from your diet:

Aged cheeses, including blue, Brie, cheddar, Swiss, Parmesan, Gouda, and feta. Cottage and ricotta cheeses are okay.

Aged or processed meats, such as bacon, corned beef, hot dogs, salami, pepperoni, and sausage. Fresh meats and fish are fine as long as they're eaten or frozen within a day of purchase.

Dried fruits and fermented foods, such as sauerkraut, soy sauce, and Asian fish sauces. Fresh, frozen, and canned fruits and vegetables contain little tyramine, but the content in fresh produce increases if it's stored for more than 48 hours.

Homemade yeast breads, sourdough bread, and yeast extracts. All commercially baked breads are safe, as are rice, pasta, and cereals.

5 Far-Fetched Migraine Relievers

A migraine treatment that works like a charm for one person may be a total dud for another. But legions of sufferers have found relief with some mighty kooky-sounding tricks. At the first hint of symptoms, try one of these remedies:

Boil a handful of cabbage leaves until they're soft. When they've cooled to a comfortable temperature, place them on your forehead and the back of your neck, and secure them with bandages. Then relax while the leaves draw out the pain.

Mix a few drops of lavender oil with a dab of moisturizer, and massage it into each temple.

Soak your feet in a basin of warm, ultra-strong black coffee until you feel relief.

Stir ¼ teaspoon of ground ginger into a glass of water, and drink up.

Take 1 tablespoon of raw honey. If you don't feel better within 30 minutes, repeat the dose, and chase it down with three glasses of water.

As many as **85%** of **migraines** are **triggered** by **food**.

Chronic Fatigue Syndrome and Fibromyalgia—All-Over Relief

➡ Not so long ago, these two mysterious but agonizing conditions were considered to be entirely separate disorders. Now, though, the medical community generally views them as essentially two faces of the same coin. While it is possible to have one without the other, most people who suffer from fibromyalgia (FM) are also clobbered with chronic fatigue syndrome (CFS). Hence, the widely used moniker CFS/FM.

An Odious Energy Crisis

The scientific jury is still out on the precise cause, or causes, of CFS/FM. But it most often sets in during or following a long illness or prolonged period of physical or mental stress, when your body uses so much energy that it overloads the generating powers of the hypothalamus. This is the part of your brain that governs the crucial

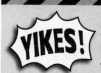

YIKES! Studies have confirmed that Lyme disease can be a trigger for CFS/FM, and the two conditions share some of the same symptoms. If you suspect that you have CFS/FM, get tested for it and Lyme both—even if you don't think you've been targeted by a tick. Because the menaces that spread this and various other infections are so tiny (about the size of a period at the end of a sentence), many people don't even realize they've been bitten. Plus, only 40 to 50 percent of victims develop the infamous bull's-eye rash commonly associated with a Lyme infection.

functions of sleep, blood flow and blood pressure, body temperature, sex drive, mood, hunger, and thirst. This cerebral dynamo regulates the pituitary gland and its production of hormones that control metabolism, energy, and immune function, too. CFS/FM can rear its ugly head in one of two forms:

FM-dominant. Your major symptoms are insomnia and intense muscle pain. At first, it may be intermittent or affect only specific parts of your body, but in most cases the pain expands, and before long, you're aching all over, all the time.

CFS-dominant. In this case, your insomnia is accompanied by debilitating fatigue that just won't go away no matter what you do.

10 Harrowing Hints That You May Have CFS/FM

Regardless of whether your condition leans toward CFS or FM, these are 10 of the most common symptoms:

1. Achiness
2. Brain fog or an inability to concentrate
3. Digestive or bowel disorders
4. Exhaustion following even mild exertion
5. Forgetfulness
6. Increased thirst
7. Low or nonexistent sex drive
8. Recurring infections or chronic low-grade fever
9. Sleep disturbances
10. Weight gain

32 million Americans have **chronic fatigue syndrome/ fibromyalgia**.

Dodge Dr. Denial

Although there is no actual cure for CFS/FM (not yet anyway), it is possible to recover from the debilitating symptoms. The key to success lies in finding a doctor who will work with you to find the most effective treatments—natural, conventional, or (more likely) a combination of both. But be forewarned: While the top players in the medical world now recognize both CFS and FM as real and highly common diseases, most physicians still are not trained in diagnosing and treating them. Some docs will actually tell you that your symptoms are "all in your head" or attribute them to a hard-charging, overachieving lifestyle. So take the time to seek out a practitioner who is keeping up with all the cutting-edge research and will help you tap into the latest and greatest. Several online sources provide searchable databases to get you started. Look for "CFS/FM trained physicians."

Your Fabulous 5-Point Action Plan

Natural health pros who specialize in treating CFS/FM recommend a five-part regimen to conquer the malevolent miseries:

Part 1. Treat any underlying infections you may have.

Part 2. Get your hormones back in balance.

Part 3. Work to restore healthy sleep patterns.

Part 4. Correct nutritional deficiencies that contribute to the problem.

Part 5. Begin getting regular exercise—but very gradually.

While it is crucial to carry out this strategy under expert medical direction, there are plenty of effective changes you can make in your daily routine to help get the parade under way.

Wake Up and Smell the Rosemary!

Jaw-Dropping DISCOVERY

When your energy flags and your brain begins to fog over, don't reach for a jolt of java—reach for rosemary instead. According to studies conducted by the Smell & Taste Treatment and Research Foundation, the herb's pungent aroma triggers the trigeminal nerve, which jump-starts beta brain waves that boost your alertness and concentration. You can put this "scentsational" power to work in one of two ways: Either set a potted rosemary plant on your desk and rub its leaves to help you focus on the task at hand, or dab rosemary oil on the pages of a report or other paperwork that you need to absorb.

The Gluten-as-Gremlin Theory

The theory: Swearing off gluten will cure your CFS/FM.

The reality: Maybe it will, and maybe it won't. Some sufferers have reported remarkable results when they eliminated gluten from their diets, while other folks have found it made no difference in their condition whatsoever. Experts speculate that if going cold turkey on the Big G is effective, it's usually because the patient has undiagnosed celiac disease or a gluten sensitivity, both of which can mimic or intensify the symptoms of CFS/FM.

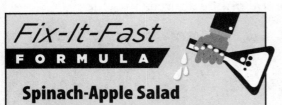

Fix-It-Fast FORMULA

Spinach-Apple Salad

The synergistic combo of spinach and apples helps ease your pain and delivers a delicious jolt to your inner engine. This recipe makes four servings.

2 apples, cored and diced

4 tbsp. of freshly squeezed lemon juice

3 tbsp. of extra virgin olive oil

2 tbsp. of raw honey

1 tbsp. of unprocessed apple cider vinegar

Salt and pepper to taste

8 cups of baby spinach leaves, washed

2/3 cup of crumbled goat cheese

1/2 cup of walnuts

Toss the apples with 2 tablespoons of the lemon juice. Whisk the remaining juice with the olive oil, honey, and vinegar, and season with the salt and pepper if desired. Combine the spinach, apples, and dressing, and divide among four bowls. Top with the cheese and nuts, and dig in!

The bottom line: If you want to try it, by all means, go ahead—but don't expect miracles.

5 Dietary Dynamos

A great many CFS/FM sufferers see one of the most horrifying results of the disease on their bathroom scales: weight gain of 30 pounds or more. But, as distressing as that baggage may be, specialists advise patients *not* to launch any weight-loss efforts until other symptoms are under control. Instead, you should focus on filling your plate with nutrients that can help put your system back on track—namely, this heroic handful:

The B vitamins. The whole clan helps improve your energy, immune function, and mental sharpness, but B_1 (a.k.a. thiamine) and B_{12} are especially important in that regard. Seafood, beef, lamb, and yogurt contain big supplies of B_{12}. Wheat germ, rice bran, peanuts, pecans, and walnuts are all excellent sources of B_1. **NOTE:** *Too much thiamine can cause nerve damage, so steer clear of high-dose supplements.*

Calcium. If you're plagued by nighttime muscle cramps that prevent you from sleeping deeply, you are most likely deficient in this important mineral. The simple solution: Keep milk in your fridge, and guzzle a glass of it every day.

Magnesium. It's a must for boosting your energy and relieving muscle pain. Prime sources include avocados, cornmeal, dried beans, lentils, spinach, and other leafy greens.

Malic acid. It jump-starts the production of adenosine tri-phosphate (ATP), your body's energy-storage molecules, and it's most effective when you team it up with magnesium. Apples are the most abundant source of malic acid, but it's also found in tomatoes and most fruits, including apricots, berries, mangoes, pineapple, and watermelon.

Vitamin C. Citrus fruits and C-rich vegetables, such as broccoli and red peppers, spur your body's production of glutathione, a powerful antioxidant that CFS/FM drains from your system. Doctors often prescribe glutathione supplements, but studies question its ability to work effectively on its own.

Rock Your Pain Away

Way back when, you went softly off to dreamland in your mama's arms as she gently "drove" the family rocking chair. Well, now that you're all grown up and battling CFS/FM, that old rocker can produce the opposite effect on your dormant muscles, waking you up instead of putting you to sleep. That's because the easy back-and-forth motion moves the fluid in your middle ear, which, in turn, stimulates the nerves in your muscles that clear out accumulated waste products. The result is a boost in energy that provides a soothing spring-board to more vigorous activities, such as walking, bicycling, and swimming.

Rout Gout Out!

➡ The prevalence of gout in the United States has more than doubled over the past 20 years. And, in fact, its meteoric rise exactly parallels the dramatic increase in obesity over that same time period. (Are you beginning to see a lethal lifestyle pattern here, folks?)

5 Curious Causes of Gout

This painful and sometimes debilitating condition results from excess uric acid in the joints. But what causes the buildup? Frequently, it's an overload of purines, which are compounds found in many fatty foods, such as anchovies, organ meats, sardines, and (attention, heavy beer drinkers!) yeast. But this handful of triggers can also launch a gout attack:

1. Crash dieting

2. Dehydration

3. Excessive use of aspirin, cyclosporine, diuretics, and levodopa

4. Injury to a joint

5. Stress

Too Much of a Good Thing Can Hurt Bad

Vitamin B_3 (a.k.a. niacin) is an absolute must for good health. In addition to being one of your body's major energy sources and a key player in metabolic processes, niacin may help prevent heart problems and Alzheimer's disease. But a steady oversupply of this nutritional hero can give you gout—big-time—along with even more serious problems, such as liver damage. So do yourself a favor: Unless your doctor has prescribed supplemental doses to treat high cholesterol or another specific condition, get your daily quota from niacin-rich foods. Avocados, eggs, legumes, milk, and whole grains are all good sources. That way, there's no chance of an overdose.

The Myth of Male Victimhood

The common assumption is that men are far more likely than women to suffer from gout. Is it true? Yes and no. Here's the nitty-gritty when it comes to gout:

- During their childbearing years, women are at far lower risk than men, but after menopause, the tables start to turn and the gals become a little more vulnerable.

- After age 60, the disease targets both genders equally.

- Beyond age 80, women are actually more gout-prone than men.

Gout Reality Check: The Bad and the Good

First the bad news:

- There is no cure for gout.

- The condition can run in families (about 20 percent of cases are hereditary).

- About 62 percent of people who have a gout attack for the first time will suffer a repeat performance within a year, and 95 percent will be clobbered again within five years.

Now the good news:

- Contrary to rumors you may have heard, gout is not contagious.

- It does not spread from one joint to another.

- Even if your genes predispose you to gout, there is plenty you can do to help prevent trouble (see "3 Startling Ways to Bar the Gate on Gout," below).

Obesity quadruples your **risk** of developing **gout**.

3 Startling Ways to Bar the Gate on Gout

Just because you have a family history of gout doesn't guarantee that you'll get it—but it does mean that you'd danged well better take some commonsense precautions to head off trouble and woe. Here's your three-point to-do list:

Control your weight. In addition to all the other health hazards of weighing more than you should, hauling around those extra pounds makes you a prime candidate for gout. And the more excess baggage you pack, the more likely you are to be "elected." Numerous studies show that achieving the obesity category quadruples your risk of developing gout.

Exercise with caution. Although regular exercise is a must for good health, if you're at high risk for gout or already have it, you need to choose physical activities with care. For example, running and jogging can easily put enough strain on your joints to spur an attack. And any kind of strenuous exercise carries the potential for dehydration, which increases the concentration of uric acid in your blood. So play it safe: Opt for a milder pastime, such as walking, swimming, or biking, and always have water with you when you exercise.

Watch your diet. Even if the scales show exactly the right numbers, beware of overeating. If you're predisposed to gout, shoveling in too much food at once—especially the kinds that are high in purines—can easily launch an attack.

---

2 Freaky Fruity Gout Fighters

As strange as it may seem, a couple of delicious—and all-around healthy—fruits rank among the most effective remedies for gout. Studies have proven that compounds in the fruits neutralize the uric acid that's causing the misery in your joints. Here's how to put the dynamic duo to work:

Cherries. Either drink a cup or two (or more) of 100 percent cherry juice each day, eat 4 ounces of cherries a day (preferably fresh, but canned or frozen versions will also work), or take 1 tablespoon of cherry juice concentrate (available in health-food stores) three times a day.

Strawberries. For three or four days, eat almost nothing but strawberries. That's all there is to it. None other than the 18th-century botanist Carl Linnaeus, who devised our modern plant-classification system, came up with this "strawberry fast" solution.

Menacing Maladies

Short of moving into a single-occupancy cave at the North Pole, there is no way any of us can avoid infectious diseases altogether. But there is plenty we can do to reduce the number we fall victim to—and to lessen the severity of any that strike. And it's well worth making such an effort a top priority because in all their varied, um, glory, infectious diseases are the third-leading cause of death in America.

Bronchitis—Open Your Airways

➡ There's no mistaking a case of acute bronchitis. You have a cough that comes in one of two forms: tickling with no phlegm coming up (what doctors call "unproductive"), or deep and rumbling like a seal's bark, accompanied by gobs of mucus that may be clear, white, or yellowish gray. In either case, your muscles ache from nonstop hacking, you have a runny nose and a slight fever, and your voice sounds like a bullfrog croaking in a swamp.

The Surprising Cause of Your Cough

Acute bronchitis is a temporary inflammation of the mucous membranes of the bronchi, the main, branching airways of your lungs. These irritated passages swell and produce excess mucus, which your body attempts to clear by coughing. Contrary to previous assumptions, only a tiny percentage of bronchitis cases are caused by bacteria. The vast majority are brought on by the same viruses that cause head colds

CALL 911

In most cases, acute bronchitis responds just fine to gentle DIY treatments, but you should get medical help *immediately* in any of these instances:

▶ Your coughing continues for longer than six weeks.

▶ Your breath has a rattling sound.

▶ You wake up sweating during the night.

▶ The mucus you're coughing up turns thicker, yellow, darker green, or bloody.

▶ You become breathless or you're running a fever that's above 101°F.

You could have pneumonia or asthma, both of which demand urgent attention.

and flu, which means they do not respond at all to antibiotics. Fortunately, there are hordes of gentle, natural remedies that can send your misery into your unpleasant-memory bank. What's more, in the highly unlikely event that a type of bacteria has bashed your bronchial tubes, those same easy-does-it fixes can often send it packin', if you act quickly. At the very least, they'll make you a lot more comfortable while your doctor-prescribed meds are doing the heavy lifting.

Almost **100%** of acute **bronchitis** is **caused** by **viruses**.

An Alarming Airborne Assault

In addition to viruses and bacteria, pollen and other allergens can irritate and inflame your air passages enough to launch an attack of acute bronchitis. So can the same kinds of environmental pollutants that cause chronic bronchitis (see "Chronic Bronchitis: A Catastrophic Cough," at right). The good news is that, unlike germ-induced bronchitis, this type is not contagious. The bad news is that if the aerial bombardment continues long enough, your condition can make the potentially lethal leap from acute to chronic. Your two-part mission: Treat your symptoms using the remedies in this section, and do whatever you can to put as much distance as possible between you and your "attackers." And if you smoke, stop *NOW*!

Trouble Ahead: Keep Your Airways Clear

If you're prone to bronchitis, during either the allergy season or the winter months, this potent syrup is just what the doctor ordered. Mix up a batch or two, and keep it close at hand. Here's what to do: Put 6 tablespoons of raw honey (locally produced if at all possible) in a clean bottle, and add 3 drops of anise oil and 3 drops of fennel oil (both available in health-food stores, herbal-supply stores, and online). Cap the bottle tightly, and store it at room temperature. Take 1 teaspoon whenever you start to feel the wheezing coming on.

Clear Out with Chicken Soup

Chicken soup is renowned for its ability to fight off viruses of all kinds, including the ones that cause bronchitis. It also makes your cough more productive, which means that you can bring up and clear out the mucus that's clogging your lungs. But here's something you may not know: Simply inhaling the steam from chicken soup as it rises from your bowl, or from a pot on the stove, will help open both your nasal and bronchial passages, so you can start breathing easier. If you don't have the time or energy to make a big pot of homemade chicken soup, don't fret—for this purpose, the canned version will do just fine.

2 Potent Production-Promoting Teas

When your hacking fits fail to bring up any mucus, a couple of herbal tea blends can come to your aid by expanding your airways so the phlegm can flow. These two combos are both top-rate bronchodilators:

- Aniseed, coltsfoot, marshmallow root, and mullein
- English plantain, fennel seed, and thyme

Combine equal parts of whichever dried herbs you prefer, and keep the mixture in an airtight container away from heat and light. To make the tea, put 2 teaspoons of the blend into 1 cup of just-boiled water, cover, and let it steep for 10 minutes. Drink a cup four times a day, and your production rate should soar.

NOTE: *All the herbs are available in health-food stores, herbal-supply stores, and online.*

Chronic Bronchitis: A Catastrophic Cough

Unlike acute bronchitis, the chronic form is not contagious. Nor is it curable. It is a condition that occurs when the lining of your bronchial tubes becomes permanently inflamed and thickened. While chronic bronchitis may appear on its own, most often it teams up with emphysema in a horror called chronic obstructive pulmonary disease (COPD), which is the third-leading cause of death in the United States (see "The Cruelest Killer" on page 8). If you've been coughing for more than three months—especially when you get up in the morning—chances are that chronic bronchitis has struck. Smoking is by far the leading cause of this and other forms of COPD, but repeated or prolonged exposure to secondhand smoke or other lung irritants can also bring it on. These are some of the prime culprits:

Dust from substances like coal or grain

Fumes from chemicals such as ammonia, bromine, chlorine, strong acids, and even some organic solvents

Toxic gases such as nitrogen dioxide, ozone, and sulfur dioxide

A Curative Bedtime Cough Buster

Nothing is more crucial than sound sleep for booting bronchitis. But it's hard to get your much-needed z's if, like many folks, you launch into a convulsive coughing spell shortly after you hit the sack. This trick should help: Dilute a few drops of peppermint oil in a tablespoon or so of olive oil, and rub the mixture onto your thymus area (just below where your collarbones meet). Cover it with a cold washcloth, and top that with a dry towel. It'll cool and soothe the inflamed bronchioles that tickle your bronchi and trigger your cough. If the washcloth warms up and you start coughing again before you fall asleep, just wave the cloth in the air to cool it down, and put it back in place.

Fix-It-Fast FORMULA

Bronchitis-Bashing Bath Blend

No matter what has triggered the torment in your chest, a tub of steaming water laced with this marvelous mixture can put you on the high road to recovery.

1 cup of Epsom salts

2 drops of eucalyptus oil*

2 drops of rosemary oil

2 drops of thyme oil

Pour all of the ingredients into your bathtub as you fill it with hot (but not burning hot!) water. Then settle in, relax, and breathe deeply for 20 minutes or so. The steam will increase the flow of mucus; the molecules from the oils will dilate your internal airways, thereby easing your breathing; and the mega-dose of magnesium in the Epsom salts (absorbed through your skin) will relax your stressed-out bronchi. Repeat the process daily, as needed, until your cough has decamped.

* All the oils are available in health-food stores, herbal-supply stores, and online.

3 Quick and Quirky Torment-Tossing Tricks

When you ache all over and you're coughing up a storm, the last thing you want to do is stand in the kitchen mixing up some complex concoction. So don't do it! Instead, reach for one of these double-duty winners. They'll soothe your sore pipes and loosen the mucus with no muss and no fuss—so you can spend essential quality time in bed or your favorite easy chair.

1. Every two hours or so, mix equal parts of orange juice and warm water in a glass, and sip the drink slowly.

2. Fill a Thermos® or insulated pitcher with hot tap water, add a drop or two of either basil or spearmint oil (available in health-food stores, herbal-supply stores, and online), and sip the potion as needed throughout the day.

3. Take 1 teaspoon of anisette liqueur in 1 table-spoon of hot water every three hours.

The Daffy Dairy Delusion

We've all heard the age-old advice that when you have bronchitis or any other kind of chest or head congestion, you should avoid dairy products. Well, forget that! Numerous clinical studies, including one published in *The Journal of the American College of Nutrition*, have shown that milk and other cow-derived delights do *not* increase the amount of mucus produced by your respiratory system. In fact, docs in the know now advise their patients to go ahead and guzzle milk, and especially to gobble that formerly forbidden ice cream that feels oh-so-good on your sore throat. Besides easing your pain, it can provide essential calories that you may be missing if your appetite for "real" food has gone AWOL.

Just one note: It is true that milk products can make any mucus that's already in your throat a little thicker and more difficult to swallow (which may be the source of the old wives' tale), but chasing the moo juice with water should solve that problem in a flash.

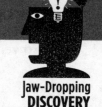

Jaw-Dropping DISCOVERY

You're Getting Drugs You Don't Need

At least there's a good chance that you will get them if you see your doctor for acute bronchitis. In a recent study, researchers at Harvard Medical School found that docs prescribed antibiotics to 73 percent of patients who paid visits for that condition. According to the scientists, the figure should have been virtually zero—for the simple fact that antibiotics are effective only against bacteria, and we now know that acute bronchitis is nearly always caused by viruses. These findings should put a firm "No, thank you!" into your medical vocabulary for two reasons:

1. When you request, and your doctor prescribes antibiotics for conditions they don't cure, you're begging for adverse drug interactions; allergic reactions; and side effects such as diarrhea, nausea, and yeast infections, with no possible benefit in return.

2. The inappropriate use of antibiotics is driving the creation of drug-resistant bacteria that pose a major public health threat (see "Tuberculosis: A Once and Future Menace" on page 228).

NOTE: *These same dangers apply when you take antibiotics for colds, flu, or any other ailment that's caused by a virus.*

Fabulous Foolproof Food Cures

Onions, garlic, and hot peppers all have astounding lung-clearing prowess, so eat 'em by the bucketful in any way that suits your fancy. Also include heaping helpings of these condiments and spices in your meals and snacks:

An acute **bronchial cough** can **last** up to **1 month**.

- Cinnamon
- Ginger
- Horseradish
- Mustard
- Pepper (red and black)
- Turmeric (the prime ingredient in curry powder)

All of these edibles contain compounds that either fight your vexing viruses or loosen and help clear out your misery-making mucus—or, in some cases, do both.

Make Flu Flee!

Every year, the influenza virus sends more than 200,000 Americans to the hospital and (depending on the strain of the year) kills up to 49,000 folks, most of them over age 65. And, ironically, although we're told over and over again to get an annual flu shot, statistics show that the effectiveness of the vaccine varies greatly from one flu season to the next—in some years protecting as few as 9 percent of inoculated seniors. Don't get me wrong, folks! I'm not advising you to shun your shot! But it does pay to have additional tricks up your sleeve.

5 Fundamental Flu Facts

Despite the fact that flu season comes around like clockwork every year, there are a lot of misconceptions floating around about its modus operandi. So let's set the record straight:

1. After you've been exposed to the flu, it can take anywhere from one to four days for the virus to take hold in your system.

2. You are contagious from the day before symptoms appear until five to ten days after your illness begins.

3. In most cases, the virus vacates your body after three to seven days, although a cough and fatigue may linger for two weeks or more.

4. Germs generally circulate most vigorously in January and February.

5. The most likely victims are people over age 65; those with a chronic health condition such as asthma, cardiovascular disease, or diabetes; and (yep—yet again) anyone who is obese.

Don't Blame It on the Weather

You hear it every March, when the numbers on the thermometer are bouncing up and down like a rubber ball: "Oh, these danged temperature fluctuations are making us all sick!" Well, according to medical science, no one—but no one—catches the flu (or even a cold) because of changes in the weather. In fact, although flu season typically extends into March, when temps are at the peak of their roller-coaster ride, you're a lot more susceptible to flu viruses in the dark, frigid depths of winter for two reasons:

1. Viruses circulate faster in cold, dry air.

2. You're spending more time indoors, in close proximity to infected people who can share their germs with you.

Every year, the Centers for Disease Control and Prevention (CDC) urges all of us to rush out and get a flu shot. Yet stats show that fewer than 50 percent of the adult population heeds that advice. Some of those needle dodgers are afraid that the vaccine may actually give them the flu (it won't), or they simply can't face the prospect of getting jabbed. Other folks (procrastinators by nature) simply put it off until it's too late to bother. Regardless of whether you fall into the "yea" or "nay" group, here are a few factoids that you may not know:

▶ The success rate—that is, the likelihood that the shot will protect you—varies wildly from year to year. At best (according to CDC statistics), the vaccine has been shown to be 67 percent effective in preventing the flu.

▶ The shot is much less effective for people age 65 and over, or for anyone who has a chronic health condition. In some years, the prevention rate is in single digits.

▶ After you've been vaccinated, it takes about two weeks for your system to develop antibodies against the flu.

The Loathsome Lives of Germs

We all know that you can pick up flu and cold viruses from touching a germ-laden surface or (more often) shaking hands with an infected person and then touching your nose or mouth. But how long do those disease-spreading organisms lie in wait for you? There's no way of knowing for sure. Studies have shown that, depending upon the particular strain, flu and cold viruses can survive on surfaces for anywhere from a few minutes to 24 hours. But these two factors also play a role in how long germs remain in attack mode:

The nature of the "dumping ground." In general, germs stay active longer on hard materials such as plastic, metal, and ceramic tile than they do on clothing, upholstery, and other soft surfaces.

Environmental conditions. The higher the temperature and humidity are, the sooner the viruses' firepower will fade away.

Between **5% and 20%** of Americans **get the flu** each year.

Your Workout Could Give You the Flu

And no, not because your fellow joggers or gym mates will share their germs—although that is always a possibility. In this case, the reason is that although moderate exercise is a must for staying in tip-top shape, overly intense exertion can actually suppress your immune system and make you more vulnerable to viruses. This is why long-distance runners often get colds after a race. Of course, what constitutes overexertion depends on your physical condition. A hike that takes every ounce of energy you've got may be a casual stroll for someone else. So before you embark on any exercise program, consult with your doctor to gauge your overall fitness level.

Deadly Doorknobs and Lethal Light Switches

Conventional wisdom has it that to protect yourself and your family during cold and flu season you need to wage a constant battle against germs that collect on all the frequently touched surfaces in your home. Is that kind of cleaning frenzy necessary? According to the most recent advice from top-tier doctors, the answer is not really. Although inanimate objects may sometimes transmit flu viruses, their sharing power can't hold a candle to human hands and breath. Still, if you want to disinfect some of the most likely germ catchers in your home and office, here's where to focus your attack:

- Computer keyboards and mouses
- Desks and tables
- Doorknobs and elevator buttons
- Faucets
- Handrails
- TV and video-game remote controls

3 Alarming Reasons to Go Anti-Antibacterial

You see the word *antibacterial* on everything from soaps and hand sanitizers to laundry detergents, shower curtains, and even clothing. Well, do yourself and your fellow humans a big favor and leave those products right on the store shelves. Why? For three reasons:

Congestion = DWI

If you think a head cold is just a nuisance, think again. Recent research shows that driving when you have a cold is just as dangerous as driving when you're drunk. That's because common head cold symptoms reduce your reaction time to the same level as drinking four beers. But that's not all! Consider these findings from a study at Cardiff University in Wales:

▶ A cold or similar minor malady reduces your overall alertness by one-third.

▶ Under-the-weather drivers tend to follow cars more closely than they should *and* take longer to stop.

▶ A single sneeze takes your eyes off the road for up to three seconds. That's long enough to travel more than 300 feet at highway speed or breeze through a stop sign on a local road.

And that doesn't take into account any meds you may be taking that make you drowsy, woozy, or light-headed. So do yourself and your fellow motorists a favor: When you're feeling under par, stay home—or at least have someone else take the wheel.

Jaw-Dropping DISCOVERY

1. This chemical assault on bacteria is performing the same dirty work as the misuse of antibiotics—it's fueling the rise of supergerms that stand up and say "Boo!" to everything medical science can throw at them.

2. Triclosan, the active ingredient in bacteria-killing products, is increasingly being linked to serious health problems, such as hormone disruption and immune system impairment.

3. According to medical pros, soaps and hand sanitizers don't need any antibacterial ingredients. While soap or sanitizer will help remove surface dirt, the simple act of rubbing your hands together for about 20 seconds destroys any germs on your skin.

The Hair-Raising Truth about Hand Sanitizers

True or false? The best way to keep from picking up flu and cold viruses is to clean your "paws" frequently with hand sanitizer.

People age **65 and over** are most likely to **die** from the **flu**.

ABSOLUTELY FALSE! According to the CDC, washing your hands thoroughly with soap and water beats sanitizing 'em hands down. Having said that, a hand sanitizer is a must for those times when you're out and about with no access to soap and water, or when you're traveling by plane, train, car, or bus and need to use (sometimes questionable) public restrooms. But keep these two facts in mind:

- A hand sanitizer will kill flu and cold viruses *only* if the formula consists of at least 65 percent alcohol that has a strength of at least 91 percent. So forget any so-called "gentle" or "natural" brands that actually boast about being alcohol-free.

- Most commercial hand sanitizers contain chemicals that not only offer zero protection against germs, but may also do more long-term harm than the maladies you're trying to prevent. In particular, steer clear of products whose labels sport any form of the terms *paraben* (for example, methylparaben, propylparaben, and/or butylparaben) and *fragrance* (a.k.a. *parfum*). These substances trigger allergic reactions in many folks and are also being implicated in major health woes, including hormone disruption, diabetes, and cancer.

Tip-Top Techniques for Germ-Free Hands

The way you wash or sanitize your hands can spell the difference between picking up a vexatious virus and sailing through the flu season in fine fettle. Here's the right way to do each job:

Washing. Simply wet your hands, work up a lather, using either bar or liquid soap, and rub vigorously for at least 20 seconds. Be sure to work the lather into the skin around and under your fingernails, between your fingers, and on the backs of your hands. (A good 20-second "timer" is to hum the "Happy Birthday" song twice.) Then rinse with clear water, and dry with a towel or air dryer. If you're using a public restroom, or if other folks in your household are sick, use a paper towel to dry your hands, and use it to turn off the faucets and open the door if it has a doorknob. (Use your elbow to push open a public restroom door.)

Sanitizing. Squirt or pump gel into your palm, then spread it around and rub-a-dub-dub until your skin is completely dry. Again, pay special attention to the areas under and surrounding your nails.

Breaking News: Alkalinity Axes Germs!

Old-timers knew a secret that the modern medical community has only recently rediscovered: Your body is best able to fend off health woes of all kinds, including infectious diseases, when your system is highly alkaline. Back in the 1920s, before fancy meds arrived on the scene, doctors routinely prescribed a solution of ½ teaspoon of baking soda mixed in a glass of cool water for patients who had come down with colds and flu (known in those days as the grippe). It works every bit as well today if you follow this schedule:

Day 1. Take six doses of the drink at roughly two-hour intervals.

Fix-It-Fast FORMULA

Heavenly Homemade Hand Sanitizer

This highly portable hand cleaner will demolish flu and cold viruses on contact—with none of the potentially dangerous chemicals found in most commercial brands.

¾ **cup of rubbing alcohol (at least 91% strength)**

⅜ **cup of pure aloe vera gel**

5 drops of cinnamon oil*

5 drops of sweet orange oil*

Pour all of the ingredients into a blender or food processor, and run it on high for a minute or two. (Don't worry: A thorough washing will remove all traces of alcohol and aloe.) Transfer the mixture to small spray or pump-top bottles, and carry them with you to use as you would any other hand sanitizer. The blend will keep at room temperature for at least six months.

* Or substitute 5 drops of one or a combination of your favorite oils. Lavender, lemon, peppermint, rosemary, and tea tree are all excellent germ-fighting choices. All the oils are available in health-food stores, herbal-supply stores, and online.

Berry Good Flu-Prevention Syrup

Generations of folks have fended off flu germs with this highly effective—and delicious—syrup. It's so tasty, you might want to take your daily dose on ice cream or pancakes!

⅔ cup of dried elderberries*

2 tbsp. of ginger (either ground or freshly grated)

1 tsp. of ground cinnamon

½ tsp. of cloves (whole or ground)

3½ cups of water

1 cup of raw honey

Pour the water into a medium-size saucepan, and add the first four ingredients. Bring the water to a boil, then reduce the heat, cover the pan, and simmer until the liquid is reduced by about half (45 to 60 minutes). Remove from the heat, and strain the mixture into a heat-proof glass bowl. Let the liquid cool to room temperature, add the honey, and stir until it is thoroughly blended. Pour the syrup into a 16-ounce glass jar or bottle with a tight-fitting lid, and store it in the refrigerator, where it will keep for several months.

To prevent the flu, take ½ to 1 tablespoon a day. If you already have the flu, take the same dose two or three times a day until you're back in the pink of health.

* Available in health-food stores, herbal-supply stores, and online.

Day 2. Take four doses at roughly two-hour intervals.

Day 3. Take one dose each morning and evening.

Thereafter, drink a glass of the solution each morning until your symptoms are gone.

CAUTION: *Baking soda has a very high sodium content. So if you're on a low-sodium diet, or you're over age 60, consult your doctor before using this or any other oral remedy that contains baking soda.*

Let's Ear It for Flu Prevention

This flu-evasion technique may sound kooky, but folks who've tried it swear it's kept them fit as fiddles even during the fiercest flu seasons. The routine: The minute you feel the first sign of symptoms, use a small eyedropper to insert four or five drops of 3% hydrogen peroxide into one ear, and keep your head tilted so that it stays in. (It may sting a little, but don't worry—that's normal.) Wait until the bubbling and stinging subside, which may be anywhere from 3 to 10 minutes. Then tip your head to drain the solution onto a tissue, and repeat the procedure with the other ear. It works because, as medical scientists first discovered in the late 1920s, the

(continued on page 218)

Pandemic! Germs Gone Berserk

Pandemics have been with us since the dawn of recorded history, and they will come again. The key to survival is to be prepared. The first step is to understand some basic public health jargon, so you know what you're dealing with:

Outbreak. A disease occurs in greater numbers than expected in a community or region, or during a particular season.

Epidemic. An infectious disease spreads rapidly to a large number of people.

Pandemic. A disease breaks out around the world. HIV/AIDS is one example. Another is the H1N1 (a.k.a. swine flu) pandemic that killed more than 12,000 Americans in 2008–2009. In contrast to the normal seasonal flu, 90 percent of the victims were under age 65.

Your First Line of Defense

Keep your eyes and ears open for alerts from the CDC and your local community's health department. Most likely, local governments will begin quarantine (a.k.a. "social distancing") measures on an as-needed basis, beginning with bans on hospital visitors, escalating to school closures, then curtailment of nonessential services, and (in worst-case scenarios) a moratorium on public gatherings.

Man Your Battle Stations

It's no secret that the best way to avoid getting sick is to stay away from sick people, so—official quarantine or not—be prepared to hunker down at home for the duration. In particular:

• Lay in enough food, cleaning, first-aid, and hygiene supplies, as well as medications (both OTC and prescription versions) to last throughout the quarantine. (For more on prepping, see "The Secret to a Safe and Sane Winter Is . . . " on page 351.)

• Because a severe pandemic could cause disruptions in public utilities, it's wise to plan for power outages. Get a generator or two, along with an emergency radio, battery-powered lanterns, propane heaters, or plenty of extra wood for your fireplace or woodstove.

airborne viruses that cause colds and flu frequently enter your body through the ear canal. As long as you've acted quickly enough, you should be able to kill the germs before they get a toe-, er, ear-hold.

A Startling, Watery Way to Fight the Flu

Drinking a solution of baking soda isn't the only way this old-time healer can speed up your exit from sick bay (see "Breaking News: Alkalinity Axes Germs!" on page 215). Believe it or not, soaking in a hot baking soda bath can also help make your viral vexations vamoose because the health-giving alkali will penetrate your system from the outside. Plus, it's perfectly safe even if you're on a low-sodium diet. Here's the routine: Just before bedtime, fill your bathtub with water that's as hot as you can stand (but not so hot that it burns you!), and mix in ½ to 1 pound of baking soda. Ease your achin' body into the tub, stay there for about 15 minutes, then immediately dry off and hit the sack. How much better you'll feel in the morning will depend on how advanced your symptoms are—but you should feel a whole lot more chipper than you did when you went to bed!

Hepatitis Ain't Hep

➡ So far, science has identified six types of hepatitis virus, tagged with the letters A, B, C, D, E, and G (don't ask me why they skipped F). They all cause inflammation of the liver, although the extent of damage varies greatly from one form of the virus to another. Regardless of type, though—and this is scary, folks—symptoms may take decades to appear. For that reason, the medical community reckons that millions of people are walking around with the potentially deadly virus without even knowing it.

More than **5 million Americans** have **hepatitis**.

6 Sinister Signs That You May Have Hepatitis

While hepatitis viruses vary greatly in their severity—and the likelihood that you'll catch them—they all share the same initial symptoms. Here's what to watch for:

- Fatigue or extreme weakness
- Jaundice (a yellow tinge to your skin or the whites of your eyes)
- Loss of appetite
- Low-grade fever (100°F or less)
- Muscle or joint pain
- Nausea and vomiting

The Appalling ABCs of Hepatitis

By far, the three most common hepatitis viruses—in order of least to most dangerous—are A, B, and C (a.k.a. HAV, HBV, and HCV). Here's what you need to know:

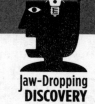

Can Getting "Inked" Get You Dead?

Jaw-Dropping
DISCOVERY

Tattoos are all the rage these days, and so is "tattoo remorse." State-of-the-art laser centers are doing a booming business removing the results of unfortunate snap decisions (or at least making them less noticeable) at great expense to the human "canvases." But there may be a lingering, deadly side effect that even the most expert technicians can't eradicate: the hepatitis C virus. A recent study by the American Association for the Study of Liver Diseases found that people with HCV were about three times more likely to have tattoos than subjects who did not have the disease. The exact nature of the link remains under investigation, but the moral of this story is clear: Think before you ink!

HAV: This is the mildest form. Medical statisticians reckon that each year it strikes about 23,000 Americans—many of whom don't even know they have it. That's because it often shows no outward signs, and when it does, they're often mistaken for the flu. There are no drugs that treat it, but fortunately, the disease generally clears up on its own within a couple of months with no permanent harm done. Nevertheless, if you're headed to an undeveloped country where food safety is dicey, it pays to get the vaccine.

HOW YOU GET IT: The virus is transmitted in three ways:

- Eating food or drinking fluids that have been handled by people infected with the virus or contaminated by fecal matter (for instance, when restaurant workers follow less-than-stellar sanitary practices)
- Eating raw shellfish from contaminated water
- Engaging in sexual or other close physical contact with someone who is infected

HBV: In the vast majority of cases, this is an acute infection that lasts six months or less and clears up on its own. But about 5 percent of those infected develop chronic hepatitis that causes permanent liver damage and sometimes cancer. Fortunately, there are powerful drugs to treat the infection—and better yet—a vaccine to prevent it.

HOW YOU GET IT: The B virus is transmitted in blood and other body fluids, and these factors put you at high risk:

- Having unprotected sex with an infected partner
- Using IV drugs
- Receiving one or more blood transfusions before 1970 (the year that blood banks began testing for the B virus)

HCV: This is the most deadly form, and most often it is diagnosed only after it's caused cancer or other permanent damage to the liver. Potent drugs can treat the infection, but they generally have severe side effects. In advanced cases, a liver transplant is usually the only option. Now for the really bad news: At least so far, there is no vaccine for HCV.

HOW YOU GET IT: The virus is almost always transmitted through infected blood in one of these ways:

- IV drug use with shared needles
- Blood transfusions given before 1992, when screening started for the C virus

- Shared toothbrushes, razors, nail clippers, or other personal gear that's come in contact with infected blood
- Nonsterilized tools used for procedures like electrolysis, manicures, pedicures, tattooing, or piercing of ears or other body parts

---

Fix-It-Fast
FORMULA

Rejuvenating Liver Tonic

This snappy cocktail is a delicious way to help rejuvenate your ailing liver—or to help head off future problems. Plus, whether you have any form of hepatitis, or you simply want to curb your alcohol consumption, it may satisfy your craving for the "hard" stuff.

5 macadamia nuts (unsalted and preferably raw)

3 medium-size, very ripe tomatoes

1 tsp. of freshly grated ginger

½ tsp. of lemon juice

Pinch of cayenne pepper

Tomato juice (if needed)

Put the first five ingredients into a blender, and mix on high speed for about 90 seconds, adding tomato juice as needed to reach the desired consistency. Then pour the potion into a glass and drink to a healthy—or at least healthier—liver.

Hot Tip: Beverages Build a Better Liver

You probably know that your liver is the only organ in your body that is capable of regenerating itself. But what you may not know is that two tasty and all-around healthy drinks can help that job along considerably. What are they? German chamomile tea and tomato juice. Whether you're suffering from hepatitis or any other liver malady, the R$_x$ from natural health experts is simple:

German chamomile tea. Sip three or four cups a day. To make it, pour 1 cup of boiling water over one chamomile tea bag or 1 to 2 teaspoons of dried chamomile (or more if you prefer a stronger brew). Cover the pot or cup to keep the herb's volatile oils from dissipating, and steep for three to five minutes. Remove the tea bag, or strain out the herbs. Add honey or lemon if you like, and drink up. **NOTE:** *Make sure to use German chamomile* (Matricaria recutita), *not Roman* (Chamaemelum nobile).

Tomato juice **regenerates liver** tissue.

Tomato juice. Toss back two or three glasses a day—preferably freshly squeezed, but the organic bottled kind is fine, too. Feel free to add hot sauce if you prefer your potions on the spicy side.

Shingles—Chicken Pox Take 2

➜ If you had chicken pox as a kid, your body is still harboring the herpes zoster virus that caused it—and it could come back to haunt you in the form of shingles. The virus can hibernate for decades in the nerve endings along your spinal cord and near your brain. It wakes up with a vengeance— and I *do* mean vengeance—when your immune system is weakened by factors like illness, stress, or nutritional deficiencies.

Calamitous Collateral Damage

As if the painful, fluid-filled blisters weren't enough, shingles can damage the nerves, resulting in a condition called postherpetic neuralgia (PHN). It most often strikes people over age 50 and causes a deep, burning pain that may linger for weeks, months, or even years, making your life miserable—to put it mildly. The good news is that, in addition to a shingles vaccine (which docs recommend for anyone over age 60), there are powerful antiviral drugs that can get rid of the blister bombardment and help reduce the chance that PHN will set in.

The Creepy Contagious Conundrum

The question of the day: Is shingles contagious?

THE ANSWER: No. However, you can spread the virus to people who have never had chicken pox, but only if they make direct contact with the fluid in your blisters. They will not develop shingles, and they may or may not get chicken pox. But play it safe by following these three common-sense guidelines:

1. Keep your pus-filled sores covered by bandages or clothing, and avoid touching or scratching your rash.

2. Wash your hands frequently to avoid transmitting the fluid that way.

3. Until all your blisters have formed solid crusts, avoid contact with people who have never had either chicken pox or the pox vaccine, as well as anyone with a weakened immune system (for instance, organ transplant recipients or people who are undergoing radiation or chemotherapy, taking steroids, or suffering from HIV).

CALL 911

If pain suddenly erupts on only one side of your body (with or without a rash, which sometimes appears after the onset of pain), get to your doctor or, if necessary, the emergency room ASAP. There's a good chance shingles has struck, and the key to avoiding PHN is to begin antiviral treatment within the first 24 to 72 hours after the onset of symptoms.

1 out of 4 people who've had **chicken pox** gets **shingles**.

Words to the Wise: When to Nix the Needle

Everyone who's had chicken pox should get the shingles vaccine, Zostavax®, right? Wrong! The CDC does recommend the injection for folks age 60 and over—but not if you fall into any of these categories:

- You have an active case of shingles.

- You are allergic to gelatin or the antibiotic neomycin.

- You have a weakened immune system, whether from a disease, poor nutrition, or medications such as steroids.

- You have cancer that affects the lymphatic system or bone marrow, such as lymphoma or leukemia.

- You are undergoing radiation or chemotherapy.

3 Simple Shingles Soothers

Here's some good news: Three of the most effective ways to ease the pain of shingles are also the simplest. Try any or all of these homemade healers and, whichever of these methods you choose, repeat the process as often as possible until your flare-up fades.

Apply a paste. Mix either baking soda, cornstarch, Epsom salts, or ground oatmeal with enough water to make a spreadable paste, and smooth it directly onto your affected skin.

Take a bath. Fill the tub with lukewarm water, and mix in 2 cups of Epsom salts; a cloth pouch filled with uncooked oatmeal; or 10 drops of either chamomile, lavender, or tea tree oil (available in health-food stores, herbal-supply stores, and online). Soak for 15 to 20 minutes, then either pat dry very lightly or (better) let your skin air-dry.

Wipe gently. Lightly dab or coat the painful spots with aloe vera gel, apple cider vinegar, honey, or witch hazel.

Give Shingles Pain the Raspberries

REMARKABLE REMEDY

For thousands of years before anyone knew what shingles was—much less had antiviral meds to treat it—the agonizing skin affliction was making people's lives miserable. This ancient remedy was a boon to befuddled blister battlers. It still can be if you grow raspberries or have friends who do. To make it, put about a cup of raspberry blossoms in a blender or food processor, and blend in enough honey to make a paste. (A tablespoon or so should do the trick, but let your eye be your guide.) Apply it very gently to the afflicted skin. Then, to keep the sticky stuff from getting all over your sheets or furniture, put on loose, clean, all-cotton pajamas or a baggy T-shirt.

NOTE: *It goes without saying (I hope!) that this pain reliever is* not *intended to replace professional medical care.*

The Amazing Amino Acid Gambit

Lysine and arginine are amino acids that perform essential, but different, functions in your body. Extensive research has shown that reducing the level of arginine compared to lysine in your system has an almost miraculous power to heal cold sores, which are caused by the herpes virus. Now, studies indicate that if you up your intake of foods that are high in lysine and avoid high-arginine edibles, your shingles may shove off sooner. Here's the rundown:

Shingles affects **1/2 to 1 million** Americans **each year**.

Foods to favor. Flounder, at 11,000 mg per pound, is far and away the most potent source of lysine. Other types of fish (but not shellfish) also rank high on the L to A scale, as do beef, pork, and poultry. In addition, cheese and other dairy products contain more lysine than arginine.

Foods to avoid. For the duration of your illness, steer clear of nuts, seeds, gelatin, and chocolate in any form. They all contain large amounts of arginine that may contribute to the severity or duration of shingles.

NOTE: *In theory, you can instigate this virus vanishing act by taking lysine tablets, but naturally occurring lysine (especially in steamed flounder) is more readily absorbed by your body. Also, the tablets typically contain large amounts of irrelevant fillers and binders, which means you have to down a whole lot of pills to get the job done.*

Stop Strep Throat Right There!

➡ A sore throat can be caused by anything from a cold or flu virus to cheering too long and too loud for your favorite team. As painful as your throat may be, the problem will generally run its course in a few days. Strep throat, on the other hand, is a different kettle of fish. It's caused by the *Streptococcus* bacteria, and unless it's treated promptly with potent antibiotics, it can lead to kidney damage or rheumatic fever, and potentially fatal heart disease. On the plus side, while you're under a doctor's care, there are plenty of natural remedies that will help relieve your discomfort and speed up your recovery.

10 Steps to a Stronger Immune System

Nothing short of sealing yourself up in a bubble can keep you germ-free. But you can make yourself a less likely target for infectious diseases—and better your chances of making a complete recovery when you do fall sick with anything from a common cold to a strep throat, or even hepatitis. How? By building and maintaining a robust immune system. Here's your to-do list:

1. Stop smoking! Of all the ways to suppress your immune system, smoking tops the list. One example: Smokers get the flu more often—and are more likely to die from it—than nonsmokers are.

2. Toss the toxins. Limit your exposure to polychlorinated biphenyls (PCBs), mercury, chemical pesticides, and secondhand smoke. They can severely compromise your immune system, and may contribute to life-threatening autoimmune diseases (more about that in Chapter 9).

3. Sleep tight. Too little, or poor-quality, sleep impairs overall immune system function and reduces the number of germ-killing cells in your body.

4. De-stress. Chronic stress causes a measurable downturn in your system's ability to fight off or recover from diseases.

5. Get happy. Even mild sadness can weaken your immune system, and the more negative and pessimistic you are, the more likely you are to get sick. Cheerful, optimistic souls have an army of battle-ready, infection-fighting T cells in their bodies.

6. Get a move on. A recent study compared people who took almost-daily brisk walks to folks who were inactive. The nonwalkers took twice as many sick days as their strolling counterparts.

7. Pal around. The more human connections you have, and the more you get out and about, the better you can fight off illnesses.

8. Eat well. Good nutrition strengthens your immune system. Poor food choices are major immunity busters.

9. Yuck it up. Laughter decreases stress hormones and raises your supply of immune-boosting hormones and endorphins.

10. Limit antibiotics. While they are sometimes necessary, they can suppress your immune system and make you more likely to become sick again.

The Untarnished Truth about Strep

As you might expect with a condition as potentially dangerous as strep, some major misunderstandings have arisen about its treatment. So let's set the record straight.

Misconception #1: If your throat is very sore for several days, it's bound to be strep.
THE TRUTH: A full 90 percent of sore throats are caused by viruses, not by the strep bacteria. Still, don't take any chances. If you even suspect that you have the infection, see your doctor for an accurate diagnosis.

90% of **sore throats** are caused by **viruses, not strep**.

Misconception #2: Strep throat is highly contagious, so when you have it, you need to avoid other people.
THE TRUTH: For the first 24 hours after you start taking antibiotics, you can still spread the bacteria to others—so, for heaven's sake, stay home! But after the first day, you can mix and mingle with no worries.

Misconception #3: If you don't stay in bed until you're fully recovered, major complications can set in.
THE TRUTH: As with any malady, getting plenty of rest will help your system kick the infection. And yes, if you feel very sick (as you might for a few days), by all means stay in bed. But once you're on antibiotics, if you feel well, it's fine to resume business as usual.

CALL 911

If your throat pain is severe, and it's accompanied by white spots in your mouth or throat and difficulty swallowing, you have a fever and chills, and you ache all over, see your doctor immediately. There's a good chance that you've been clobbered by the strep bacteria, and the longer you wait to get help, the more likely it is that your discomfort will morph into something a whole lot worse.

The Perplexing Pet Connection

If you have recurring bouts of strep throat, and you have a dog or a cat, your veterinarian may provide the answer to your problem. Just have your pet checked for streptococci. If the diagnosis is positive, once the doc makes your pal free of the bacteria, you should have no more problems—that is, after you've been treated for any current infection. Just one word of warning: When your vet prescribes antibiotics for your pet, use those meds with the same care that you would if they'd been given to you (see "4 Ways to Keep Antibiotics from Killing You," below).

Toss the Toxic Toothbrush

Whenever you're sick, these essential hygiene helpers can collect the trouble-causing bacteria and pass it right back to you. So the minute you start feeling sick, throw out your toothbrush (or the head, if you use a battery-powered brush). Dip the new one in boiling water between uses, and just to play it safe, pitch it once you're back in the pink of health. From then on, follow dentists' standard advice, and replace your brush every three months.

3 Vivacious Vinegar Soothers

Apple cider vinegar (ACV) is one of Mother Nature's most potent sore-throat relievers (whether the pain is caused by strep or a virus). You can put this valiant vanquisher to work in three ways:

Drink it. Mix 1 tablespoon each of ACV and raw honey in 1 cup of warm water, and sip the potion slowly. Repeat as desired once or twice a day.

Gargle it. Mix 2 teaspoons of ACV in 8 ounces of warm water, and proceed as follows: Gargle a mouthful
(continued on page 229)

4 Ways to Keep Antibiotics from Killing You

Antibiotics are an absolute must for treating strep throat and other serious bacterial infections. But when used in an inappropriate fashion, these same miraculous meds that can save your life can also weaken your immune system so much that you succumb to fatal diseases, including drug-resistant forms of tuberculosis. The key to ensuring that antibiotics will work when you really need them is to use them properly. In addition to shunning antibacterial products (see "3 Alarming Reasons to Go Anti-Antibacterial" on page 213), follow these commonsense guidelines:

1. Take antibiotics *only* when they're prescribed by a doctor to treat bacterial infections.

2. Always take the entire R_X—even if you're feeling just fine again before the bottle is empty.

3. Never use antibiotics in the hope of preventing infection.

4. Don't share your meds with anyone else, and don't save antibiotics, no matter how you might have come by them.

Tuberculosis: A Once and Future Menace

If you think tuberculosis (TB) is a once-deadly disease that you no longer need worry about, think again. Although there are few active cases in the U.S. (roughly 6 per 100,000 people), you need to know two frightening facts:

1. Thanks in large part to the overuse of antibiotics, some strains of the TB bacteria have become resistant to many of the drugs that were formerly used to treat it. Someone who has a strain that is receptive to antibiotics—and who gets prompt treatment—has an excellent chance of making a full recovery. On the other hand, between 40 and 60 percent of people who get an antibiotic-resistant form of the disease die from it.

2. The bacterium that causes TB (*Mycobacterium tuberculosis*) is highly contagious, and it's spread through the air by coughing, sneezing, and (yes) even speaking or singing. That makes people in close quarters, such as nursing homes, dormitories, airplanes, or even tightly packed offices, especially vulnerable.

But there is good news—TB cannot be contracted by touching germ-laden surfaces or by shaking hands or making other physical contact with infected people.

The Weird Ways and Means of TB

Being exposed to the TB bacterium does not mean that you'll get the disease. If you're basically healthy, the germs will hunker down in your body, where they will cause you no harm and cannot be passed on to anyone else. But, if your immune system has been, or becomes, weakened by age, chronic disease, or any of the other usual suspects (see "10 Steps to a Stronger Immune System" on page 225), the bacterium will begin to multiply and morph into an active—and contagious—disease.

The most obvious symptom is a bad cough that lasts for three weeks or longer and may bring up blood or sputum. You may also experience chest pain, chills, fever, weakness, and night sweats.

If you think you've been exposed to TB, have yourself tested ASAP. Treating the latent form will prevent an active outbreak down the road.

of the solution, and spit it out. Then swallow a mouthful. Keep alternating until the glass is empty. Wait 60 minutes, and go at it again. Continue as needed until you've put your pain out to pasture.

Wear it. Just before bedtime, saturate a soft cotton cloth in a solution made from 2 tablespoons of ACV mixed with ⅔ cup of warm water. Ring out the cloth, put it on your throat, and secure it with a strip of dry gauze or an elastic bandage, and leave it in place overnight. By morning, your throat should feel much better. Repeat as necessary.

Untreated **strep** can lead to **heart failure**.

NOTE: *For this and any other medicinal purpose, always use raw, organic, unfiltered apple cider vinegar (available in health-food stores and in the health-food sections of most super-markets). The clear, filtered kind that's generally found with the salad dressings in the main grocery aisles has been stripped of the enzymes and friendly bacteria that give ACV its miraculous healing power.*

Give Your Pain a Blue Pop

Blueberry juice is one of the most effective sore-throat relievers you can find. And its pain-relieving power is even more potent in frozen form. Simply pour 100 percent blueberry juice (preferably organic) into ice-pop molds, and tuck 'em into the freezer. When the treats are solid, simply bite off small pieces, and let them melt in your mouth. But don't suck on the 'sicle. The sucking action may irritate your throat even more.

NOTE: *If you can't find 100 percent juice in your local supermarket or health-food store, liquefy a couple handfuls of blueberries with a table-spoon or so of water in a juicer, blender, or food processor.*

Mustard Cuts the Mustard

This remedy won't win any awards for good flavor, but it'll put your throat back in the swing of things fast: In a mug, combine 1 table-spoon each of prepared mustard, salt, and honey with the juice of half a lemon. Then pour in ½ cup of boiling water, and mix thor-oughly. When it's cooled to lukewarm, gargle with it two or three times. (But don't swallow it!)

Your Autopilot Gone Awry

CHAPTER 9

The human immune system is a highly sophisticated mechanism. It's naturally programmed to detect any substance that does not belong in your body—and then to whip the daylights out of it. Unfortunately, on occasion, your inner army mistakes your own tissue for a mortal enemy and launches into full battle mode. The result is what medical science calls an autoimmune disease. Like many other horrific illnesses, these self-inflicted disorders are reaching epidemic proportions in the United States and other developed countries. The precise reason is under debate in scientific circles, but the scale of the problem is clear: So far, researchers have identified about 100 different autoimmune diseases, and they suspect that at least 40 more have an autoimmune connection.

The Toxic Battlefield

➲ **Autoimmune disease is not a brand-new phenomenon. There have always been people whose immune systems have turned on themselves for one reason or another, and there is no single factor that makes it happen. The difference today is the ever-escalating number of victims. And more and more experts are pinning that spiraling epidemic on one inescapable bugaboo of modern life: a constant stream of toxins pouring into our bodies from every direction.**

The Freaky Family Connection

While it does appear certain that toxic overload is fueling the phenomenal rise in autoimmune diseases, these disorders have always run in families. But it's a genetic connection with an uncommon twist because related folks are not hardwired for the same particular disease. Rather, they share a tendency for autoimmune problems in general. For example, let's say Mary has inflammatory bowel disease. Her mother might have lupus, while Aunt Martha has celiac disease, cousin Bob has rheumatoid arthritis, and Grandma had psoriasis. The reason? Nobody knows—not yet, anyway.

Human Anatomy 101: A Quick Refresher Course

In the natural scheme of things, the human body operates a continuous exchange process. For example, when you take in food and drink, your system absorbs the nutrients it needs, deposits the material it can't use into your feces and urine, and expels it from your body before it can turn toxic and make you sick. For thousands of years, this mechanism generally ran smoothly because, for the most part, the potential toxins were things like harmless food residue and hormones that had served their purpose and been broken down for disposal. When something did hang around so long that it became dangerous, your trusty immune system would step up to the plate.

Fast Forward . . .

To the post–World War II years, when scientists began cooking up scads of miraculous new chemical formulas that were supposed to make our lives easier, safer, more fun, and (yes) even healthier. Today, more than 80,000 synthetic compounds are floating around in our environment and flowing into our bodies in the air we breathe, the food we eat, and the products we use in our

YIKES! If there is any doubt in your mind how serious the autoimmune epidemic is, consider these factoids from the American Autoimmune Related Diseases Association (AARDA):

▶ The National Institutes of Health (NIH) estimates that 23.5 million Americans suffer from some type of autoimmune disorder. AARDA puts that figure at 50 million and rising. The reason for the difference: The NIH numbers include only the 24 diseases for which detailed epidemiology studies have been performed—not the 80 or more that the white-coated number crunchers have not yet examined with a fine-tooth calculator.

▶ More women suffer from autoimmune diseases than they do from breast cancer and heart disease combined.

▶ The annual direct health-care costs for autoimmune diseases ($100 billion) are second only to those for heart disease and stroke ($200 billion). By comparison, cancer racks up a measly $57 billion in yearly charges.

▶ While medical science has found cures for most infectious and many chronic diseases, so far, there are no cures for autoimmune disorders. Even the most highly skilled doctors can only treat the symptoms, generally using powerful immunosuppressant drugs, which can eventually lead to devastating side effects.

(continued on page 233)

The Internal Battle: The Major Players

A full-scale discussion of the various autoimmune diseases is beyond the scope of this chapter, but coming up, we'll talk about two of the most prevalent: inflammatory bowel disease and psoriasis. And here's a brief overview of other catastrophes that can befall your innards:

Celiac disease occurs when the immune system overreacts to gluten, a protein found in barley, rye, and wheat. The reaction damages tiny, hair-like projections called villi that line your small intestine and prevents them from absorbing the nutrients from the food you eat. The only way to avoid having your vital organs deprived of nourishment is to follow a strict gluten-free diet. (For more on gluten, see "The Great Gluten Rip-Off" on page 69.)

Graves' disease results from an overproduction of thyroid hormones. Left untreated, it can cause problems ranging from glaucoma to heart disease.

Lupus can affect many parts of the body, including your blood cells, brain, heart, lungs, and joints. It can be tricky to diagnose because most of its symptoms mimic those of other ailments.

But there is one distinct sign that appears in many cases of lupus: a facial rash that resembles the wings of a butterfly unfolding across both of the victim's cheeks.

Multiple sclerosis (MS) strikes when the immune system attacks your body's myelin, the protective coating that covers nerves. The resulting damage disrupts communication between your brain and the rest of your body, and may ultimately cause the nerves themselves to deteriorate. The severity of the problem varies greatly, depending on which nerves are affected and the degree of damage. Many victims enjoy long periods of remission between flare-ups. Skilled medical treatment is essential to help manage symptoms, and speed up recovery from attacks.

Sjögren's syndrome (pronounced *show-grins*) frequently accompanies other immune system disorders, such as lupus and rheumatoid arthritis. The initial targets are usually the glands that produce tears and saliva, so the first symptoms are likely to be dry eyes and a dry mouth. But the attack can include your skin, joints, kidneys, and other organs.

homes. Unfortunately, many of those chemicals bear a strong resemblance to hormones and other biochemicals that our systems produce naturally. As you can imagine, this massive onslaught of sort-of-familiar stuff confuses the dickens out of your immune system. And, sometimes, in its eagerness to defend the fort, it mistakes your body's own organs and tissues for foreign invaders, and charges into battle.

Don't Push the Panic Button

We all know people who are so freaked out by our century's colossal chemical overload that they've turned "detoxing" and "green living" into an obsession. They forbid themselves to ever enjoy so much as a bottle of pop or a hot dog at the ballpark. They spend countless hours—and a bundle of bucks—trying to rid their homes of every synthetic chemical and every scrap of plastic. Well, don't do that, friends. For one thing, in this day and age, it's Mission Impossible. (For instance, have you ever tried to find a computer with a wooden cabinet or hand lotion that comes in a glass bottle?) For another, in their own way, fear, anxiety, and stress are every bit as toxic as many of the unnatural nuggets that you're fretting about. Don't get me wrong! I'm not suggesting that you

50 million Americans **suffer** from an **autoimmune disease.**

The Easiest Toxin to Toss

REMARKABLE REMEDY

Natural health gurus tell us that one of the toxins that appears to trigger autoimmune disorders is acid—and the modern American diet (MAD) is chock-full of it. Your simple acid-reduction plan:

▶ Cut back on acidic edibles such as processed foods, red meat, sugar, and other refined carbohydrates, and watch your intake of alcohol and coffee.

▶ Up your intake of alkaline-rich fruits, vegetables, nuts, and seeds.

The healthiest pH balance is slightly on the alkaline side—just a shade above 7 on a scale of 1 to 14 (with 1 being completely acid and 14 being completely alkaline). If you want to see where your system ranks, pick up a supply of Hydrion® paper at your local drugstore, or order it on the Internet, then check your urine or saliva first thing in the morning, before you've had anything to eat or drink. The color of the paper will show your pH level. (Complete instructions and a color chart come with the paper.)

should sit back and pretend that everything's just hunky-dory—far from it! Just use this two-point commonsense strategy:

Step 1. Give the cold shoulder to as much toxic stuff as you can without making a second career out of it. (We covered the waterfront on edibles and their ilk in Part 1; coming up in Part 3, I'll lay out the groundwork for making your home ground—indoors and out—a body-friendlier place.)

Step 2. Stay—or get—in good shape because a healthy body is better able to fend off any kind of trouble that comes its way. Your best plan here is simply to follow the "10 Steps to a Stronger Immune System" on page 225.

13 Clues That Your Immune System Has Gone Haywire

Once autoimmune diseases kick into high gear, their symptoms, and the degree of danger involved, can vary greatly. But in the early stages, they all tend to show similar warning signals. If you experience any of these symptoms—or, especially, a combination of them—see your doctor. And be quick about it. The sooner you get help, the more likely it is that you and your doc will be able to contain the collateral damage.

1. Abdominal pain, diarrhea, or blood or mucus in your stool

2. Blood clots or multiple miscarriages

3. Constant tiredness or fatigue

4. Dry eyes, mouth, or skin; hair loss

75% of people with **autoimmune** diseases are **women**.

5. Insomnia, or trouble getting to sleep

6. Intolerance to heat or cold

7. Muscle tremors or rapid heartbeat

8. Numbness or tingling in hands or feet

9. Pain or weakness in joints or muscles

10. Recurrent hives, rashes; sun sensitivity

11. Trouble concentrating or focusing

12. Unexplained weight gain or loss

13. White patches on your skin or inside your mouth; mouth ulcers

Inflammatory Bowel Disease— Douse the Fire in Your Plumbing

➡ **Inflammatory bowel disease (IBD) occurs when your immune system mistakenly attacks all or part of your digestive tract. There are two major types: Crohn's disease and ulcerative colitis. Both are painful and debilitating— and can lead to life-threatening complications, including colon cancer. Neither condition is curable, but a combination of skilled medical care and savvy lifestyle maneuvers can reduce the frequency of flare-ups, the severity of symptoms, and the likelihood of more serious damage.**

Two of a Terrible Kind

The internal fire known as IBD may occur in one of two forms:

1. Crohn's disease (CD) can affect any part of the gastrointestinal tract, from the mouth to the anus, but most often it strikes the end of the small intestine (the ileum) and the beginning of the large intestine (the colon). The inflammation tends to appear in patches, with healthy bowel tissue in between.

2. Ulcerative colitis (UC) affects only the large intestine. It appears as a continuous sheet of inflammation on the intestinal lining, generally beginning at the anus and reaching into the colon.

IBD does not limit its dirty work to the digestive tract. It can also cause a host of wide-ranging problems—for example, arthritis, kidney stones, gallstones, inflammation of the eyes or skin, and clubbing of fingernails. Over the long haul, it frequently results in osteoporosis and increases the risk for colon cancer.

Felonious Foods

Jaw-Dropping DISCOVERY

More and more studies are fingering food sensitivities as major players in the ugly drama related to IBD. That only stands to reason, given the way your body's digestive process works: When you eat a food to which you're sensitive, your small intestine cannot completely digest it, and your immune system attacks the "villainous" nugget that's left. The collateral damage can manifest in all manner of ugly forms—including the onset of IBD.

N O T E : *Don't confuse digestion-disrupting food sensitivities with classic food allergies—for instance, to peanuts or strawberries—that produce acute symptoms, such as swelling or hives. They're two different matters altogether.*

7 Sobering Signs of Trouble

Only a colonoscopy and biopsy can determine for sure whether you've got IBD and, if so, which kind. If you experience any combination of the following seven symptoms, see your doctor for a firm diagnosis and a referral to a gastroenterologist. And be quick about it because the longer the disease goes untreated, the more likely it is to affect other parts of your body (see "Two of a Terrible Kind" on page 235). These are your calls to action:

- Abdominal pain and cramping
- Constipation and/or diarrhea
- Fever
- Frequent, urgent need to move your bowels
- Nausea
- Rectal bleeding*
- Weight loss

* *If you do not experience rectal bleeding, there is a good chance that you've been clobbered not by IBD, but by the equally painful but far less serious irritable bowel syndrome (see "IBD vs. IBS: The Dramatic Difference," at left).*

IBD ups your likelihood of **bone fractures** by **40%**.

IBD vs. IBS: The Dramatic Difference

Do not confuse inflammatory bowel disease (IBD) with irritable bowel syndrome (IBS). While IBS (a.k.a. spastic colon) can deliver agonizing symptoms, including abdominal pain, bloating, gas, and alternating bouts of constipation and diarrhea, it is not an actual disease—much less one that could threaten your life. Rather, IBS is a digestive problem with diagnosable, treatable causes. These are the most common:

▶ Bacterial, parasitic, or yeast (*Candida albicans*) infection

▶ Celiac disease

▶ Food allergies or sensitivities

▶ Underactive thyroid

Finally, according to both conventional and naturopathic doctors, it appears that (again unlike IBD) IBS can be—and very often is—caused by anxiety. So if intestinal cramps and spasms are getting you down, don't suffer silently. Get medical and, if necessary, psychological help ASAP!

An Inflammatory Fable Bites the Dust

Contrary to popular belief, IBD is not caused by anxiety, stress, or other psychological problems. So far, no one has pinpointed the precise factor that turns your intestines into a battlefield. Some scientists think that an as-yet-unidentified bacterium or virus may be the culprit that sends your immune system into a frenzy. One thing is certain, though: Both anxiety and stress can greatly intensify IBD symptoms, such as abdominal pain and diarrhea, and may increase the frequency of flare-ups.

The Dismaying Diet Dilemma

One of the most common side effects of IBD is malnutrition, for three reasons:

1. The inflammation of your intestinal lining prevents your body from absorbing all the nutrients from the foods you eat.

2. Some of the drugs prescribed to treat IBD can inhibit your ability to absorb specific vitamins and minerals.

3. It's impossible to work up an appetite for anything when you're writhing in the throes of abdominal pain, cramps, and diarrhea.

Which nutrients you need to supplement, and in what quantities, depends on numerous factors, including the frequency of flare-ups, the severity of symp-

Fix-It-Fast FORMULA

Grilled Rainbow-Pepper Salad

One of the most important tools in treating any disease—or fending it off—is the rich array of antioxidants and fiber found in fruits and vegetables. But when you've got IBD, fiber can intensify cramping and diarrhea. The simple solution: Always cook your produce. Roasting, broiling, or grilling helps break down the fiber, making it easier to digest. This colorful, tasty salad is rich in nutrients and easy on your delicate system. The recipe makes four servings, but feel free to multiply the ingredients.

4 medium bell peppers, halved and seeded*

¼ cup of oil-cured black olives, sliced

¼ cup of oil-packed, sun-dried tomatoes, rinsed and chopped

1 tablespoon of balsamic vinegar

1 tablespoon of extra virgin olive oil

⅛ tsp. of salt (optional)

Grill the peppers on medium-high heat, turning once, until they're soft and charred in spots (about five minutes per side). When they're cool enough to handle, chop them into 1-inch squares (give or take), and toss them in a large bowl with the remaining ingredients. Serve the salad with fish, chicken, or grilled burgers.

* For the maximum antioxidant boost, choose a colorful combination of red, orange, and yellow peppers.

toms, the types of medications you're taking, and what foods disagree with you (see "The Myth of the Magic Bullet," below). So don't play guessing games—confer with your doctor and/or a professional nutritionist, who can help formulate the supplement plan that targets your particular circumstances.

The Myth of the Magic Bullet

Regardless of what anyone might tell you, there is no such thing as "the right" diet for someone with IBD. A food that sets off a four-alarm flare-up in one person may be perfectly harmless to someone else. Your best bet: Keep a food diary listing every single thing you eat or drink, and note which ones cause problems, and when. Some may be troublesome only during flare-ups; others may give you discomfort even when you've been symptom-free for months. Common problem foods include anything that's deep-fried, spicy, high-fat, or high in fiber.

Astounding Healing Power—Naturally

When IBD is first diagnosed, or during serious flare-ups, you will probably need to take some mighty powerful drugs. But once the disease is under control, many natural remedies can alleviate your symptoms and help fend off such horrendous complications as colon cancer and osteoporosis—with none of the dangerous side effects the big guns can deliver. So do your body a favor: If your own gastroenterologist is not familiar with alternative therapies, add a highly skilled naturopathic or homeopathic physician to your health-care team so that you can all work together to formulate the best long-term treatment plan for you. To find a superstar teammate near you, check out the American Association of Naturopathic Physicians at www.naturopathic.org or the Homeopathic Academy of Naturopathic Physicians at www.hanp.net.

The Malevolent Moo Juice Mystery

Calcium plays a vital role in any healthy diet, but it's especially important that IBD sufferers keep their bodies well stocked with this bone-building mineral. That's because one of the most common complications of the dastardly disease is osteoporosis. Unfortunately, though, in many folks with IBD, dairy products cause pain, gas, or diarrhea. That's the bad news. The good news is that frequently, those symptoms are triggered not by IBD, but by lactose intolerance. To find out for sure, get yourself tested. If you are lactose intolerant, Lactaid® supplements or Lactaid-branded dairy products can solve the problem lickety-split—at least between flare-ups. Be quick about your detective work because IBD-related bone loss is nothing to take lightly. In fact, studies show that it may raise your risk for spinal and other bone fractures by 40 percent or more.

Psoriasis—The Painful Skin You're In

➜ Psoriasis is a case of your immune system turning a simple bodily function into a speed demon. As we all learned back in high school biology class, our bodies are constantly growing new skin cells and shedding the old ones. Normally, the process occurs in a smooth 28-day cycle, in which new cells gently shove the ones above them to the surface of your skin, where they're sloughed off. But in people with psoriasis, the "assembly line" ramps up its production schedule to such an extent that cells begin to pile up, causing thick, red, scaly patches that are not only unsightly, but also itchy and often excruciatingly painful.

Terrible T Cells

7.5 million Americans **have psoriasis**.

Most scientists pin the blame for psoriasis on a naturally occurring type of white blood cell called T lymphocytes, or T cells. Their job is to cruise through your body in search of alien invaders like viruses and bacteria and to fight them off, thereby healing a wound or preventing infection. No one knows why they sometimes attack healthy skin cells instead of stricken ones, but when they do, bingo—psoriasis erupts. There is no cure, but trouble tends to occur in cycles, with flare-ups lasting for weeks or months, then going into remission for a time. The secret to living with psoriasis without losing your mind is to make those time-outs as long as possible and to find treatments that minimize the discomfort when the T cells go on a rampage.

The Sinister Spillover

As if what an old TV commercial used to call "the heartbreak of psoriasis" weren't enough, having the condition increases your risk

YIKES! In addition to sprouting loathsome lesions from the tops of their heads to the soles of their feet, between 10 percent and 30 percent of psoriasis sufferers (depending on whose statistics you read) are hit with a double-pronged demon: psoriatic arthritis, which causes inflammation in the joints, spine, eyes, lung lining, and even the aorta. Because the two sets of symptoms are so different, doctors treat them separately. In severe cases of psoriatic arthritis, surgery may be necessary.

of developing other autoimmune disorders, including IBD and celiac disease. But that's not all! Psoriasis also raises the odds that you'll contract any number of other serious health problems, including these:

• Cardiovascular disease

• Eye disorders

• High blood pressure

• Kidney disease

• Parkinson's disease

• Type 2 diabetes

And the collateral damage doesn't stop there. The discomfort of psoriasis, coupled with its unattractive appearance, can also lead to health-threatening psychological issues, such as depression, low self-esteem, and social isolation.

The Prime Hit List

While anyone can fall victim to psoriasis, these factors all increase your chances of being clobbered:

Family history. This is the number one risk factor. If one or both of your parents had psoriasis, you're much more vulnerable than someone whose nearest and dearest did not have the problem.

Compromised immune system. You're a more likely target if, for instance, you're undergoing chemotherapy or radiation treatments, you have another autoimmune disease, such as lupus or celiac disease, or you're prone to recurring infections, such as bronchitis or strep throat.

Obesity, smoking, and stress. Yep—this trio again. Any one of these plants you firmly in the red-alert category for developing psoriasis, as well as triggering flare-ups and increasing the severity of symptoms. And when that terrifying triad teams up . . . well, you can guess what that does to your inner workings.

Of course, the good news here is that while you may be stuck with the first two risk factors, when it comes to that last, three-part item on the list, you're in the driver's seat. So get a move on *now*! See Chapters 1 and 5 for some terrific tactics that can help you quit smoking and shed pounds. As for stress, it may be an unavoidable fact of life, but you don't have to let it get the upper hand. In Chapter 2, you'll find a treasure trove of tricks that'll help you lighten your load—and cope in a healthy manner with the stress that you simply can't avoid.

5 Sneaky Psoriasis Starters

While the underlying cause of psoriasis lies within your immune system, a number of factors can launch an attack or make symptoms worse when a flare-up is raging. Here's a handful of triggers to beware of:

Cold, dry weather. On the other hand, sunny skies, hot temps, and high humidity appear to control psoriasis symptoms in many people.

Heavy alcohol consumption. Primarily men are affected; alcohol does not seem to cause problems for women. (I hasten to add, ladies, that I am *not* implying that you should start hitting the bottle to nurse your sore skin!)

Infections. Strep throat and tonsillitis are two examples. On the bright side, flare-ups often calm down once the infection has cleared up.

Skin injuries. These include cuts, bruises, bumps, burns, and bug bites.

Medications. Some drugs are troublesome, such as those used to control

Needles Can Be Nasty

Jaw-Dropping **DISCOVERY**

A kitchen cut or a skeeter bite that would be a minor nuisance for most folks can kick off a major flare-up in a psoriasis sufferer. But it's not only accidental skin invasions that can cause trouble. Needles traumatize your skin, too. So consult with your doctor before you get any shot or undergo acupuncture treatment because the risks may outweigh any benefits. Above all, don't even think of getting a tattoo! The process of repeatedly piercing the skin and injecting it with dyes is highly invasive and likely to launch legions of lesions—although they may not appear until 10 to 14 days after the job is done.

arthritis, heart disease, high blood pressure, malaria, and psychiatric conditions (specifically lithium, which is a common treatment for bipolar disorder).

Aloe Axes Psoriasis

Aloe vera is renowned for its healing powers, and both clinical research and firsthand reports from sufferers ("anecdotal evidence" as it's known in scientific circles) have shown it to be one of the most effective treatments of all for psoriasis. The two-part treatment plan:

- Gently smooth pure aloe vera gel onto your lesions three to five times a day.

- Drink 8 ounces of pure, unsweetened aloe vera juice every day. You can buy it in health-food stores, many supermarkets, and even discount chain stores. Be forewarned, though: This stuff has a bitter taste, so you may want to mix it with your favorite fruit juice. Or whip it up into a smoothie like the Aloe-Blueberry Smoothie (at left).

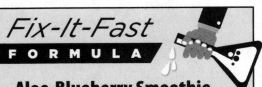

Fix-It-Fast
FORMULA

Aloe-Blueberry Smoothie

This delicious drink combines the potent healing power of aloe with antioxidant-rich fruits to deliver a knockout punch to psoriasis woes.

1½ cups of fresh or frozen blueberries

1 large apple, peeled and chopped

1 medium banana, peeled

2 oz. of pure, food-grade aloe vera gel*

1 cup of water

Liquefy all of the ingredients in a blender, pour the potion into a glass, and drink to healthier skin!

* This is equivalent to 8 ounces of aloe vera juice. You can buy food-grade aloe vera gel online, as well as in health-food stores and many supermarkets. Or, if you have an aloe vera plant, remove the spiky edges from a leaf, then slice it in half lengthwise, and use a spoon to scrape out the gel. Repeat until you have 4 tablespoons of gel.

The Food-Flare-Up Fraud

A lot of folks (especially, it seems, the currently trendy anti-gluten crowd) would have you believe that anyone who has psoriasis, or is at high risk of getting it, should avoid certain foods at all costs. Well, as in the case of IBD (see "The Myth of the Magic Bullet" on page 238), it just ain't so. At least, no credible scientific research has confirmed any connection between specific foods and the frequency, severity, or duration of flare-ups. However, that is *not* to say that food doesn't play a role in psoriasis. It's simply that food sensitivities are a highly individual matter: What sets off major eruptions in one person may pose no trouble for someone else. So just use your common sense, and follow this three-part plan:

1. Keep track of what you eat, and if you find that something bothers you, don't eat it again.

2. Eat a healthful, well-balanced diet that's rich in all the essential nutrients we discussed in Chapter 3.

3. If you must avoid particular foods that are major sources of key nutrients (for example, iron-rich red meat, which causes flare-ups in many people), confer with your doctor about supplements— but don't go dosing yourself!

Bath-Time Bonanzas

Although bathing in Dead Sea salt water is a slam-dunk way to heal psoriasis lesions (see "Stop Psoriasis Dead in Its Tracks," below), it's not your only excellent option for soothing relief. Just pour any of these easy-to-come-by healers into a tub of warm water, and soak for 20 minutes or so. Repeat as often as needed to minimize your misery.

▶ ¼ cup of extra virgin olive oil mixed into 8 ounces of milk

▶ 2 to 4 cups of buttermilk

▶ 2 cups of raw, unfiltered apple cider vinegar

▶ 10 drops of either bergamot, cedarwood, or geranium essential oil

Stop Psoriasis Dead in Its Tracks

Scads of controlled, peer-reviewed scientific studies have shown that 80 to 90 percent of psoriasis sufferers who took regular dips in the Dead Sea for three to four weeks sent their problem-producing patches packin' pronto. What's that? You say that your schedule doesn't allow you to jaunt off to Israel for a month or so? Not to worry: The miracles of modern transportation can bring that therapeutic water right to your doorstep. Just pick up a supply of Dead Sea salt at your local health-food store, or order it from one of a gazillion websites. Then, before bedtime, toss about 2 pounds of the salt into the tub as you fill 'er up with warm water (the exact temperature is your call). Soak for 20 minutes or so. Then rinse off, and wrap yourself up in a thick terry-cloth bathrobe or big beach towel to intensify the healing power while you dry off. When you're thoroughly dry, toddle off to bed. Repeat the procedure three or four times a week, and your scales should soon hit the trail to the land of forgotten nightmares.

Up to **30%** of psoriasis sufferers **develop psoriatic arthritis**.

Head for Psoriasis Relief

When psoriasis has flared up on your scalp, chances are you'd rather not soak your head in a bathtub for 20 minutes. Nor, most likely, do you want to risk messing up your hair with aloe vera gel or any other topical healer—at least not unless you're headed off to bed rather than out the door. Enter this shower-time treatment that's as easy as pie and neat as a pin: Pour 1 cup of olive oil into a bowl, and mix in 1 drop of oregano oil and 2 drops of calendula oil. Massage the mixture into your scalp, and shampoo as usual. Rinse with a half-and-half solution of apple cider vinegar and water, dry and style your tresses as usual, and go on your merry way. Repeat daily, or as needed, until your scales have scurried off.

3 Steps to Scale-Free Hands and Feet

Psoriasis lesions can be especially troublesome on hardworking hands or feet. But you can say good-bye to them with this simple, three-step process:

Step 1. Just before bedtime, soak for 15 to 20 minutes in a bath laced with about 2 cups of Epsom salts.

Step 2. Pat your itchy skin areas dry, and massage them with warm peanut oil (do not substitute any other kind).

Step 3. Cover the oil with a paste made from baking soda and castor oil, then pull on clean white cotton gloves and/or socks, and hop into bed.

Repeat this treatment every few days as needed, and your scales should soon sail away.

NOTE: *Needless to say (I hope!), you should not even think of using this remedy if you are allergic to peanuts.*

PART 3

Is Your Home Toxic Territory?

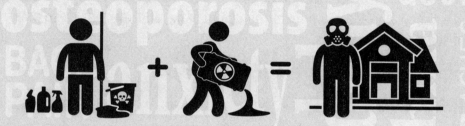

The chemical industry would have you believe that in order to maintain clean surroundings, you need to rely on hundreds of products that didn't exist 50 years ago. Most of us have bought into that myth hook, line, and sinker—at least judging from the fact that every year, Americans use more than 300 million pounds of synthetic chemicals to spiff up their homes, indoors and out. And many of these compounds have been linked to health woes ranging from allergies to deadly diseases. While there is no way to escape these poisons entirely, I'm here to show you how to greatly minimize their impact on your life.

Housekeeping Horrors

In earlier chapters, we covered many of the dangerous toxins in our food and personal-care products. But that's only a drop in the cesspool. Research scientists reckon that there are anywhere from 80,000 to 100,000 potentially deadly chemicals coming at you from every angle in your home sweet home. They're used to manufacture everything from computers, furniture, and kitchen appliances to the clothes you wear, the flooring you walk on, and—ironically—the products you use to make all that stuff clean and free of disease-causing germs.

Clean but Deadly

➡ Like antibiotics and other potent medicines, most of our modern "miracle" cleaning products began arriving on the scene shortly after World War II. They took the country by storm, and for good reason: For the most part, they work every bit as well as the TV commercials claim they do. Unfortunately, the vast majority of them contain ingredients that can hand you a whole lot more trouble than the dirt and germs you're aiming to banish. The good news is that a whole lot of safer options exist, and you'll find some of the best of the bunch right here.

Unquestionably Clean

It's no secret that the synthetic compounds in cleaning products are far from harmless. In fact, as far back as 1985, a report by the Environmental Protection Agency (EPA) announced that the toxic chemicals in household cleaners are three times more likely than outdoor air pollution to cause cancer. And yet—and this is really scary, folks—the federal government does not demand premarket testing for any chemicals used in consumer products. But that's not all! While regulations do mandate that labels identify "hazardous" substances, the verbiage only needs to specify in what way the formula could do harm: for instance, that it's combustible, corrosive, or poisonous. Manufacturers are not required to disclose the full list of ingredients on product labels because the recipes are considered trade secrets.

Pristine and Perilous

No doubt you've noticed that the labels of many cleaning and deodorizing products sport scenes of pristine beaches at sunset, shady pine forests, lemon groves on a sunny summer day, or bunches of pretty flowers. Well, those images aren't there just because some graphic designer thought they looked nice. Savvy marketers know that those peaceful, bucolic pictures subconsciously evoke visions of what we all want our homes to be: serene, beautiful retreats from the frantic, noisy world outside our doors. Their reasoning works, too: Consumers drop billions of dollars a year on these pretty packages—rarely stopping to even read any ingredients listed on the label, much less ponder the possible damage they could cause.

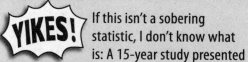

YIKES! If this isn't a sobering statistic, I don't know what is: A 15-year study presented at the Toronto Indoor Air Conference found that women who are full-time homemakers or who work from home have a 54 percent higher risk of dying from cancer than those who are employed elsewhere. The reason? They're exposed to more toxic cleaners and other household chemicals in the home.

3 Sneaky Ways Cleaning Chemicals Are Killing You

Every year, hundreds of thousands of people (and pets) are injured or even killed by ingesting household cleaners or splashing the caustic solutions onto their skin. But you don't have to take a swig of the stuff or douse yourself with it to suffer serious harm. Here are three other ways that these scoundrels can sneak into your body:

Aerial bombardment. Liquid cleaners that you just spray and wipe are convenient all right. The problem is, not all of the fluid reaches the surface you were aiming at. Small amounts of the stuff are also released into the air and (of course) into your nearby nose. Aerosol sprays are even worse because they release a superfine mist that instantly vaporizes and spreads throughout your home, so every time you inhale, you take in some toxins.

Skin contact. While some cleaning products—especially any that contain ammonia, lye, or chlorine bleach—can cause immediate damage to the surface of your skin, other types act in more subtle ways. Even though you may display no visible reaction, the toxins penetrate your body whenever you (let's say) use a cleaner-soaked sponge or scouring pad, or wring out a mop using your bare hands.

The **#1 cause** of household **poisoning** is **dishwasher detergent**.

Surface residue. Whenever you use a cleaning product on anything, from kitchen countertops, cutting boards, and carpets to hard-surface floors and toilet seats, trace amounts of the cleaner or polish remain behind. Then, for example, food that's prepared on newly washed counters or cutting boards gets gobbled up. As for those other supposedly pristine surfaces, anytime you touch them with your bare hands, feet, or other body parts, the toxic residue goes onto—and right through—your skin.

4 Clues to Toxic Overload

When you're taking in too many toxins—whether they're coming from your surroundings, your food, or both—your body can show symptoms that mimic those of many early-stage diseases. If you're experiencing any of this handful of annoyances, and you've ruled out underlying health conditions, clean up your act *now*, before serious trouble sets in.

CALL 911

Mixing bleach with a cleaner that contains ammonia (as many products do) produces a highly toxic gas that can cause coughing, loss of voice, a burning sensation, suffocation—or death. So don't take chances: If you or anyone in your household inadvertently combines these two high-voltage substances, head for the ER *immediately*.

- Aches or pains in muscles or joints
- Constant fatigue or sluggishness
- Mood swings
- Recurring headaches

The Harrowing Hazards of Hormone Disrupters

It seems as though every time you turn around, a new study comes out linking yet another common cleaning product to hormone (a.k.a. endocrine system) disruption. So what's the big deal, you may ask? Here's the big deal: Your endocrine system is made up of glands, positioned throughout your body, that make hormones, which in turn trigger particular responses from your various organs. When chemicals interfere with this finely tuned routine, chaos breaks loose. (Think of what happens when a member of a symphony orchestra plays the wrong notes.) But in this case, what you get is worse than musical discord. Endocrine-disrupting chemicals appear to lie at the heart of many, if not most, of our escalating health problems, including diabetes, auto-immune disorders, heart disease, and both breast and prostate cancer (not to mention premature puberty in children, and infertility in both men and women).

4 Fiendish Felons

Cleaning ingredients vary greatly in the type and degree of hazard they pose. Some cause acute reactions, ranging in severity from watery eyes to chemical burns, while others have been linked to chronic diseases, such as diabetes and cancer. These are four of the worst offenders:

A Little Dab'll Do You In

Jaw-Dropping DISCOVERY

Scientists have known for quite a while that even low doses of certain hormone disrupters, like phthalates and bisphenol A (BPA), can cause serious and permanent harm in both laboratory animals and people. Well, now an analysis of more than 800 peer-reviewed studies suggests just about all chemicals that interfere with your hormones can perform their dirty work even at low doses—the levels deemed "safe" for human beings as opposed to the massive loads of the substances pumped into animals in the testing labs. The damage done by these small amounts of toxins may take time to show diagnosable effects, but as they accumulate in your body, they are forming a monster of a wrecking ball that's gearing up for a devastating whack!

Air fresheners work in one of two ways: They either give off nerve-deadening compounds that hamper your ability to smell, or they coat your nasal passages with a film of oil—most often methoxychlor, a pesticide that builds up in your fat cells. Other common ingredients are formaldehyde (a known carcinogen) and phenol, which can cause your skin to burn, swell, peel, and break out in hives.

Carpet and upholstery shampoos rout out tough stains by blasting them with such heavy artillery as perchlorethylene, a known carcinogen that can damage your liver, kidneys, and nervous system; and ammonium hydroxide, a corrosive chemical that irritates your eyes, skin, and breathing passages.

Oven cleaners contain lye and ammonia, both of which eat your skin and emit fumes that damage the respiratory system. Furthermore, the next time you turn on the oven, you intensify the release of the residue.

Chlorine was first used during World War II as a **chemical weapon**.

Toilet bowl cleaners generally pack a highly corrosive duo of hydrochloric acid and hypochlorite bleach, which can damage your liver and kidneys and burn your eyes, skin, and respiratory tract. As if that's not enough, when these products come in contact with other chemicals, the combo can produce potentially deadly chlorine fumes.

Help for Harried (and Hurried) Homemakers

Believe it or not, there are some safe cleaning products on your supermarket shelves—but it can take a lot of time to find them if you have to read the fine print on every label. Enter the Environmental Working Group (EWG), the same folks who issue the annual Dirty Dozen and Clean 15 produce lists featured on page 112. EWG has also analyzed almost all the brand-name products on the market and graded them for safety on a scale of A through F. Check out the Guide to Healthy Cleaning at www.ewg.org.

Living with the Enemy

Laundry detergents are formulated from countless chemicals, including phosphorus, ammonia, naphthalene, and phenol—not to mention various enzymes and fragrances. They can trigger symptoms ranging from watery eyes to rashes, respiratory irritation, sinus problems, and headaches. And, as you might imagine, they're especially problematic for asthma sufferers. Even a thorough rinse cycle doesn't get rid of the detergent residue. It remains on your clothes and your bed linens, and from there it moseys right on into your body.

Softness to Die For

Would you say that soft, static-free clothes are worth dying for? No? Then do yourself a favor: March into your laundry room, grab the fabric softener and the dryer sheets, and take 'em both to the closest toxic waste facility. They're chock-full of dangerous chemicals, including these three that are actually on the EPA's Hazardous Waste List:

Chloroform was used as an anesthesia until the early 1900s, when docs discovered that (whoops!) it can cause fatal cardiac arrhythmia. In addition to its intended purpose of causing loss of consciousness, chloroform can aggravate heart, kidney, and liver problems, and it's classed by the EPA as a "probable human carcinogen." Plus, its effects are worsened when the gas is subjected to heat (like the hot air in your dryer).

Ethanol can cause disorders of the central nervous system (CNS).

Ethyl acetate irritates the eyes and respiratory tract and can cause severe headaches, loss of consciousness, and damage to the kidneys and liver.

And that's only the trio of terrors the EPA has targeted as toxic. The laundry list includes more than half a dozen other dangerous chemicals, the most deadly being alpha-terpineol (a.k.a. a-terpineol), which has been closely linked to just about every CNS disorder under the sun, including stroke, multiple sclerosis, and both Alzheimer's and Parkinson's diseases.

Clear the Air—Naturally

The marketing hype for commercial air fresheners would have you believe that these things actually remove unpleasant odors from the air. Baloney! All they do is cover up the aromas with

REMARKABLE REMEDY

Safer Ways to Soften

Besides being highly toxic, both liquid fabric softeners and dryer sheets are entirely unnecessary. There are scads of safe—and less expensive—ways you can make your laundry soft and static-free. Like this handful, for instance:

▶ Add ½ cup or so of either vinegar or baking soda to each wash load.

▶ Spray vinegar on a piece of all-cotton cloth, and toss it into the dryer.

▶ Throw an old wool sweater into the dryer with your laundry. Besides reducing static, it'll cut drying time.

▶ Buy a supply of wool dryer balls (available online).

▶ Forget synthetic fabrics (and blends, too). Instead, buy clothes and linens that are made from 100 percent cotton, silk, linen, wool, or combinations thereof. Natural fabrics are, well, naturally soft—and naturally nonclinging.

fake (and dangerous) fragrances, and mess up your smelling mechanism (see "4 Fiendish Felons" on page 249). Fortunately, you have many terrific, safe alternatives that actually *do* banish unpleasant odors. Take these, for instance:

Act with vim and vinegar. Just pour some of it into bowls, and set them around the problem areas. The acidic liquid will banish the unwanted smells pronto.

Burn your troubles away. Throw slices of dried citrus peel (your choice of aromas) into the fireplace. They'll fill the whole house with a wonderful fragrance.

Light a candle. Better yet, light several. But don't bother with the fancy scented kind. Like spray air fresheners, they'll add dangerous odor-masking chemicals to the air (see "4 Steps to Stop Diabetes" on page 154). On the other hand, a pure soy or beeswax candle flame will simply burn away foul-smelling gases (even the ones that occur in bathrooms every now and then).

"Adopt" some houseplants. The more of them you have around your house, the cleaner and fresher your air will be. That's because green plants naturally absorb and neutralize air pollutants. What's more, they do an especially good job in small, enclosed rooms, where the air quality is usually worse. Any kind of plant can perform this feat, but according to NASA scientists (who know a thing or two about tight spaces), these are the air-cleaning superstars:

- Aloe vera
- Chrysanthemums
- English ivy (*Hedera helix*)
- Spider plants
- Weeping fig (*Ficus benjamina*)

1,300+ chemicals have been proven to **disrupt** your **endocrine system**.

Rout Out Rust

There's nothing more frustrating than reaching for a favorite tool, kitchen knife, or cast-iron pan and finding that it's splotched with rust. Well, don't fret—and don't rush out and buy a corrosive commercial rust remover. Use one of these ultra-safe kitchen-counter "cures" instead:

The quick method. Make a paste from 2 parts salt and 1 part lemon juice. Rub the paste onto the metal until the spots vanish, and rinse with clear water.

The slower but easier way. Soak your "stricken" pieces overnight in full-strength vinegar. The rust will dissolve like magic.

An inside job. When the trouble spots are on the inside of a pan or skillet, put 3 cups of sliced rhubarb into it, and pour in just enough water to cover the rusted areas. Cook the rhubarb over low heat, stirring occasionally until the rust drifts off the metal surface. (How long this takes depends upon the thickness of the rust layer.) Toss the contents into your compost bin, or bury it in a flower bed; then wash the pan and dry it thoroughly.

Through a Glass Clearly

If you live in a cold-winter climate, you know that a few months of blustery weather can make a grimy mess of your windows. The simple solution: Come spring, thoroughly mix 3 tablespoons of cornstarch and ½ cup of water in a bowl. Dip a soft, 100 percent cotton cloth into the mixture, and rub it onto each pane. A film will develop at first, but as you keep rubbing, the glass will become crystal clear.

A Cleaning Crew in a Box

One of the safest—and most effective—cleaners comes in a bright orange box. It's none other than baking soda, of course! It's been

---

The Great "Green" Brainwash

Jaw-Dropping DISCOVERY

You might think that when a product label sports terms like *natural*, *green*, or *environmentally friendly*, the stuff is bound to be perfectly safe to use. Well, think again, my friends! Here are just two sobering cases in point, courtesy of the Environmental Working Group:

Citra Solv® Cleaner & Degreaser contains d-limonene, which, when sprayed into the air, reacts with ozone to form formaldehyde (a known carcinogen) as well as other tiny, harmful lung-penetrating particles.

Simple Green® All-Purpose Cleaner contains a solvent by the tongue-twisting name of 2-butoxyethanol, which can seep through your skin and damage red blood cells. What's worse, when folks buy the spray version, many of them assume (quite naturally) that it's fine to shoot the stuff straight from the bottle, and they never stop to read the fine print warning users to "dilute before use."

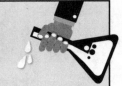

Fix-It-Fast
FORMULA

All-Purpose Household Cleaner

Who needs cupboards full of harsh, toxic (and expensive) cleaning products? This simple formula combines the workhorse power of baking soda and vinegar with the antiseptic and clarifying properties of witch hazel and tea tree oil. The result: a super-strength, antibacterial cleanser that wipes up cleanly—no rinsing needed.

½ **cup of baking soda**

½ **cup of water**

½ **cup of white vinegar**

¼ **cup of witch hazel**

1 **tsp. of tea tree oil***

Mix all of the ingredients together in a handheld spray bottle, and use the mixture to clean all of your bathroom fixtures and kitchen appliances (inside and out), as well as countertops and ceramic-tile surfaces throughout your house.

* *Available in health-food stores, herbal-supply stores, and online.*

helping folks keep their houses clean and fresh-smelling since long before anyone even heard of hormone disrupters. You can use it straight from the source, as you would any scouring powder, to clean grungy ovens, small appliances, or scuffed floors. To spruce up painted-wood surfaces, wash them with a solution of 1 teaspoon of baking soda per gallon of hot water, and dry 'em with a soft cotton cloth. Got a smelly drain? Just pour a cup of baking soda into the opening, and flush with hot water.

Cut Those Clogs

It's no secret that commercial drain cleaners are among the most toxic products on the market— just ask any plumber. Fortunately, there is a powerful and much gentler way to dissolve stubborn gunk in your kitchen *or* bathroom drain. How? Simply pour ½ cup of baking soda into the drain, and follow up with ½ cup of either white vinegar or lemon juice. Let it sit for about 15 minutes. (The acid-alkaline combo will make a *lot* of noise, but don't be alarmed—this dynamic duo won't do any harm to your plumbing.) Rinse with hot tap water, and you're good to go! Just one word of caution: Do *not* use this method if you've already tried a commercial de-clogger. The vinegar or juice can react with the drain cleaner to create dangerous fumes.

To prevent future buildups, pour a cup of white vinegar down the drain every month or so.

When the Going Gets Tough . . .

Team up baking soda with some other heavy hitters, and turn the combos loose on your most challenging cleaning jobs. Here's the roster:

Heavy-duty cleanser. Combine equal parts of baking soda, salt, and borax, and store the mixture in a closed container. It'll get grease and grime off pots and pans, appliances, tile floors, bathroom fixtures, and just about every other surface.

Scouring powder. Mix equal parts of baking soda and salt in a container with a tight-fitting lid, and keep it close at hand. Use it as you would any other scouring powder. It's strong but gentle enough for colored-porcelain bathroom fixtures, kitchen counters, and other easily scratched surfaces.

Silver polish. Find a pan that's big enough to hold the silver, and fill it with water. Add your treasures, along with 1 tablespoon each of baking soda and table salt and three 12-inch sheets of aluminum foil. Let the mixture sit for an hour or so. Like magic, the tarnish will be pulled from the metal onto the aluminum, creating a rotten-egg smell in the process (so don't be concerned!). Your silver will come out as bright and shiny as a full moon!

Soft-scrubbing cleanser. Mix ⅛ cup of baking soda with enough natural dish liquid to get a creamy consistency. Apply the mixture with a sponge or soft brush, and rinse with clear water.

Toilet bowl cleaner. Sprinkle ¼ cup of baking soda into the bowl and drizzle ¼ cup of vinegar over the soda. Add a few drops of your favorite essential oil if you like (any aroma that suits your fancy is fine). Then grab a long-handled brush and scrub-a-dub-dub!

> Each year, Americans use more than **300 million pounds** of **toxic chemicals**.

Magic Carpet Deodorizer

Whether Fido or Fluffy has left aromatic residue on your rugs, or you simply want to get rid of that stale smell that builds up in the wintertime, reach for this remarkable (and remarkably safe) recipe. It's quick and easy to create a batch: Pour 1 cup of baking soda into a glass jar. Then mix in 10 drops of ginger essential oil and 10 drops of grapefruit essential oil, stirring well. Sprinkle the contents over your carpet. Wait for 60 minutes or so, and vacuum as usual. Then close your eyes, and take a good, deep sniff—you'll swear you'd been whisked away to a sea-breezy island!

Fatally Flawed Furnishings

➡ Although cleaning products account for the majority of toxins floating around our homes, they're far from the only health destroyers in our midst. Everything from the rugs you walk on to the shower curtain you stand behind each morning could be bombarding you with trouble.

A Slippery Devil

90% of Americans have **flame-retardant chemicals** in their **bodies**.

Perfluorooctanoic acid (PFOA) is one of a class of highly questionable chemicals called perfluorochemicals (PFCs). PFOA is best known as an ingredient in nonstick coatings used on cookware and microwavable food containers, but its sinister slickness extends far beyond the kitchen. It's also used to manufacture stain-resistant finishes for carpets and upholstery fabrics as well as scads of other everyday products, including phone cables, computer chips, and disposable coffee cups. Medical science labels PFOA as a "possible" human carcinogen (it has been proven to cause several types of cancer in laboratory animals), and it has been linked to thyroid disease, heart disease, stroke, and peripheral artery disease in humans. And here come a couple of really chilling tidbits:

- Once this stuff gets into your body, it hangs around for years. In scientific terms, it has a half-life of more than four years (that's the time it would take for your system to expel half of any dose it consumed).

- PFOA has been found in the blood of more than 98 percent of people tested for it.

A Monstrous Moving Target

Phthalates (pronounced "THAL-ates") are dynamic hormone disrupters (see "The Harrowing Hazards of Hormone Disrupters" on page 248). They're key ingredients in hundreds of household products, most prominently those made from polyvinyl chloride (PVC). That familiar roster includes everything from vinyl flooring, shower curtains, and automobile interiors to food-storage containers and product packaging of all kinds. So where does the "moving target" angle enter the picture? In these two ways:

1. Small, but highly toxic, doses of phthalates migrate from PVC to anything that touches it, whether that's food or drink, skin lotion—or even your bare feet on a vinyl floor.

2. Congress has banned a number of specific phthalates, and manufacturers have voluntarily ushered others out of their factories and pledged to phase out many more. This now-you-see-it-now-you-don't process means that choosing safe products is something of a crapshoot. And here comes the really scary part: In many cases, the new ingredients may be every bit as dangerous as the old ones.

The Flame-Retardant Fraud

True or false? Products that have been treated with flame-retardant chemicals make your home a safer place.
ABSOLUTELY FALSE! Despite the hype you hear, these chemicals do not make anything fireproof. In fact, when (let's say) a cigarette or a lighted candle falls on flame-retardant upholstery fabric, the flames are only delayed by a few seconds. What's more, when the chemical-drenched material does burn, it releases higher levels of carbon monoxide, smoke, and soot than nontreated fabric does. And, as any firefighter or EMT will tell you, those—not flames—are the leading causes of fire-related deaths.

Meanwhile, flame-retardant chemicals have been directly linked to a variety of health problems, including cancer, hormone disruption, infertility, learning disabilities, and birth defects.

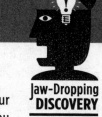

Smelling Trouble

Jaw-Dropping DISCOVERY

Phthalates don't just enter your body through your mouth or skin. You also breathe them in every day, in two ways:

▶ The compounds in vinyl floors and furnishings break down and float through the air—right into your nose, either solo or as part of household dust particles.

▶ In addition to their role as softening agents for plastics, phthalates are used as carriers for fragrances added to cosmetics, personal-care products, and household cleaners. And the chemicals don't have to be identified individually. Under current law, they can simply be included in the "fragrance" listing on the label—despite the fact that they often make up 20 percent or more of the contents.

Fire the Fire Retardants!

Or at least lessen their intrusion into your life. Let's face it: In this day and age, there is no way you can completely divorce yourself from flame-retardant chemicals. But you can reduce your exposure. Whenever you're shopping for new furniture or electronics, simply ask the folks on the sales floor if the items you're interested in contain any of these deadly additives and, if so, which ones. If they can't answer your question, call or e-mail the manufacturer. As in the case of phthalates (see "A Monstrous Moving Target" on page 256), the status of flame retardants is in a constant state of flux. What's here today could be banned tomorrow—but possibly replaced by something just as bad, if not worse.

4 Ploys to Protect Yourself from Polyurethane

There's no telling for sure what particular perilous poisons may be escaping from the polyurethane products at your place, but these four measures will help minimize the risk to you and your family:

- Use a vacuum cleaner that's fitted with a high-efficiency particulate air (HEPA) filter. These are designed especially to trap small toxic and allergenic particles of all kinds. For good measure—especially if anyone in your household is very sensitive to airborne contaminants—consider getting a HEPA-filter air cleaner.

- Replace anything with a torn cover or filled with old foam that's beginning to deteriorate.

- Do not reupholster foam-filled furniture. If buying new isn't an option, go with slipcovers in cotton, linen, or wool.

- When you're removing old carpet, proceed with caution. Most likely, the padding contains fire-retardant chemicals—as well as volatile organic compounds (see "Villainous VOCs," below). After the job is done, clean the floor thoroughly with a HEPA-filter vacuum, followed by a damp mop to pick up as many offending particles as possible.

65% of the **air** we breathe comes from **inside** our homes.

Villainous VOCs

Volatile organic compounds (VOCs) are chemicals used to manufacture or maintain just about every kind of household item you can think of, including building materials, furniture, electronics, hobby supplies, insecticides, paints, and finishes, as well as cleaning and personal-care products. The term *volatile* means that at room temperature, they evaporate or otherwise cut loose from their parent products and escape into the air. *Organic* means that they're carbon-based—so, technically speaking, they are "natural" ingredients. And there's no escaping them. Studies show that anywhere from 50 to hundreds of individual VOCs may be in the air of your home, office, or friendly neighborhood shopping mall at any given time, and they've been shown to cause a slew of problems, ranging from relatively minor woes, such as headaches, nausea, and skin irritation, to major miseries, like asthma, cancer, and damage to your central nervous system.

Out of the Jammies and into the Cushions

Jaw-Dropping DISCOVERY

In the 1970s, the flame-retardant chemical chlorinated tris (a.k.a. TDCPP) was banned for use in children's pajamas because of adverse health effects, including cancer. Well, guess what? TDCPP is still one of the most common additives in car seats, mattresses, and other baby products—and in the polyurethane foam used in upholstered grown-up furniture and pillows. Your trouble-avoidance mission here is simple: Take a pass on stuff that's stuffed with polyurethane. Instead, go with cotton-, wool-, polyester-, or down-filled furniture and cushions. Ditto when you're shopping for baby gifts. When in doubt, pick up the phone, call the manufacturer, and ask the customer service folks exactly what's in your future purchase. If you don't get a clear bill of goods, take your business elsewhere.

Furniture in Attack Mode

As you know if you've shopped for new wooden furniture lately, a lot of it is actually made of particleboard or fiberboard with a thin veneer of real wood. Unfortunately, both particleboard and fiberboard often contain urea formaldehyde (UF), which releases VOCs. To avoid trouble, look for versions that are guaranteed UF-free. Better yet, opt for solid wood.

NOTE: *To save money, check out flea markets, thrift shops, and "junktique" stores, as well as local artisans. Even actual antique pieces are sometimes less expensive than any all-wood versions coming out of the big manufacturing facilities in North Carolina.*

The Vile Wiles of VOCs

While some VOCs produce instantly recognizable odors, even at very low levels, many of them have no detectable aroma at all. At high concentrations, some VOCs are toxic, and long-term exposure can lead to cancer and other chronic diseases. Here's a dirty dozen of the most common offenders in homes, offices, retail stores, and public buildings:

- Butoxyethanol
- Chloride
- Decane
- Formaldehyde
- Isopentane
- Limonene
- Methylene
- Perchloroethylene
- Styrene
- Toluene
- Vinyl chloride
- Xylenes

Escape from Trouble Underfoot

Two factors go into determining the toxicity of carpeting. The first is the fiber it's made from. The second is the materials used in the backing and the adhesives used to fasten the carpet to the floor. Often, these materials contain VOCs. So whenever you're in the market for new floor coverings, consider these two options:

Go organic. Just search online for "organic carpets" or "organic furnishings." Dozens of sites will pop up, including some retail outlets that might not be too far from home. But be forewarned: The prices won't be cheap (although they're coming down fast). Also, you can often find big bargains, especially if you need to cover only a small area. For instance, if a dealer has some special-order pieces left over from a recent job, you may be able to snatch them up for a song (or two).

Opt for natural-fiber area rugs on bare floors. Cotton, wool, sisal, jute, and sea grass are all good choices—and they come in a range of prices.

It's Only Natural

Carpeting is not the only source of VOCs (see "Escape from Trouble Underfoot," at left). Upholstered furniture, table linens, bedding, and anything else that's made from synthetic fabrics can give off unhealthy gases, or even release chemicals into your skin. Don't get me wrong—I'm not suggesting that you run out and replace all of your worldly goods! Just keep in mind that when you *are* shopping for new soft goods, natural fibers like cotton, linen, wool, and hemp are a whole lot healthier to have around the old homestead.

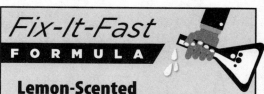

Fix-It-Fast
FORMULA

Lemon-Scented Furniture Polish

When you go to the trouble to seek out all-wood furniture, it only makes sense to use an equally safe, natural furniture polish. This one is just the ticket.

1 cup of olive oil
½ cup of water
2 tbsp. of white vinegar
1 tsp. of lemon oil

Mix all of the ingredients together in a dark glass jar with a tight-fitting lid, and store it, firmly closed, at room temperature. Shake well before using. Pour a small amount onto a soft cotton cloth, and wipe it onto your furniture. Buff with another clean, dry cloth. Then stand back and admire yourself in the shiny surface!

3 Steps to Safer Carpeting

If you have your heart set on wall-to-wall carpeting, and the organic version is beyond your means, take these three steps to minimize the danger to you and yours:

1. Ask the retailer to air it out in the store or warehouse for 24 to 48 hours before it's delivered to your home.

2. Insist that the installer use the lowest-VOC adhesives possible or—much better yet—none at all.

3. During the installation process, make sure the area is well ventilated, with all windows wide open and your ventilation system or fans turned on full blast.

Plastic by the Numbers

According to some health experts, it's likely that no kind of plastic is entirely safe, but some types pose far greater health risks than others. Here's a roster of the players.

The 3 Worst Offenders

This is the trio that you should boot out of your life ASAP:

Polyvinyl chloride (#3). Found primarily in flexible products ranging from garden hoses to squeezable bottles, they're phthalate minefields (see "A Monstrous Moving Target" on page 256).

Polystyrene (#6). Found in egg cartons, disposable coffee cups, take-out food containers, packaging for meats and cheeses, as well as (in nonfoam form) in disposable cutlery, some yogurt containers, and the transparent containers used for baked goods. The key ingredient is styrene (a.k.a. vinyl benzene), a suspected carcinogen that can be toxic to the kidneys, respiratory system, and gastrointestinal tract.

Polycarbonates (#7). Found in sports drink and watercooler bottles, food-storage containers, kitchen appliances, telephones, compact discs, plastic lumber, and the coatings on the insides of many food and drink cans. The problem: The #7 crowd contains BPA, which like phthalates, is a potent hormone disrupter.

The Safer Bunch

These plastics are free of BPA, phthalates, and PVC and do not pose any known health hazards:

Polyethylene terephthalate, a.k.a. PET or PETE (#1). Found in most clear water and soda bottles. Just bear in mind that they are intended for one-time use only; with repeated use, bacteria can build up on the plastic.

High-density polyethylene, a.k.a. HDPE (#2). Found in many containers, including detergent, shampoo, and milk bottles.

Low-density polyethylene, a.k.a. LDPE (#4). Found in shopping and sandwich bags, some types of cling wrap, and wrappers for toilet paper and paper towels.

Polypropylene (#5). Found in storage boxes, plastic buckets, rope, construction materials, carpeting, mats, and furniture.

Menacing Materials

➡️ We all like to think of our homes as safe-and-sound shelters from the hubbub of the outside world. But, ironically, many of our major health threats come from the walls around us and the floors we walk on. The good news is that you can fight back.

The Mounting Menace of VOCs

Volatile organic compounds have been with us since the dawn of time. And many of the products that contain them have been around for decades. So why, you may wonder, has the situation suddenly gotten worse? Well, the major reason goes back to the energy crisis of the 1970s, when airtight construction became all the rage. Commercial builders and home-owners alike did their best to eliminate any openings in homes through which heated or cooled air could leak out and fresh, untreated air could come in. That maneuver saved energy all right. Unfortunately, it also ensured that noxious fumes given off by building materials, furnishings, office chemicals, and cleaning products could not escape as they used to. Neither could the dampness and tiny organisms that create mold. The result has been an epidemic of environmentally triggered illnesses and allergies, in homes as well as schools, hospitals, and office buildings. (Remember the hoopla about "sick building syndrome" a number of years back? Well, this is what caused it.)

Annual **PVC flooring** production in North America totals **14 billion pounds**.

Healthy Things from Sick Buildings

As the old saying goes, behind every dark cloud there's a silver lining. In the case of sick building syndrome, there are two silver linings:

1. Because we now know just how much and what kind of damage seemingly harmless things can cause, a whole lot of companies are hard at work creating and marketing healthier alternatives. For instance, all of the major paint companies, including Benjamin Moore® and Sherwin-Williams®, are producing paints that emit no

VOCs (and no odor) during application and drying. And at least two famous makers of plastic-laminate countertops (Formica® and Arborite®) have switched from "off-gassing" adhesives to nontoxic versions.

2. We've all realized how important it is to keep fresh air flowing freely. Simply by opening some windows and letting the balmy breezes blow, you'll make the great indoors a whole lot healthier. If your house was built with non-opening windows, replace at least some of them with functioning versions. And for good measure, ease off a little on the weather stripping. This is especially important if you live in a climate where you tend to move from heating season into air-conditioning season, with little or no time for an open-window respite.

VOC levels may be up to **1,000 times higher indoors** than outdoors.

Fix-It-Fast
FORMULA

Ultra-Safe Wood Stain

If you're a do-it-yourselfer, this simple recipe belongs in your tool kit. It's perfect for furniture, planters, children's toys, or anything else that's made of unfinished wood—whether you've built it from scratch or bought it.

1 part food coloring

5–6 parts water

Mix the food coloring and water together (the more coloring you use, the darker the shade will be). Saturate the wood surface, wait about five minutes, and wipe with a soft cloth. Let the wood dry overnight, then wipe again. Repeat the process if you want an even darker color.

Your Floors Are Flooring You . . .

And lots of your fellow earthlings, too! That is, they are if you have vinyl tile or other types of vinyl flooring. This stuff is popular because it's inexpensive, easy to install, and easy to replace. For that reason, 14 billion pounds of PVC flooring is produced each year in North America. But because of the toxins involved in manufacturing, using, and disposing of it, it poses monumental health risks—even for people who don't have it in their own homes.

What Goes Around Comes Around

Linoleum was invented by an Englishman named Frederick Walton in the 1860s, and with its easy-to-clean, water-resistant surface, it took the world by storm. It remained a hands-down favorite until the late 1940s, when it was largely overshadowed by the new, cheaper, more colorful, and (we now know) highly toxic vinyl tile. Well, now Mr. Walton's "baby" is back in full force—and not only on floors. It's also turning up on countertops, and even walls, from coast to coast. And it's still made from the same natural, nontoxic ingredients that Mr. Walton used— namely, linseed oil (from the flax plant), cork dust, wood powder, resins, ground limestone, and mineral pigments, all mixed together and rolled onto a jute backing. Plus, there are no toxins involved in either the production of linoleum or its disposal processes.

Where the Rubber Meets the Floor . . .

And the crud meets the air. Recycled rubber is widely touted as a brilliant "green" flooring material because it saves millions of pounds of cast-off tires from being dumped into landfills (or simply abandoned in vacant lots and roadside ditches). That's an admirable objective, but the fact is that from a health standpoint, "green" does not mean "go." These former tires give off VOCs and other toxins galore. So do most products that are made from synthetic rubber, recycled or otherwise. Some brands are safer than others (or at least claim to be). If you're considering this soft-on-the-feet option for your kitchen or bathroom, search online for "nontoxic rubber flooring."

Jaw-Dropping DISCOVERY

4 Ways Linoleum Can Light(en) Up Your Life

In addition to not releasing toxins into the air, linoleum has four other advantages you might want to consider when it's time to choose flooring materials:

1. While most vinyl patterns are merely printed on the surface of the tile, the true colors of linoleum go all the way through. So if your floor or countertop gets scratched, a light sanding will send the mark packing. To mend a deeper gouge (say, one from a dropped knife), simply scrape some shavings from a leftover piece, mix them with wood glue, and work the paste into the crack. Bingo—end of blemish!

2. Speaking of colors, the muddy tones you may remember from your grandma's linoleum floor have been replaced by a palette worthy of a crayon box. And new factory-applied sealers keep those colors bright and stain-free.

3. Linoleum has natural antibacterial qualities. That's one big reason it's become a popular choice in hospitals, day-care centers, and heavily trod retail stores.

4. Linoleum is tough and durable, and it commonly holds its good looks for 30 to 40 years or more in high-traffic commercial environments. So just think how well it will perform at your house!

Go With a Real Corker

Cork is another earth- and body-friendly material that's been around since long before anyone started to fret about unhealthy household materials. In fact, although cork made its flooring debut in 1889 (more than a quarter century after linoleum hit the scene), it's been used in one form or another since 2500 B.C. Early products included fishing floats, bottle stoppers, and shoe soles. Among the more recent uses are anti-vibration joints in NASA's space shuttle boosters.

From a purely practical standpoint, cork feels comfortable on the feet and legs, reduces noise, and insulates floors against both heat and cold. It also has remarkable staying power. One case in point: A church in Chicago installed cork flooring in 1890, just a year after the material came on the market. Today, well over 100 years and millions of footfalls later, that same floor is still going strong!

A Glass Act

If you're hankering for a real touch of nontoxic elegance in your kitchen or bathroom, look for recycled glass terrazzo. As the name implies, it's made from irregularly shaped bits of recycled, glittering glass mixed with a binder, such as epoxy resin or portland cement. It comes in two forms: slabs that are great for countertops, and individual tiles that work better for walls and floors. You could even use them to make decorative planters or add colorful accents to a garden wall. An Internet search for "recycled glass terrazzo" will bring up a number of manufacturers, most of them small local companies.

NOTE: *Find a supplier within a few hundred miles of your home, or the shipping could cost more than the product. (This stuff is* heavy!*)*

Catastrophic Closets

➡ **More and more, clothing shoppers are opting for fabrics that are designed not just to feel comfortable or look attractive, but to make life easier. Chances are, you've got a whole lot of garments in your wardrobe that are wrinkle-free, stain-resistant, water-repellent—or even ones that repel insects or have built-in sunscreen. Well, the folks who make that stuff are pulling the wool over your eyes because those "miraculous" materials spew out tons of VOCs and other toxins that go directly into your body, both through your skin and from the air you breathe.**

The Potent Perils of Polyester

If you're like most folks, you've got a whole lot of this stuff hanging in your closet and tucked into your dresser drawers. And for good reason: Just about every item of clothing that you see in a store or on a website contains polyester and many other threads made from synthetic polymers, which, in turn, are made from esters of dihydric alcohol and terephthalic acid, both of which are highly toxic. They remain in the fabric after the manufacturing process and migrate into your body through your skin (especially when it's moist, from either rain or perspiration). Regular wearing of polyester and polyester-blend materials has been shown to generate problems ranging from rashes and other skin irritations to severe respiratory infections and some forms of cancer. What's more, the toxins used in the production of polyester and related fabrics wind up in the water and air, where they cause even more trouble.

Wearing polyester clothes can make you **sick**.

It sounds like a dream come true: the comfort and breathability of pure cotton combined with the convenience of no-iron polyester. Well, it's more like a nightmare. In order to get that easy-care nature, clothing manufacturers treat the cotton with the same perfluorochemicals (PFCs) that give nonstick cookware its slippery finish. Not only does this toxic stuff go into your skin, but it also eliminates the soft feel and breathable nature that we all expect from cotton. So the next time you see a clothing label or catalog description touting a natural-fiber garment as "wrinkle-resistant," "wrinkle-proof," or "easy-care," forget it. Also, cast a cold eye on terms like *permanent press*, *stain-resistant*, *static-resistant*, and *insect-repellent*. They all indicate that the fabric—whether natural or not—has been thoroughly doused with chemicals.

Forgo These Fabrics!

Although polyester and its high-tech offshoot fabrics are by far the most dangerous clothing ingredients, these are the top-four runners-up:

1. Acrylic is made from polymers (forms of plastic) by the tongue-twisting name of polyacrylonitriles (a.k.a. PAN). In addition to being highly flammable—potentially explosive during the manufacturing process—acrylic fabric has been fingered by the EPA as a likely cancer causer.

2. Rayon is manufactured from recycled wood pulp or bamboo cellulose. In order to survive routine wearing and washing, it must be treated with such chemicals as acetone, ammonia, carbon disulfide, caustic soda, and sulfuric acid. The toxins released from the fabric can cause nausea, headache, vomiting, chest and muscle pain, and insomnia. But that's not all! Regularly wearing rayon clothing has been linked to anorexia, Parkinson's disease, and tissue necrosis.

3. Acetate and triacetate undergo much the same chemical processing that rayon does, with the same potential dangers. The major difference is that these two related synthetics are made from fresh cellulose (a.k.a. wood fibers) rather than recycled pulp.

Fumes from **dry-cleaned clothes** can float to **your lungs**.

4. Nylon is made from petroleum. In addition to being treated with caustic soda, formaldehyde, and sulfuric acid during the manufacturing process, the finished fabric is doused with a combination of bleaching and softening agents, such as chloroform, limo-nene, pentene, and terpineol. Related health issues may include skin allergies, dizziness, and headaches, as well as cancer, spinal pain, and nervous system dysfunction.

The Colossal Clothing Conundrum

Let's face it: Just as there is no way to completely escape less-than-healthy ingredients in your diet, there is no way to build a wardrobe that is 100 percent pure and free of toxic chemicals. Even natural-fiber fabrics like cotton, linen, silk, wool, and cashmere nearly always get their colors from chemical-based dyes. Plus, most cotton and the flax that linen is made from are grown with the use of synthetic pesticides and fertilizers. And there's no telling what the silkworms, sheep, and cashmere goats are eating. Furthermore, can you imagine trying to find (much less wear) underwear that does not have elastic in the waistband? So what's a health-conscious clothing shopper to do? Simply use your common sense, and follow these guidelines:

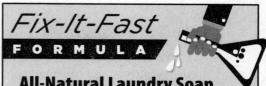

Fix-It-Fast FORMULA

All-Natural Laundry Soap

Laundry detergents are specially formulated for use on synthetic materials like polyester and acrylic. (In fact, like the fabrics themselves, most of these products are made from petrochemicals, too.) But natural fibers, such as cotton, linen, silk, and wool, keep their good looks longer when you wash them with a soap-based formula. This is one of the best.

1 cup of grated soap*
½ cup of borax
½ cup of washing soda**

Combine all of the ingredients thoroughly, and store the mixture in a lidded container. Use 1 tablespoon of the soap for a small or lightly soiled load of laundry and 2 tablespoons for a large or heavily soiled load. For a sink full of hand-washable items, use about 2 teaspoons.

* Fels-Naptha®, Octagon®, and Ivory® are all good choices.

** Available online and in the laundry products aisle of your supermarket.

- Opt for natural fabrics whenever possible, especially for garments that directly touch your bare skin. (For example, a nylon or polyester rain slicker is likely to do far less damage than a rayon blouse or a cotton-poly-blend shirt.)

- If you want to go the extra mile, seek out organically grown cotton, linen, silk, and wool. But be forewarned: It's all but guaranteed that the stuff will cost you a pretty penny.

Deadly Storage

If you're like most folks, the clothes in your closet aren't the only culprits on the toxin team. It's a good bet you've got shoes, belts, handbags, and backpacks that are made, at least in part, from vinyl, synthetic rubber, or synthetic fabrics. But you also, no doubt, own plastic clothes hangers and storage containers. The most problematic of these organizers are made of vinyl, such as hanging shoe bags and the zippered boxes commonly used to store out-of-season garments. Well, do yourself a favor and replace these holdalls with ones made of healthier materials. If budget is a factor, you don't need to do the trade-off in one fell swoop, but when you do add new gear to your collection, look for versions made with any of these body-friendlier options:

- Acid-free cardboard
- Cotton or other natural fibers
- Leather
- Metal
- Rattan or sea grass
- Wood

3 Secrets to Safe Clothing Storage

REMARKABLE REMEDY

While choosing unhealthy materials in which to store your clothes and accessories can have an impact on your health, it can have an even more immediate effect on your duds—not to mention your bank account—when you need to replace the damaged goods. To keep your wearables in tip-top condition, keep these three guidelines in mind:

1. Pass by plastic bags. Moisture will be trapped inside the plastic and can eventually damage the fabric beyond repair. Instead, either invest in garment bags made of breathable material, or make your own dust deterrents from old sheets. Simply cut a hole in the middle for the hanger, and drape the sheet over your clothes.

2. Forget wire hangers. They'll stretch your garments out of shape, or send them slipping off onto the floor, where they then lie in a wrinkled heap.

3. Use acid-free cardboard. The acid found in most cardboard containers will damage anything made of fabric, leather, or paper.

Vexatious Vapors

When it comes to causing bodily harm, the synthetic fabrics in your closet can't hold a candle to the fumes that float from any garments that you've had dry-cleaned. The problem lies in a chemical called perchloroethylene (a.k.a. PCE or PERC). People who are exposed to the stuff, even for brief periods, often experience confusion or dizziness; fatigue; headaches; and irritation of the eyes, lungs, mucous membranes, and skin. Repeated exposure (like that experienced by people who work in dry-cleaning establishments) has been linked to kidney, liver, and central nervous system damage. PERC is also classed as a "possible carcinogen" by the EPA. Here comes the scary part: While some cities and states are beginning to phase out this demon, as of this writing, PERC is still being used by 85 percent of dry cleaners in the country.

The Dastardly "Dry-Clean-Only" Lie

When you see the words *dry-clean only* on a garment label, it's natural to think that if you ignore that admonition, you'll wind up with a wardrobe that would fit a two-year-old. Well, it ain't so, folks! If you follow these guidelines, you can do the job yourself, and your clothes will come out just fine.

Critter-derived fabrics, including alpaca, angora, cashmere, mohair, and wool

- Gently hand-wash in lukewarm (100°F) water with mild soap.

- Rinse in cool water with a teaspoon or so of white vinegar added to it.

- To dry the garment, lay it flat, and stretch it to its original shape and size.

Silk

- Fill a basin with 100° to 120°F water, and mix in a little gentle castile soap, which has a neutral pH.

- Swirl the article around in the soapy water, then rinse with clear, cool H_2O.

- Hang the item up indoors to dry. Never hang silk outdoors because the sun's UV rays can damage it badly.

- Once it's dry, you can hang the garment in a steamy bathroom to smooth out any wrinkles, or iron it on low, using a piece of 100 percent cotton to cover the silk.

Launder with Care

Although most garments made of silk or wool (and its close relatives) can be safely washed by hand, always play it safe: Before you plunge a favorite skirt or blouse into the drink, practice on a few expendable pieces following the techniques in "The Dastardly 'Dry-Clean-Only' Lie" (at left). Also, before you wash any item for the first time, test it for colorfastness by swishing an inconspicuous piece of the fabric in warm water.

Clutter Causes Calamities!

➡ We've all read about compulsive pack rats who died when they were buried under toppled mountains of decades-old newspapers. Well, freak accidents like that are far from the only negative effect of clutter on your health. Conversely, ridding your home of excessive stuff is one of the simplest ways you can give your physical *and* mental well-being a great big boost.

On average, people spend **1 year** of their lives **looking** for lost **stuff**.

CALL 911

Believe it or not, clutter can be a life-threatening situation: You could have so much junk piled up that an EMT crew would have difficulty reaching you in the event of an emergency. Or maybe, like a whole lot of folks, you have to keep your car outside—the garage is so full of stuff, you can't park the vehicle indoors. On some wintry day or night, you may need to hightail it to the ER, or evacuate your home because of a looming disaster. The time you spend scraping ice and snow off your windows—or getting the engine to crank over in the cold air—could easily spell the difference between life and death.

4 Ways Clutter Harms Your Health

There's no doubt that even moderate amounts of clutter can send your stress level soaring sky high (see "Clutter Kills" on page 46). But a junk-filled, disorganized home or office can also take a toll on your physical health. Here are four ways you may be doing your body a big disservice by letting a lot of possessions pile up throughout your home:

1. The more stuff you have lying around, the more handy hiding places you provide for germs of all kinds.

2. The more dust collectors you have, the more exposed you are to the toxins released by PVC and other plastics.

3. All kinds of health aids, ranging from nutritional supplements and must-have medications to your walking shoes and exercise mat, can easily get lost under the piles of clutter you have.

4. A cluttered home can make you embarrassed to invite folks over—so you deprive yourself of stress-busting social interaction.

Clutter Busts Your Bank Account

That, in turn, not only raises your stress level, but also reduces the amount of cash you might spend on health-giving ventures such as a health- or swim-club membership, or active vacations or weekend getaways to (let's say) hike, sail, or ski. Not convinced? Consider these places where your junk may be costing you big bucks:

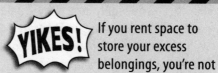

- You eat out frequently because your kitchen is such a mess that you don't want to prepare dinner or pack yourself a lunch.

- You have to keep buying more clothes because you're gaining weight from either too many fast-food meals or clutter-caused stress—or both.

- You're continually buying duplicate stuff—ranging from food and clothes to tools, lightbulbs, and office supplies —because you can't find the ones you have.

YIKES! If you rent space to store your excess belongings, you're not alone: The storage-rental business rakes in about $154 billion a year. That's more than the Hollywood film industry generates! And here's another sobering statistic: One in 11 American households rents a self-storage space at a cost of more than $1,000 a year.

- You're constantly paying late fees because you misplace your checkbook, your bills, or even the stamps to mail them. These penalties will damage your credit rating to boot.

- You have so much stuff that it won't fit in your home, which means that each month you have to shell out rent for a storage locker (or two or three).

Divide and Conquer

If your home is buried in stuff, there's no way you're going to sort it all out in one day—or even one week. And don't even try. If you do, you'll only send your stress level higher than it is already. Instead, start by choosing a single room to focus on. Which one is your call, but from a health standpoint, the bedroom is an excellent option. That's because a clutter-free bedroom will not only provide a peaceful place to start your day and a restful haven at the end of it, but it'll also promote better sleep (and more health-giving sex). Plus, by tackling this important room first, you'll realize just how wonderful de-cluttered surroundings can be, and that will keep you motivated to conquer the rest of the house.

Set a Winning Strategy

A lot of de-cluttering "experts" lay down didactic—and highly unhealthy—rules about what to keep and what to pitch. Well, ignore them. Remember: Your goal is to simplify your life and reduce your stress—not to deprive yourself of treasures you hold dear. For example, if you truly love and appreciate the rich, natural sound of your LP records (as every professional musician I know does), don't let anyone talk you into transferring your collection to digital format and tossing your treasured vinyl in the interest of freeing up shelf space. Instead, follow this golden rule for every item you own: If you need it, use it, or love it, keep it. Otherwise, deal with it according to category 1, 4, or 5 in "Clear the Deck!" (at right).

Start Small

Especially if you're a natural-born pack rat, take that "Divide and Conquer" tip (see page 273) one step further: Begin your de-cluttering campaign with the smallest drawer in your chosen room. Let's say it's your bedroom. Whether your target is the drawer in the nightstand, or the top one in the dresser, it shouldn't take more than 10 or 15 minutes—max— to sort through the contents and put back the stuff that really belongs there. And once you see how neat and orderly it looks, you'll be all fired up to tackle the rest of the room.

Clear the Deck!

As you move from room to room (or from drawer to drawer), make enough space for five boxes (or piles if you prefer). As you grab each item, think carefully, then assign it to one of these categories:

1. Trash

2. Keep Here

3. Elsewhere (see the note below)

4. Donate or Sell

5. Recycle

NOTE: *Bear in mind that some of the things in "Elsewhere" may remain in the current room—but simply not in their current drawers.*

Downsizing without Losing Your Mind

Even if you've relocated many times, moving from larger quarters to smaller ones is never easy. And when the place you're moving out of has been your family's home for decades, downsizing can be a very stressful experience. But don't think of it as casting off generations' worth of cherished possessions. Instead, consider it a golden opportunity to weed out all the extraneous clutter in your life and focus on things that really matter.

It's Never Too Soon to Start

If you and your spouse have decided that you'll move to smaller quarters when you retire in a few years, the time to begin downsizing is now—not a few weeks (or even a few months) before the moving van arrives. Here's why:

- The sooner you start getting rid of things you don't really need or want—or at least deciding what you'll do with them when the time comes—the less you'll have to deal with as moving day approaches. The result: a *big* reduction in your stress level.

- The less stuff you have to pack up and transport, the simpler— and less expensive—your move will be.

- It's a whole lot easier on your physical *and* mental health. Just the thought of clearing out an entire house on a tight deadline can make your whole body ache and your stress hormones hit the stratosphere.

Start High or Low

The best place to begin your weeding-out campaign is the attic or the basement because that's generally where most clutter piles up. And much of it is probably useless junk that you can easily toss. The instant results should spur you on to tackle the rest of your house. If you don't have a basement or an attic, or you're simply not ready to face those areas yet, start in whatever other space meets these two criteria:

1. It contains a lot of items that are being stored rather than displayed or used on a regular basis.

2. For the most part, the contents have little sentimental value.

Insidious Invaders

In earlier chapters, we covered the dangers of things that you intention-ally bring into your home, ranging from the food you eat to the products you clean with, and even the clothes you wear. In these pages, I'll clue you in on some big-time, unintentional troublemakers—living and otherwise—that can put your health, your sanity, and your bank account at high risk.

Invisible Killers in Your Midst

➡ Some of the biggest domestic dangers to your health and well-being are airborne toxins that you can't see—or, in most cases, even smell. Here's the scoop on the most diabolical dirty workers of 'em all.

Speak Up!

Even if you don't use toxic pesticides in your home or yard, poisons used by other folks can sail right in through your windows. Fortu-nately, while you may not be able to stop the spraying, you can cut the amount of the stuff that winds up in your house. If you have neighbors who insist on using this noxious stuff on their lawns, gardens, or farm crops, ask them to alert you before they spray, so you can close your windows and leave them closed for a few days (or longer, if it's windy outside). Likewise, find out if and when your town plans to spray roadsides, parks, or vacant lots near your house. With a little advance warning, you can head off a whole lot of trouble!

5 Horrific Home Crashers

The Environmental Protection Agency (*EPA*) has found DDT and chlordane in homes (see "The Tummy-Turning Truth about Banned Pesticides," at right) and has detected this fistful of still-legal toxins:

Chlorpyrifos is a nerve-blocking agent, formerly sold under the name Dursban®. In 2000, it was banned for residential use, except as bait in contained traps. But it's still permitted—and used extensively—in agriculture, on golf courses, and for control of public health menaces like fire ants.

Cypermethrin is a bug killer classified by the EPA as "moderately toxic." It's used extensively in and around homes, businesses, schools, and nursing homes—and by veterinarians to control external parasites on livestock and pets.

Fipronil, an EPA-labeled "possible carcinogen," is used in ant and roach baits. It's also an active ingredient in many flea and tick treatments, including the highly popular Frontline®.

Permethrin, a "likely human carcinogen," is an ultra-common—and widely advertised—repellent and insecticide for fleas and ticks, as well as mosquitoes, chiggers, and slews of other bugs. In cream form, it's used to treat scabies.

Piperonyl butoxide (PBO) is an ingredient in insecticides galore, including those sprayed on fruits, vegetables, and other crops, as well as products designed to kill fleas, ticks, mosquitoes, and head lice. So far, the EPA still lists it as only "slightly toxic." But that designation could change soon because PBO has been fingered as a potential hormone disrupter, and as of this writing, more testing appears to be on the horizon.

Boot the Horrid Stuff Out!

Your best defense against any pesticide residue that is already in your home is the same as it is for fighting

The Tummy-Turning Truth about Banned Pesticides

Jaw-Dropping **DISCOVERY**

If, like many folks, you think that once a particular pesticide has been banned, you don't need to fret about it anymore, think again. When one of these poisons finds its way into your home—no matter how it got there—the residue hangs on. And on . . . According to a recent report by the EPA, the dust in nearly every one of 500 homes studied contained measurable levels of insecticides, including remnants of compounds such as DDT, which was banned way back in 1970, and chlordane, which was added to the EPA's no-no list in 1983. And here's the *really* scary part: Scientists estimate that "retired" pollutants like these dinosaurs that are, to this very day, still lingering in our air, soil, and water are responsible for nearly half of our increased risk for cancer.

volatile organic compounds (VOCs) and other toxins emitted from household cleaning products:

- Open your windows as often as you can for as long as you can to keep air flowing freely. (Studies have found the quality of indoor air to be anywhere from 2 to 10 times worse than it is outdoors.)

- Vacuum at least twice a week, using a vacuum cleaner that has strong suction and a high-efficiency particulate air (HEPA) filter. Then immediately clean the filter(s) and the tank (or dispose of the bag), so dust isn't spewed back into the air.

- Dust frequently using a damp cloth. Wipe firmly, making sure you pick up all the dust particles. Then rinse the cloth thoroughly, and continue the process.

Don't Drag the Demons through the Door!

On average, an astonishing 85 percent of household dirt is tracked in from outdoors, primarily on your shoes and your pets' paws. And that crud includes just about every kind of noxious substance you can name, from viruses and bacteria to mold spores, pesticides, animal waste, insect eggs, construction debris, and even heavy metals. The list goes on. The good news is that while you can't avoid picking up a little bit of everything from the surfaces you walk on, these three simple ploys will help you keep most of that stuff outside:

Ploy #1. Leave your shoes at the door, and have everyone in your family do the same. What you

> **Pesticides** can **linger** in your home **for decades** after use.

do once you're inside is your call. You can walk around barefoot or in your stocking feet, as many folks like to do, or trade your outdoor footgear for versions you keep for indoor use only. Likewise, you can decide whether to extend the shoes-off demand to visitors, or simply have them comply with Ploy #3 below.

Ploy #2. Wipe your dog's paws thoroughly after every outing, preferably using a glove or mitt that's specially designed for the purpose. (You can find them in pet-supply shops, both online and in brick-and-mortar versions; just do a quick search for "paw cleaning gloves.") And if you know the pup has been walking on a toxic surface—for instance, a lawn that's been treated with pesticides or weed killers—give his paws a soak in a povidone iodine bath (see "Detox the Doggone Paws," at right).

Ploy #3. Invest in a high-quality doormat for every exterior entrance in your home. Make sure it's the kind specially designed to trap and retain dust, dirt, and water. (One brand widely used in health-care facilities and other public buildings is the Waterhog™ line.) Whatever you do, be sure to avoid any of the materials described in "3 Astonishing Doormat Duds" (below).

3 Astonishing Doormat Duds

You might expect that the same natural materials recommended for

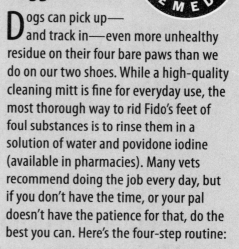

Detox the Doggone Paws

REMARKABLE REMEDY

Dogs can pick up—and track in—even more unhealthy residue on their four bare paws than we do on our two shoes. While a high-quality cleaning mitt is fine for everyday use, the most thorough way to rid Fido's feet of foul substances is to rinse them in a solution of water and povidone iodine (available in pharmacies). Many vets recommend doing the job every day, but if you don't have the time, or your pal doesn't have the patience for that, do the best you can. Here's the four-step routine:

Step 1. Fill a tub, sink, or basin* with just enough lukewarm water to completely cover the dog's foot pads.

Step 2. Add enough povidone iodine to get a solution that's the color of iced tea.

Step 3. Soak the pooch's feet for at least 30 seconds, and preferably from two to five minutes if the soakee will tolerate the procedure for that long.

Step 4. Pat the paws dry—no need to rinse because povidone iodine is organic and nontoxic.

* If your pet refuses to have all four feet submerged at once, mix up the solution in a container big enough to accommodate a single paw, and soak one at a time.

a healthier indoor environment would be just the ticket for grime-grabbing doormats. Not so. In particular, don't let anyone talk you into any of this trio—indoors or out:

Cotton retains moisture like there's no tomorrow, and a damp environment is the ultimate home for germs and mold spores. Plus, cotton mats have little or no traction, so if you don't wipe your feet very gingerly, you could wind up on your fanny.

Fibrous materials—like coir, sea grass, and sisal—do not effectively capture the crud that you're aiming to get off your footgear. In fact, they're infamous for kicking up dust—which defeats the whole purpose of using a doormat.

Metal and wood are trendy mat makings because well-made versions look as classy as all get-out. The problem is that they, and any other hard materials, do next to nothing to rid your shoes of dirt, dust, and grime-laden water.

Multilegged Marauders

➡ Contrary to what some folks would have you believe, bugs can show up in even the cleanest of homes. Most of them are harmless, but a few kinds can cause major trouble. Fortunately, though, you can get rid of them and keep them from coming back without resorting to poisonous chemicals.

Wily Ways to Fence 'Em Out

Regardless of what kinds of troublesome insects ride the range in your neck of the woods, these simple, savvy strategies will help ensure that they don't saunter into your house.

Cockroaches spread 33 types of **bacteria** and 6 kinds of **parasitic worms**.

Outdoors

• Use heavy-duty caulk to seal up exterior entry points, including cracks in or around your home's foundation.

• Push foam insulation snugly into openings around pipes.

- Add weather stripping to all doors and windows, but make sure you don't close up the openings so tightly that toxic odors can't escape (see "Villainous VOCs" on page 259).

- Deter flies and other airborne pests by keeping screens on windows and doors that stay open in warm weather.

Indoors

- Dust or squirt boric acid into all indoor cracks to kill bugs that may be lurking there. Then seal up the openings thoroughly.

- Fill gaps around kitchen countertops with caulk.

Creepy, Crafty Cockroaches

CALL 911

Unlike many insects, cockroaches don't bite or sting, but they can deliver fatal trouble in other ways. If the revolting roaches have ridden into your home, and you suddenly experience symptoms such as abdominal pain, severe stomach cramps and tenderness, diarrhea, nausea, and vomiting, head for the ER. There's a good chance that your unwelcome houseguests have handed you either the *E. coli* or *Salmonella* bacteria, and if one of them spreads to your bloodstream, it can cause a life-threatening infection.

Although cockroaches are most prevalent down south and in densely populated cities like New York, they can show up virtually anywhere. And contrary to what you may think, they are not simply hideous-looking nuisances. Various species of cockroaches have been directly implicated in the spread of 33 types of bacteria, including *E. coli* and *Salmonella*, as well as six kinds of parasitic worms, seven other types of human pathogens, and allergens that can trigger severe asthma attacks—especially in the elderly.

Your five-part elimination strategy:

1. Keep all of your food in airtight containers.

2. Clean up food and drink spills immediately.

3. Thoroughly—and frequently—vacuum any cracks and crevices that you can't seal up.

4. Make sure all of your trash cans have tight lids.

5. Set out baited traps. (It's easy to make your own; see "2 Remarkable Roach Traps" on page 282).

2 Remarkable Roach Traps

Either of these tricks will send cockroaches to their just reward without a trace of toxic residue—and with no risk to children or pets. As with any DIY tactic, you probably won't get immediate results, but whichever method you choose, you should see a dramatic downturn in the offending population within a few days.

- Fill a small jar or old drinking glass with moistened coffee grounds and set it inside a larger bowl that's filled about a quarter of the way with water. Place the trap against a wall in your kitchen or anyplace else where roaches are lingering. The irresistible coffee aroma will lure them to the jar, but before they get there, they'll fall into the water and drown.

- Mix equal parts of sugar and baking soda, and leave small piles of the mixture in kitchen cupboards and any other places roaches might go in search of food (including crumbs) or water. The bugs will be drawn to the sugar, and when they gobble the combo, the baking soda will produce enough gas to kill the varmints.

Hellish Houseflies

Houseflies have been been on the scene for as long as humans have been living in houses—and most likely, before that, the obnoxious buzzers were called caveflies. Unfortunately, these pests do more than simply put a crimp in your summertime peace and quiet. They also carry a gazillion ghastly germs on their feet and in their gut and deposit the makings of who-knows-what diseases on your food, kitchen counters, and elsewhere in your humble abode.

Your first line of defense is outdoors: Make sure your yard is free of favorite fly-breeding places such as pet poop, food scraps, and food wrappings. Keep your garbage cans tightly closed between pickups, and wash them weekly, or at least sprinkle the insides with boric acid, so that any residue the flying felons eat will kill them. Finally, if you make your own compost, use a securely covered bin rather than an open version.

Fabulous Fly Catchers

You can buy commercial flypaper and reusable traps, but it's a snap to make your own. Here's how:

More than **200 bacteria** are known to be **carried by houseflies**.

Don't Give Them a Free Ride

There's no telling what kinds of insect eggs, larvae, or even full-grown bugs may be lurking in furniture or other possessions that have been stored in a basement, garage, shed, or locker. So before you bring anything into your house from any of these places, vacuum the item thoroughly or (depending on the nature of the object) wipe it down with a damp rag. If you're dealing with something that's been kept in a cardboard box, unpack the contents and dispose of the carton before it gets even remotely near your living quarters—or your car. From a bug's point of view, corrugated cardboard is the ultimate in home-construction material.

NOTE: *To play it extra safe, also follow this procedure with whatever fabulous finds you've snagged at yard sales or flea markets. You never know where the stuff may have been residing before you spotted it.*

Flypaper. Mix 1 cup of corn syrup, 1 tablespoon of brown sugar, and 1 tablespoon of white sugar. Cut strips from a brown paper bag, poke a hole in the top of each strip, and put a string through it. Brush the syrup mixture on your strips, and hang them wherever flies are bugging you.

Reusable traps. Grab an empty plastic jug that has a narrow neck. Cut off the top third of the bottle, and toss fruit peels or other food scraps into the bottom part. Invert the top piece and shove it into the bottom portion of the jug so that

Give Pests a Deadly Dusting

REMARKABLE REMEDY

Diatomaceous earth (DE) is one of the best—and safest—substances you can find for eradicating fleas (see "A Down-to-Earth Way to Say, 'Flee, Fleas!,'" at right). And it's just as lethal for plenty of other household pests, including ants and cockroaches, as well as outdoor earwigs, grasshoppers, and slugs. Plus, it's perfectly safe to use around pets and people. But before you rush out and buy a bag, there are two things you need to keep in mind:

▶ Make sure you get DE that's intended for pest-control purposes. The type used in swimming pools has been heat-treated to form crystals, which don't cut the mustard when it comes to killing insects.

▶ Although DE is nontoxic to both humans and pets, it is a fine powder that can irritate your lungs if you breathe it in. So before you use it indoors, make sure there are no fans turned on or breezes blowing through open windows. Outdoors, choose a calm day to dust your troubles away. (In Chapter 12, you'll find the whole nine yards on natural pest control for your lawn and garden.)

it forms a funnel. (Tape the seam if there are any gaps.) The flies will mosey down through the funnel to feast, but they won't be able to get back out. **NOTE:** *If you want to make darn sure they don't survive, sprinkle a little boric acid on the bait.*

A Down-to-Earth Way to Say, "Flee, Fleas!"

The folks who keep such statistics tell us that for every flea lurking on your dog or cat, there are 30 or more in your house. So to solve the problem, you need to do more than simply get rid of the crew that's bugging your pet. You need to make a clean sweep of your home sweet home. Here's how to do just that—without resorting to toxic chemicals, which, besides harming you and your pets, are also fueling the rise of chemical-resistant fleas and other superbugs:

1. Steam clean your carpets to kill any flea eggs.

2. Thoroughly vacuum carpets, bare floors, and furniture at least once a week to pick up eggs, larvae, and pupae. Then immediately wrap the vacuum cleaner bag (or the contents of a bagless tank) tightly in a plastic bag, and toss it into your outdoor garbage can.

3. Wash your pets' bedding in hot, soapy water at least once a week.

4. Sprinkle a light dusting of diatomaceous earth (DE) throughout your house, paying particular attention to areas near your pets' beds;

> **A flea** can live for 90 days, laying **60 eggs per day**.

under your stove, cupboards, and furniture; cracks between walls and baseboards; and similar hiding places. You can even rub DE into your cat's or dog's fur. And keep it up, even after you think all the felons have flown the coop, because hibernating fleas can survive in their cocoons for up to a year without food.

2 Fantastic Flea Traps

No matter what kind of fleas have crashed the gate at your place, these two utterly harmless traps can wipe out a big segment of the adult population:

- Set dishes of soapy water under nightlights in areas where your pet sleeps or tends to hang out. If you don't have a pet, randomly place the traps throughout your house.

- Buy a few lighted electric flea traps (available in hardware stores and online), and put them in strategic places. They work on the premise that fleas are drawn to the light and—bingo!—they wind up on a reusable sticky pad beneath it. Every day, clean off the pad (each one lasts for three to six months), and set the trap back in place. Repeat the process until no more tiny dead bodies appear.

It goes without saying (I hope!) that if some of the fleas in your house are camped out on your dog or cat, you will need to use these traps in conjunction with whatever debugging treatment your vet recommends. Your safest bet: Seek out a naturopathic vet, who can recommend nontoxic remedies for your pal(s).

CALL 911

Although the vast majority of flea bites are merely annoying, in some people, they can trigger anaphylaxis, a potentially life-threatening allergic reaction. If you've been bitten, and you experience general flu-like symptoms, or any of the signs listed below, get medical help immediately:

▶ **Difficulty breathing**

▶ **Dizziness**

▶ **Fever**

▶ **Joint pain**

▶ **Light sensitivity**

▶ **Muscle aches**

▶ **Palpitations**

▶ **Paralysis**

▶ **Severe headache**

▶ **Swollen lymph nodes**

NOTE: *Bites by fleas that are carried by rats or mice are a whole different ball of wax. For the lowdown on those lowlifes, see "Wretched Rodents" on page 292.*

2 Tiny Terrors

A couple of the most common household gate-crashers are completely harmless, but many folks let loose with potent poisons at the first sign of one of the little guys. Well, don't you do it! Instead, do 'em in—or keep 'em out—with these safe and sane maneuvers:

Ants. You can usually keep these bugs at bay simply by storing food in tightly closed containers and immediately cleaning up any spills. Also, consistently wipe down counters, floors, and other surfaces where you've spotted ants. That way, you'll eliminate the scent trails their pals could follow. For good measure, sprinkle cloves, ground cinnamon, or dried mint in entry areas to stop any invaders in their tracks. If the situation gets desperate, mix equal parts of confectioners' sugar and borax with enough water to make a syrup. Pour it into jar lids or shallow disposable pie pans, and set them where the ants are raising a ruckus. (But keep the containers where pets and youngsters can't get at them.)

Fruit flies. The good-riddance method for these guys is simple: Make a fly trap like the one described in "Fabulous Fly Catchers" (see page 283), and bait it with an inch or so of fruit juice, soda pop, or leftover wine. The pesky pests will fly into the drink and drown.

REMARKABLE REMEDY

Stop Ants in Their Tracks

When ants are swarming into your kitchen from a nest outside the house, use this simple trick to stop them before they get anywhere near the door: Put a piece of duct tape over the hole in the bottom of a flowerpot, and set the pot upside down on top of the anthill. When the little fellas emerge from the nest, they'll scramble up the sides of the pot. Then all you have to do is pick it up and dunk it into a bucket of boiling water.

The Hole Truth about Clothes Moths

Although clothes moths can't harm your body in any way, they can put a gaping hole in your bank account when you have to replace your damaged goods. And contrary to what many folks think, these marauders don't confine their egg-laying activity to wool clothing. Any natural-fiber item in your house can become a moth maternity ward. So can furs, down pillows or bedding, pet hair, and even human hair in off-duty wigs or forgotten hairbrushes. Here's how to get rid of them without exposing your family and pets to mothballs or other toxic pesticides:

Cook 'em or freeze 'em. Either soaking infested fabric in hot water (above 120°F) for 20 to 30 minutes or running it through a dryer, set on high, for an hour or so will kill moths and their eggs. So will tucking your clothes into the freezer for three or four days, at a temperature that's below 18°F. The key is dropping the temperature as rapidly as possible, so the emptier the freezer is, the better.

Get 'em on a clean sweep. Thoroughly vacuum every single nook and cranny in closets, dressers, armoires, and upholstered furniture, as well as places where any wall-to-wall carpet meets the baseboard. Then immediately seal up your vacuum cleaner bag, and toss it in the outdoor garbage can.

Iron 'em to death. If you suspect that larvae may be lingering in your carpet, saturate a bath towel with water, wring it out, and spread it out on the rug. Then grab your steam iron, set it on high, and press the towel until it's dry. You don't need to push down hard; the steamy heat will kill the pests.

Trap 'em. Buy some commercial (and perfectly safe) pheromone-baited clothes-moth traps, and hang them throughout the house to catch any culprits your DIY tactics may have missed. Then keep a trap or two hanging in your closet.

Fix-It-Fast FORMULA

Easy Herbal Moth Repellent

You'll love the aroma of this all-natural blend—but moths hate it. Feel free to either cut or multiply the recipe, depending on how many protectors you need to put on guard duty.

1 cup of cedar shavings*
1 cup of dried lavender**
1 cup of dried lemongrass
1 cup of dried peppermint
1 cup of dried rosemary
1 cup of dried tansy
Cheesecloth or muslin sacks

Mix all of the ingredients together in a large bowl. Stuff ¼ to ½ cup of the mixture into each sack, and (if they don't have drawstrings) tie each one closed with twine or ribbon. Then hang them in closets, tuck them into drawers, and set them on shelves or anyplace else you're storing clothes, bedding, or other potential moth targets. The repellents will remain effective for about a year; then you'll need to whip up a new batch (but it's fine to reuse the fabric bags).

Available in hardware stores and most supermarkets.

**All the herbs are available in health-food stores, herbal-supply stores, and online.*

Create a Moth-Resistant Climate

REMARKABLE REMEDY

One of the most effective moth-deterring strategies is to make the living conditions in your closets as uninviting as possible. The mother moths prefer the humidity to be on the high side—between 70 and 80 percent. Your ultra-simple mission: Put a dehumidifier in every place you have clothing stored. You can buy a mini version for less than the cost of an average sweater and a whole lot less than a high-quality wool or cashmere version.

Stay Moth-Free with 4 Savvy Strategies

Once you've gotten rid of the moths in your life—or if you simply want to keep the holey terrors from moving in—develop these four defensive habits:

1. Clean or wash all of your winter *and* summer clothes and linens before you store them away. Moths zero in on anything sporting food or dirt stains, and even body oils that your eyes or nose can't detect.

2. Whenever you buy a piece of clothing or any other natural-fabric item at a resale shop or garage sale, wash it or have it dry-cleaned immediately. Or simply give it some quality time in your dryer or freezer (see "The Hole Truth about Clothes Moths" on page 286).

3. Vacuum your closets, drawers, and other storage areas frequently and thoroughly.

4. Get rid of garments and accessories you no longer wear. The less moth-enticing stuff you have in your closets or drawers, the fewer havens you'll provide for expectant moth mamas.

Beastly Bedbugs

Until not so long ago, most of us thought "Sleep tight, don't let the bedbugs bite" was just a catchy rhyme originating in earlier times, before potent pesticides wiped the buggers out. Well, now we all know that not only are these diminutive demons still around, but they're on a coast-to-coast rampage. The reason is twofold:

A **bedbug** lays up to **10 eggs** per **day**.

• American-born bedbugs that survived the onslaught of now-banned pesticides in the years following World War II have gradually rebuilt their populations.

- Thanks to today's nonstop movement of people and goods around the globe, bedbugs that have never been eradicated in other countries can hitch free rides to here, there, and everywhere—and they're taking full advantage of the opportunity.

Like mosquitoes, bedbugs dine mostly on human blood, and they leave similar-looking welts that itch like crazy. The good news is that although some people do have allergic reactions to the bites, bedbugs do not transmit diseases—at least, according to the Centers for Disease Control and Prevention (CDC), none that we know of yet. The bad news is that the pesticides in use today have very little effect on the beastly buggers.

4 Actions to Bid Bedbugs "Bye-Bye"

While bedbugs cause the most trouble in apartment buildings, where they move readily from one unit to another, they can show up in any home, from a country cottage to a suburban McMansion. If they've come a-calling at your place, follow this four-part good-riddance plan:

1. Get help. Bedbugs are as clever as all get-out, and they're highly creative at finding seemingly unreachable hiding places. They also move at lightning-like speed. So at the first sign of trouble, call an exterminator who uses integrated pest management (IPM) techniques. These pros know where to look for the wily devils, and they will use the least toxic methods possible to

They're Pulling the Green Wool over Your Eyes

Jaw-Dropping DISCOVERY

Stores and websites are doing a brisk business in detergent- and essential-oil-based sprays that are formulated to kill bedbugs safely. Unfortunately, according to a recent study published in the *Journal of Economic Entomology*, these products are a waste of money. The researchers, based at Rutgers University, evaluated 11 brands and found that 9 of them had no effect whatsoever. One type killed more than 90 percent of the nymphs it was used on. Another wiped out just as many nymphs plus 87 percent of the eggs. But here's the clincher: These results were generated in a laboratory setting, where the pesticides were sprayed directly on the targets. In a home, it's extremely difficult to spray anything directly on bedbugs because of their ability to hide in teeny-tiny cracks and crevices to lay their eggs. And when you are able to make direct contact with the enemy, plain old alcohol works fine. It doesn't have any residual power—but neither do any of the pricier commercial concoctions.

actually get rid of them—not merely send them scurrying to other hard-to-reach hidey-holes, as any DIY attempts are likely to do.

2. Go on a cleaning spree. To minimize the amount of pesticides the IPM crew will have to use, give your bedroom a thorough cleaning. Take your bed frame apart, and scrub it with a stiff brush to dislodge eggs. Before you reassemble the frame, clear out everything that was stored under the bed. Clean the items thoroughly, and take them elsewhere (the location is your call, but don't put them anywhere near your bed). Vacuum carpets and furniture, including the inside and underside of each piece. Vacuum and seal cracks in walls and floors that allow the bugs to move from room to room. Wash your bedding in hot water, and dry it on high heat.

3. Seal up your mattress. Online and in many home-furnishing stores, you can buy casings that will kill any bedbugs inside your mattress and box springs and keep their relatives from moving in. If you decide to ditch your infested ones, guard against future invasions by encasing their replacements before you bring them home from the store.

4. Make your bed an island. Move your bed to a spot where no part of it touches a wall, and keep it isolated until you're absolutely certain that all the bedbugs are gone. If you have a bed skirt, remove it, and tuck your sheets and blankets securely under the mattress so they have no contact with the floor.

Order a Suit of Armor

The bedbug stampede has reached such huge proportions that several companies make travel products specifically designed to "fence" the varmints out. So do yourself a favor: Before you hit the road for business or pleasure, do a quick Internet search for "bedbug travel protection." It'll bring up sites that sell luggage liners, laundry bags, pillow encasements, and other protective gear to keep your belongings and your body safe from the little bloodsuckers wherever you may ramble.

Keep Bedbugs at Bay

If you live in a single-family home, it's highly unlikely that bedbugs will simply march into your living quarters—but there is an excellent chance you could pick them up in your travels and cart them back with you. These globe-trotters routinely appear in airplanes, trains, cruise ships, rental cars, and every kind

(continued on page 292)

3 Sinister Spiders

All spiders deliver venomous bites—that's how they subdue their prey. In most cases, a spider bite is merely annoying for humans. But a few kinds can be deadly. If you spot any of this trio, don't even think of going after them yourself—call an exterminator *immediately*. And if you're bitten, hightail to the ER, pronto!

Black widow. This is the deadliest of all American spiders. Males are harmless, but the female injects venom that attacks the central nervous system, and even a small dose can be fatal. Adult females are generally about ½ inch across, with a leg span of approximately 1½ inches. They are shiny black, with a mark on the underside of the abdomen that is usually a red hourglass, but may be a dot ranging in color from yellowish orange to red. They're found throughout the United States. Indoors, they favor sheds and garages, as well as crawl spaces and undisturbed areas of cluttered basements.

Brown recluse. Both genders are aggressive and deadly. Adults are ¼ to ¾ inch long, with a leg span of 1 to 1½ inches. They are light brown, with a darker, violin-shaped marking on the back, just behind the eyes. Young spiders don't have the marking, though, so look for key identifiers: Instead of the eight eyes of a normal spider, these guys have six. Also, the legs are smooth, not spiny or banded. They're found primarily in the South and southern Midwest. They can turn up in any dark, undisturbed place such as heating ducts, cracks and crevices, or stacks of seldom-worn clothes and boxes of junk.

Hobo spiders. Although their venom (delivered by both sexes) is not usually lethal, it can cause trouble ranging from nausea and temporary memory loss to vision impairment. Adults measure ⅓ to ⅔ inch in length, with a leg span of ⅔ to 2 inches, and they have several chevron-shaped markings on the abdomen. Males have two swollen mouth parts, called palpi, that resemble boxing gloves. Females have smaller palpi and a larger, rounder abdomen. Hobos live primarily in the Pacific Northwest and Intermountain West. You'll find them in the basement or at ground level in dark, quiet places.

of lodging from roadside motels to world-famous resorts. There is no way to guarantee you won't encounter the foul things, but following these three guidelines will lessen the chance that they'll use you as a mode of transportation:

- If you're taking off on a cruise, or headed for a specific hotel or resort, call ahead, and ask whether they encase their mattresses.

- While you're on the go, once you've reached your destination, and before you depart for home, keep an eagle eye out for any signs of bedbugs, living or dead, including their molted shells, which will be translucent and bug shaped, and black fecal spots. In hotels, look at mattress seams, the top of the box spring, and behind the headboard.

- When you get back home, or before you get into your car at the airport—but definitely before you cross over your doorstep—inspect your luggage and its contents thoroughly. If you find any multilegged hitchhikers, you may want to simply toss the whole shebang into a trash can rather than carry trouble into your house or vehicle.

Wretched Rodents

➡ Beginning with the 1928 debut of Mickey Mouse in *Steamboat Willie*, mice and rats have played starring or supporting roles in scads of Hollywood movies and TV shows because—let's face it—they are clever, crafty, and just about as comical as critters can get. On-screen, that is. In real life, the devastation these rodents can deliver is anything *but* funny. Each year, they cause millions of dollars in damage to homes all over the country, and they spread some of the most despicable diseases on the planet. In this section, you'll find a roundup of slick—and safe—tricks for protecting your place and your loved ones from the filthy villains.

In **1 year**, 1 pair of **rats** and their offspring **produce 1,500+ youngsters**.

Fire!

According to the CDC, fires and burns are the third-leading cause of fatal home injuries. In many cases, the source of the conflagration is clear, but often the damage is officially attributed to a "fire of unknown origin." Well, statistics suggest that more (possibly *many* more) than one-fifth of those mystery blazes are started by rodents chewing on household wiring or on matches that they've collected and dragged back to their nests.

A Terrifying Tool Kit: 6 Ways Rodents Make You Sick

It doesn't take much to pick up trouble from a rat or mouse. Any of these half-dozen actions can do the trick—sometimes without your knowing a thing about it:

1. Being bitten or scratched by the critter

2. Being bitten by a rodent parasite, like a flea or tick

3. Breathing in dust contaminated with rodent droppings or urine

4. Consuming food or water contaminated with rodent feces or urine

5. Making contact with droppings, urine, or other rodent bodily fluids

6. Touching an infected mouse or rat, living or dead

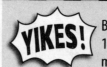

YIKES! Back in the 14th century, millions of people in Europe died from the bubonic plague (a.k.a. black plague or black death). That horrible disease was transmitted by rat-borne fleas, and it still is. Despite all of our sophisticated rodent-control methods, every year, 6 to 12 cases of bubonic plague are reported in New York City alone.

Serve a Dinner of Death

When mice or rats are driving you crazy, mix equal parts of flour and plaster of paris, and spoon the powder into jar lids or similar shallow containers. Add a pinch or two of chocolate cookie crumbs or chocolate drink mix to each one, and stir it in. Then set out the bait where *only* the rodents can get to it (not children or pets), and put a saucer of water nearby. The varmints, being bona fide chocoholics, will gobble up the bait and chase it with a swig of water. That will activate the plaster of paris, which will form a big, hard lump inside the critters' tummies. End of story!

No plaster of paris on hand? Not to worry: Set out out shallow containers of instant mashed potatoes, with a dish of water close at hand. The munchkins will eat, drink, swell up, and die.

8 Steps to Safe Rodent Cleanup

Cleaning up rodent droppings, nesting material, or dead bodies is not a matter to be taken lightly. If the area or the amount of debris is extensive, or if the stuff is inside your home's heating system, vents, or other hard-to-reach places, have a pest-control company do the job. If you opt to tackle the project yourself, wait for seven days after all signs of the critters are gone—for example, if you've seen no fresh damage or droppings, and all your traps have remained clear. Then follow these steps:

Step 1. About an hour before you start, open all doors and windows (with screens in place!) in the area, and turn on fans to provide maximum air circulation.

Step 2. While the airflow is building, dress for the occasion. You'll need long, thick rubber gloves with no tears or holes; a dust mask; disposable shoe covers; and sturdy (preferably expendable) long pants, thick socks, and a long-sleeve shirt.

Step 3. Saturate the crud and surrounding area with either a commercial disinfectant, a mix of 1 part household bleach to 10 parts water, or 3% hydrogen peroxide followed by white vinegar. Wait five minutes for the homemade solutions to work; if you're using a commercial product, follow the instructions.

Step 4. Use paper towels or rags to wipe or pick up the debris, including contaminated material, such as papers, insulation, or cardboard boxes. Put everything into sturdy plastic bags (double bagging any dead rodents), and seal them tightly.

Step 5. Thoroughly clean the area with the solution you used in Step 3, and wipe down any plastic, glass, or metal containers.

Step 6. Put all discards in an outdoor trash can.

Step 7. Disinfect your gloves, and wash your clothes in hot, soapy water—or, better yet, seal up all the items and throw them out. Then hop in the shower and scrub vigorously with hot, soapy water and shampoo your hair.

Step 8. Steam clean or wash any upholstered furniture, carpets, clothes, or bedding where you've found urine or droppings.

CAUTION: *Do not vacuum or sweep up droppings or debris. It will spread the contamination.*

7 Dreadful Diseases Spread by Mice and Rats

If there is any doubt in your mind that a rodent invasion is cause for concern—and fast action—take a gander at the following list of potentially fatal ailments spread by contact with mice or rats (dead or alive) or with their waste products.

- Bubonic plague*
- Hantavirus
- Human taeniasis (a parasitic infection spread by mouse-borne tapeworms)
- Leptospirosis
- Lymphocytic choriomeningitis (LCM)
- Rat-bite (a.k.a. mouse-bite) fever
- Salmonella infection

Bubonic plague is also spread by rat-borne fleas infected with the disease.

2 Types of Trouble Once Removed

Deer mice are notorious for hosting deer ticks, which transmit Lyme disease, but these mostly outdoor pests aren't the only rodent-plaguing parasites that can make you sick. Both mice and rats (primarily urban Norway rats) play host to a flea that transmits murine typhus. While the disease is treatable with antibiotics, it can result in death, most often in the elderly and people whose immune systems are compromised. (You'll find the lowdown on ticks—the deer variety and otherwise—in Chapter 13.)

An adult **rat** can slip **through** a **1/2-inch gap**.

CALL 911

If you live in or are visiting an urban area that has a large rodent population and you're bitten by a flea, don't panic—but do be alert for signs that could indicate serious trouble ahead. If you experience any of the symptoms below, get medical help immediately:

▶ Fever, vomiting, cough, headache, and muscle pain—These could signal a typhus infection.

▶ Fever, severe headache, shaking chills, and swollen, painful lymph nodes—These are typical early symptoms of bubonic plague.

Trapping 101

Folks have been trying for years to build a better mousetrap, but as professional pest controllers will tell you, you still can't beat the

Fix-It-Fast
FORMULA

Ultra-Safe Mouse and Rat Poison

This dilly of a killer formula works on the same principle as the roach poison in "2 Remarkable Roach Traps" (see page 282), but it has a third key ingredient that's especially enticing to rascally rodents.

1 cup of baking soda
1 cup of flour
1 cup of sugar

Mix all of the ingredients in a bowl, and put a tablespoon or so of the mixture into jar lids or similar containers, and set them where you've seen droppings or other signs of rodent visitations. The baking soda will mix with their stomach acids to create carbon dioxide. Because the critters can't burp, their tummies will swell up and squash their lungs.

old-fashioned snap trap. But to get the very best results, you need to stage a full-scale blitz. Rather than setting out a few traps each night over a period of time, invest in as many as your budget will allow, and set them out all at once. Mice normally travel close to walls, so put plenty of traps along those routes and any places where you've seen evidence of mice. Repeat the process until your bait has no more takers. And speaking of bait, this trio is tops:

• Chunky peanut butter
• Cucumber pieces with the rind left on
• Dryer lint (The tiny tykes covet the soft, fluffy stuff as nest-building material.)

3 Ways to Dodge Rampaging Rodents

Mice and rats are a determined bunch, and it can take some fancy footwork to keep them out of your abode. In some cases, it may take help from a pest-control pro, but here's the basic routine:

Close the restaurant. Put your cleaning routine on steroids. Even a few stray cookie crumbs in the space between a counter and your fridge can bring mice running from near and far (along with rats, if they're in the neighborhood). And pet food, wild bird food, and even cardboard boxes are all gourmet chow, rodent style. Ditto plant seeds and even organic mulches and fertilizer that you may have in your garage or shed. Seal all of these potential menu items in solid containers—not bags. Sturdy plastic bins or tubs will usually keep mice out, but rats will chew right through them. Only metal will deter these gluttons.

A **mouse** can get **through** a **1/4-inch opening**.

Reduce the nearby habitat. The less enticing you make the area next to your house, the less likely it is that mice and rats will venture close enough to break inside. Trim trees and shrubs so they don't make contact with your walls. Clean up leaves, brush piles, and other debris that provides shelter. Keep compost bins and garbage cans tightly closed. If you have a woodpile, site it as far away from your house as your yard size and climate allow. (The standard recommendation is 100 feet, but in a tiny yard or a far-north location, that might not work for you.)

Seal up all openings. And I do mean *all*. The average mouse can jump 18 inches and squeeze through a space as small as ¼ inch across. Rats often jump 4 feet or more and can get through a ½-inch gap. And both imps can climb up just about any kind of surface. (For the simple closing procedure, see "Bar the Door on Mice and Rats," below.)

Bar the Door on Mice and Rats

The most effective way to close potential rodent entry "doors" depends on the size of the opening. Here's the rundown:

Holes less than 3 inches in diameter. For a quick but temporary fix, tightly pack steel wool, wire screening, or copper gauze into the opening. (Beware, though, that steel wool may leave rust stains, so if you must go that route, replace it with another material as soon as you can.) For permanent protection, mix a quick-drying patching plaster or similar anchoring material into a wad of

(continued on page 299)

It's Not a Job for Fluffy

If you're a current or former cat owner, you can ignore this not-news-to-you tip. But if you've got rodents in the house, you've never had a cat before, and you're thinking of enlisting one to help solve the problem, take my advice: Don't bank on this strategy. In the first place, contrary to folklore, not all cats are mousers. I have known quite a few that would simply sit there and watch in amusement as rodents romped around the room. Second, many of the cats that do catch mice have an, um, disconcerting habit of proudly laying the quarry on their owners' pillows in the middle of the night. As for rats, a deter-mined adult can actually kill the average house cat. Finally, cats (and other pets) can pick up the same rodent-transmitted diseases that you can—and in some cases, pass them on to you.

Bats in the Belfry

Because they eat so many insects, bats do a lot more good than harm—outdoors, that is. Indoors it's a whole different ball game. The danger lies not so much in rabies, which they can (but don't often) transmit. Rather, the problem is histoplasmosis, a respiratory disease you can catch if you inhale fungal spores found in bat droppings. It is not contagious, and in many cases the flu-like symptoms are quite mild. But histoplasmosis can be serious for the elderly, people with compromised immune systems, and (surprise!) smokers. It can lead to a chronic illness resembling tuberculosis, and left untreated, can even be fatal.

Terrible Trouble Ahead?

As you might expect, people who are exposed to bat droppings on a regular basis, such as roofers, HVAC contractors, and chimney sweeps, are at far higher risk for histoplasmosis than the average homeowner whose home has recently been invaded by bats. Still, don't take chances. If you think you've been exposed, and any of the symptoms listed below set in about 10 days later, call your doctor:

- Chest pain
- Dry cough
- Fever
- Headache
- Impaired vision
- Loss of appetite
- Muscle or joint pain
- Shortness of breath

Your Anti-Bat Action Plan

First, don't panic! Call a local wildlife-control professional who can safely and legally relocate your unwelcome houseguests. Not only can this process be physically risky for untrained amateurs, but a slipup could also land you in legal trouble because many states have strict laws against harming bats in any way. Once the gang is gone, depending on the nature of your home's construction, the location of any openings, and your handiness with tools, you may be able to rig up your barriers to prevent further trouble. The contractor you hire can advise you on that score, too.

copper gauze before shoving it into the hole. Then smooth more plaster over the outside.

Holes 3 inches or more in diameter. Fit sturdy, ¼-inch woven, welded hardware cloth into the gap. Then fill the opening with a high-quality patching compound. You can also buy a commercial-grade, galvanized steel product called Strong Patch®. It has an adhesive backing and roughed-up mesh on the surface, allowing for better adhesion of the patching compound, and it comes in various sized squares.

Trouble in the Air

➡ Pesticide residue isn't the only airborne menace posing a major threat to your health. In this section, we'll talk about some potentially deadly (and invisible) substances that may be floating through the air in your house.

Radon: The Stealthiest Intruder of All

Unlike most of the dangerous substances we've been discussing in this book, radon is not produced as, or used in, any commercial products. Nor is it a living organism that you can kill or repel. Rather, it is a naturally occurring gas that comes from the breakdown of uranium in soil, rock, and water, and it's the second-leading cause of lung cancer in the United States. You cannot see, smell, or taste radon, so unlike the number one cause of lung cancer (we all know what that is!), this menace could be doing you in, and you won't have a clue. Radon typically moves up through the ground into the air, and then into your home. What's more, any house—old or new, well sealed or drafty, with or without a basement, in any part of the country—can have radon trapped inside. The only way you can rest easy is if you live at least three stories above ground level.

Radon causes at least **21,000 cancer deaths** per year.

3 Fiendishly Frightful Facts about Radon

Radon levels are measured in picocuries per liter, or pCi/L, and the EPA considers 4 pCi/L to be in the high danger zone. If that single-digit figure doesn't sound very dramatic, consider these three petrifying particulars:

1. If your home has radon levels of 4 pCi/L, you and your family are exposed to about 35 times as much radiation as the Nuclear Regulatory Commission allows at the fence of a radioactive-waste site.

Radon is the **#2 cause** of **lung cancer**.

2. At the 4 pCi/L level, radon carries roughly 1,000 times the risk of death as any other EPA-designated carcinogen.

3. Nationwide, at least 1 in 15 American homes has a radon level above 4 pCi/L, but that's only the average figure. In many parts of the country, the number is 1 in 3 or higher. At www.EPA.gov, you can find a map that will show you where your home county ranks.

The Ultra-Simple Way to Cut Your Radon Risk

If you glance at the EPA radon map and see that you live smack in the middle of a county shown in red (which denotes the highest levels), don't panic. Conversely, if your home ground is yellow (the lowest on the scale), don't think you can just sit back and rest easy. Remember: These survey numbers are county-wide averages. The amount of radon coming out of the ground varies greatly within very small areas—even between houses that are right next door to each other. So do yourself a favor, and test your house. Many home-improvement stores and websites sell DIY kits, complete with simple instructions for setting up the measuring device and where to send it to get your reading. After that, your action plan depends on the numbers, but no matter what they are, a qualified contractor can help you get them down to a safer level. Your official state radon contact can point you to a pro in your area (see www.EPA.gov for those details).

 Unlike living pests and most airborne toxins, radon does not depend solely on cracks and crevices as entry points to your home. Because it is a single-atom gas, it easily penetrates common building materials such as Sheetrock®, concrete block, mortar, tar paper, wood paneling, and insulation, as well as most paints, paper, leather, and even some low-density plastics (like the kind used for plastic bags).

Carbon Monoxide: A Silent Killer

Carbon monoxide (a.k.a. CO) is a prime example of the fact that a "natural" substance is not necessarily good for you. Just in case you don't remember the details from high school chemistry class, CO is an odorless, colorless gas formed during the incomplete combustion of organic substances, ranging from dead leaves to fossil fuels. And it can kill you, or any other living organism, because it interferes with the normal intake of life-giving oxygen.

In large doses, CO is a quick and highly efficient killer (which is the reason a running car in a closed garage is such a common venue for suicide). And inhalation of CO-laden smoke is the most common cause of death in house fires. Lower concentrations of the gas can cause flu-like symptoms that are easy to ignore until it's too late (see "Is It the Flu or CO?" on page 302).

Common Sources of CO Poisoning

Aside from motor vehicles and fires, any of this bunch can also emit dangerous levels of the demonic gas:

- Camp stoves and charcoal grills
- Fireplaces and woodstoves
- Gas clothes dryers, cooking stoves, furnaces, and water heaters
- Gas furnaces
- Gas- and kerosene-fueled space heaters
- Lawn mowers
- Portable generators
- Power tools that have internal combustion engines

Back Up with Caution

Jaw-Dropping DISCOVERY

Each year, more and more folks are buying portable generators as backup power sources so they can keep their homes functioning on an even keel during outages. Well, that domestic comfort comes with a potentially huge price tag: These devices can produce carbon monoxide (CO) levels several hundred times higher than those emitted by modern car exhaust. Those fumes can kill people in no time flat, and they do so frequently. According to the U.S. Consumer Product Safety Commission (CPSC), since 1999, the number of generator-related CO deaths has increased more than 1,000 percent. The sobering takeaway: *Never* use a portable gas-powered generator indoors or in your garage! The CDC recommends keeping portable generators at least 25 feet away from and downwind of your house.

10 Clues That You May Have a CO Problem

If you have a leak in your gas furnace or incoming gas lines, you'll know it immediately because natural gas used in heating systems is treated to emit a somewhat skunk-like aroma. But any of the following signs could also indicate trouble:

CALL 911

The signs of carbon monoxide poisoning may seem mild, but the condition is a life-threatening emergency. If you or anyone you're with experiences any of the symptoms below after exposure to CO, get medical help immediately:

▶ **Blurred vision**

▶ **Confusion**

▶ **Dizziness**

▶ **Dull headache**

▶ **Loss of consciousness**

▶ **Nausea or vomiting**

▶ **Shortness of breath**

▶ **Weakness**

Streaks of soot around fuel-burning appliances

Orange or yellow flames, rather than blue ones, in your furnace, oven, or other combustion appliances

Excessive rust on appliance jacks, flue pipes, vent pipes, or other piping connections

Excess moisture on windows, walls, or other cold surfaces

Lack of an upward draft in your chimney

Fallen soot in your fireplace

Small quantities of water leaking from the base of your chimney vent or flue pipe

Discolored or damaged bricks at the top of your chimney

A general smoky smell that hasn't set off your smoke alarm(s)

Flu symptoms when you don't have the flu (See "Is It the Flu or CO?," below.)

Is It the Flu or CO?

CO poisoning in homes most often occurs during the flu season—for the simple reason that it's the time when most folks are turning on their furnaces, snuggling down by their cozy fireplaces, and generally spending more time indoors trying to keep warm. Fortunately, there are some simple ways to tell

CO poisoning **kills 2,000+** people each year.

whether you've got the yearly bug, or something that could be far worse. Suspect CO poisoning—and get help quickly—in any of (or more likely a combination of) these seven instances:

1. Several people in your home fall sick at the same time.

2. You feel better when you're away from your home.

3. Your symptoms appear or worsen shortly after you turn on a fuel-burning device (like your gas furnace, fireplace, or oven).

4. Your pets have symptoms similar to yours.

5. You don't have a fever or the all-over achiness typical of a flu virus.

6. Symptoms appear at the same time as indications of a CO leak (see "10 Clues That You May Have a CO Problem," at left).

7. The people who are most affected are the ones who spend the most time indoors.

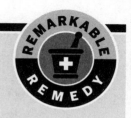

Common Sense Counteracts Catastrophes

The secret to preventing CO tragedies boils down to a few simple measures: Properly vent and maintain all fuel-burning appliances. Have your furnace checked by a qualified heating contractor every year. Use your devices properly—for example, never cook with a barbecue grill in any enclosed space, and don't try to heat your house with an oven that's designed for cooking. Last but not least, install and maintain CO alarms in your home. You can find them in virtually all home-improvement stores. Make sure the ones you buy conform to the latest Underwriters Laboratories (UL) standards, and follow the manufacturer's instructions for placement and operation. Also, change the batteries once a year, or as stipulated in the product instructions.

The Surprising Truth about Asbestos

Common assumption: If there is any asbestos in your house, you need to get it outta there *yesterday*!

THE FACTS: While it is true that asbestos can cause major health problems, including lung cancer, the damage occurs only when you inhale the fibers over an extended period of time. (The vast majority of people who have contracted asbestos-related diseases have worked for years in factories, shipyards, and other places where the tiny, sharp particles filled the air all day long.) If you've recently bought an older house that has now-banned asbestos insulation—especially if it's covered up by plaster or drywall—getting rid of it could actually cause a lot more harm than good because the removal process would release the fibers into the air and send them flying.

THE BOTTOM LINE: If you know or suspect there is asbestos in your home, or one that you're about to acquire, definitely have a reputable contractor perform a thorough inspection and take whatever mitigating steps are deemed necessary. But don't insist that the stuff be removed—and whatever you do, don't try any DIY tricks!

2 Simple Steps to Controlling Mold and Mildew

We've all heard about the dangers that lead paint and asbestos can present in older homes. But mold and mildew can raise a royal ruckus in even the newest construction, and we're learning more about how perilous these fungi can be when they get into the air in your home. The worst by far is toxic (a.k.a. black) mold. But exposure to any form of mold or mildew can compromise your immune system and bring on allergic reactions or flu-like symptoms. Over the long haul, it may lead to chronic respiratory infections, liver disease, and cancer. If the foul fungi have moved into your place, here's your game plan:

Step 1. If you find mold or mildew on porous materials such as wallboard, carpets, or insulation, remove, discard, and replace them immediately (or have a pro do the job).

Step 2. To clean nonporous surfaces such as pipes, ceramic tile, and bathroom fixtures, use either straight white vinegar or a solution made from ¾ cup of household bleach per gallon of water. Open up as many windows as possible throughout your house, and (especially in the bathroom) keep the fan running. Also, clean all shower and tub drains using the formula in "Cut Those Clogs" (see page 254).

Great Grimy Grout Cleaner

REMARKABLE REMEDY

To get stubborn mold or mildew out of the grout between ceramic tiles, soak three or four paper towels in white vinegar, and lay them over the grout. Press the towels firmly to ensure full contact, and leave them in place for about eight hours. If the paper begins to dry out, spray or splash it with more vinegar to keep it saturated. When time's up, remove the towels, and use an old toothbrush to scrub away any remaining crud. Then rinse with cool, clear water.

An Unseen Danger

One of the biggest risks to your and your family's well-being is not anything that may come into your home but, rather, something you've banished from it—that is, if you're like a lot of folks these days. What is it? A traditional landline telephone. Don't get me wrong! I know a cell phone is a mighty handy thing to have, especially when you're traveling. But relying on one of these gadgets as your only way of contacting the outside world can literally endanger your life. If that statement sounds extreme, consider these two "adventures" that actually happened to good friends of mine (let's call them Bob and Mary).

True story #1. Bob took off for work as usual one rainy morning. His wife and kids had already left. A short way down the road, he realized he'd forgotten some papers he needed for a meeting. He hightailed it back home and leaped out of his car, leaving his cell phone on the seat. As he dashed toward the kitchen door, his feet picked up some wet leaves, which he didn't even notice. When he got inside, still moving fast, he slipped on the terra-cotta tile floor, came crashing down, and (he later learned) broke his hip. Somehow, he managed to drag himself to the wall-hung telephone, knock the receiver off, and dial 911. Had there been no phone, he'd have lain there in agony until someone came home many hours later.

True story #2. Mary went to bed early one evening, hoping to fend off a cold that she felt coming on. Her cell phone was in her purse downstairs. A short time later, she was awakened by a crashing sound at her front door, followed by footsteps moving up the stairs toward her bedroom. She leaped to her feet, leaned against the door, and dialed 911 on her bedside phone. The dispatcher immediately signaled for a cruiser and told Mary to stay on the line and keep talking. The footsteps kept coming, and a man bashed against the door with a crowbar, hurling Mary into the room. Still holding the phone, she shouted, "You better get out of here! The cops are on the way!" Suddenly, a siren wailed outside, and the intruder ran off. If that phone hadn't been there . . .

Chapter 12

Pretty . . . but Perilous

Throughout this book, we've talked about the ways that noxious chemicals are making us sick—or worse—and I've laid out some dynamic strategies for minimizing their impact on your life. In this chapter, we'll take aim at the toxic territory just outside your door (a.k.a. your yard). Now, this is not a gardening book, so you won't find instructions on growing plants of any kind. But you will discover some terrific tips, tricks, and tonics to help you fight off pests and diseases and keep your lawn, flowers, and woody plants at the peak of health without using chemicals that may be hazardous to yours!

Lush but Lethal Lawns

➡ As an American icon, the lawn ranks right up there with Mom, baseball, and apple pie. It's the quintessential playground, where we watch our children take their first steps, romp with our dogs, and host neighborhood barbecues, among other things. And each year, it's the recipient of millions of tons of highly toxic weed killers, bug killers, and manmade fertilizers. But here's the good news: You can pitch those poisons and still keep that beloved turf green, thick, and weed-free, for less money than you'd spend on a "conventional" lawn-care regimen.

Your Lawn's Deadly Diet

Every time you turn around, you hear about another scientific study confirming the diabolical dangers of chemical pesticides, and we've talked about many of them in earlier chapters. But what you don't hear quite so much about is the fact that the ultra-potent ingredients in nonorganic fertilizers can also cause major health problems, both directly and as a result of running off into our groundwater and open waterways. To add insult to injury, studies have shown that, contrary to marketing hype, some of these souped-up nutrients aren't exactly doing wonders for your lawn—in fact, they can actually hinder plant growth.

4 Frightening Facts about Chemical Lawn Foods

Here's a creepy quartet of reasons that you'll be doing yourself, your family, and everyone else on the planet a big favor if you trade those pseudo-foods for a healthier natural diet for your lawn—and all of the other plants in your yard.

1. The nitrogen in chemical fertilizers (identified as N on the package label) is generally processed from ammonia, which is far from the mildest stuff on the planet.

What's much worse, though, is that to make slow-release lawn fertilizers, the folks in the factory mix ammonia with urea and formaldehyde, or they encase it in sulfur or a synthesized polymer— some of which are being fingered as possible endocrine disrupters and carcinogens. And all of that crud gets tracked into your house on the shoes (or paws) of anyone who has walked on chemically fertilized turf. (For some dynamic damage-control tactics, see "Don't Drag the Demons through the Door!" on page 278.)

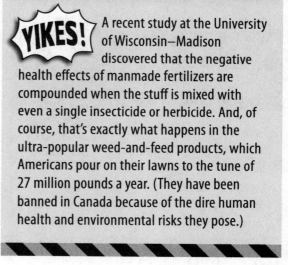

YIKES! A recent study at the University of Wisconsin–Madison discovered that the negative health effects of manmade fertilizers are compounded when the stuff is mixed with even a single insecticide or herbicide. And, of course, that's exactly what happens in the ultra-popular weed-and-feed products, which Americans pour on their lawns to the tune of 27 million pounds a year. (They have been banned in Canada because of the dire human health and environmental risks they pose.)

2. Studies have shown that airborne and waterborne nitrogen from fertilizers may cause respiratory ailments, cardiac disease, and even several types of cancer.

3. The runoff from the phosphorus in manmade fertilizers contains toxic heavy metals, fluoride, radon, and other radioactive components. And it all goes into your drinking water and the drinking water of any livestock you might eat—not to mention the water that fish live in.

4. On top of all that, besides wrecking your health, using synthetic lawn fertilizer isn't doing your grass any favors. Many of these chemical cocktails supply only nitrogen (N), phosphorus (P), and potassium (K). But they actually *deplete* the other nutrients and minerals that are naturally found in truly fertile soil—and that all plants, including turfgrasses, need to grow strong and healthy enough to fend off pests and diseases.

Ditch the Dreadful Runoff

Even if you don't use a speck of chemical fertilizer in your yard, the stuff can still cause torrential trouble if it runs off into your soil from your neighbors' lawns or—worse—an adjacent golf course or nonorganic farm field. Fortunately, there's an easy way to solve the problem. Just dig a ditch about 12 inches wide and 6 inches deep between your turf and the adjacent territory. Line it with woven landscape cloth. (Don't use plastic of any kind because water must be able to drain through the material.) Then fill the trench with gravel. Use a decorative version if you're concerned that a bare-bones-basic barrier may not be a welcome sight in your neighborhood.

Fertilizer Can Give You the Blues—Literally!

Jaw-Dropping DISCOVERY

Excessive use of synthetic high-nitrogen fertilizers has been linked to methemoglobinemia, a blood disorder that damages hemoglobin, the oxygen-carrying molecule found in blood cells. When this frequently fatal condition occurs in infants, it's known as "blue baby syndrome" because it turns their skin blue as it starves their body tissues of life-giving oxygen. But babies aren't the only victims of this tongue-twisting and potentially fatal condition. It can also strike adults, with the same gruesome results.

2 Safer Ways to Feed Your Lawn

There are plenty of organic lawn fertilizers on the market that will enable you to maintain a great-looking lawn without putting your health at risk—or your family's.

But you can accomplish the same feat in either of these simple (and cheaper) ways:

• Use my Super-Safe Lawn Fertilizer recipe (at right).

• Spread a layer of top-quality compost across the turf twice a year, in the spring and again in the fall. If you want to try this approach, you'll need a minimum of 50 pounds of compost for each 1,000 square feet of lawn area. As for the maximum, well, the sky's the limit—there's no such thing as an overdose of black gold! You can buy compost at any good garden center, and most likely that's what you'll want to do if you have even an average-size lawn. But if your grassy area is tiny, and you prefer the DIY approach, you can make your own supply following the simple instructions in "The Phenomenal Feats of Compost" (see page 323).

A Bonus Benefit of Banishing Chemical Fertilizers

Believe it or not, simply by leaving the grass clippings in place when you mow your lawn, you can supply up to half the nitrogen your grass needs—without spending a dime! Of course, there is one catch: This trick works only if you don't use nasty chemical fertilizer on your turf. Studies have proven that because these potent formulas kill off significant numbers of underground organisms (including earthworms, good fungi, and beneficial bacteria) that break down organic matter, they stall the decomposition of the grass blades.

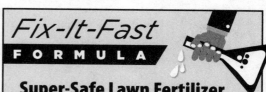

Fix-It-Fast
FORMULA

Super-Safe Lawn Fertilizer

This easier-than-pie recipe will provide all the nutrients your turf needs, with none of the dangers of synthetic lawn foods.

2 parts alfalfa meal

1 part bonemeal

1 part wood ashes

Mix all of the ingredients together, and apply the mixture at a rate of 25 pounds per 1,000 square feet of lawn area first thing in the spring, and again last thing in the fall. Then watch your grass grow green and healthy—and your neighbors grow green with envy!

Go Cold Turkey on Toxins

In Chapter 4, I clued you in on the horrors of chemical pesticides in the foods we eat, but the amount of poisons used by farmers is small potatoes compared to the load that homeowners pour onto their yards. Statistics show that each year, up to 90 million pounds of insecticides, herbicides, and fungicides are applied to lawns in the United States. Acre for acre, that's more than 10 times the amount used on American farmland. The good news is, while you have no control over the way agribusinesses deal with their trouble-makers, you can eliminate toxins in your yard in one of two ways:

1. If you do your own turf tending, simply use the safe, natural methods (coming up in this chapter) to get rid of both bad bugs and destructive weeds.

2. If you let a lawn-care company handle the chores (as upwards of 30 million households do), and they're using chemical pesticides and/or fertilizers, switch to an all-organic outfit. There are more and more springing up all across the country, so search online for a company near you.

The Lethal Lawn-Care Snow Job

In their quest to keep up with the Joneses—or simply to take the least-possible-effort approach to maintaining a lawn that comes up to snuff in suburbia—a whole lot of folks are in denial about the true danger of the products they're using. Here are some of the major misconceptions out there:

Misconception #1: Once lawn chemicals have dried—and those little warning flags are taken away—it's safe to romp and play on the grass.
THE TRUTH: Those sinister substances can continue to release toxic vapors for anywhere from 30 days to more than a year

Talk about sobering statistics! Scientists have studied the health risks of the 30 most commonly used lawn pesticides, and when the numbers were crunched, here's how the products stacked up:

▶ 26 of them were linked to kidney or liver damage

▶ 21 to reproductive problems

▶ 19 to cancer

▶ 15 to nerve damage

▶ 13 to birth defects

▶ 11 to hormonal disruption

On top of that direct damage, humans suffer indirect consequences of these poisons because 23 leach into drinking water, 17 are present in groundwater, 24 are toxic to fish and other aquatic organisms that are vital to maintaining our ecosystem (or that we eat!), 16 are toxic to birds, and 11 are toxic to bees—and we need both birds and bees to pollinate our food crops.

after they've been applied. Plus, while children and pets are most susceptible to the poisons, you don't have to get down and roll on the turf, as they do, to suffer dire consequences. Just mowing or walking on contaminated grass, picking up a dropped toy (or golf tee), or even breathing in fumes that drift from neighbors' yards can make you sick.

Misconception #2: If a product is allowed on the market, then it must be safe.

THE TRUTH: The Environmental Protection Agency (EPA) makes no attempt—and no claims—to keep harmful pesticides from being sold. In fact, it is a violation of federal law to use terms like *safe*, *harmless*, or *nontoxic to humans or pets* on any pesticide label. The vast majority of insecticides and herbicides on the market today have not even been tested for their effects on anyone's health or safety. The simple solution: Don't rely on the government to protect you—use your own common sense!

Misconception #3: If a pesticide has been banned, it can't possibly hurt me now.

THE TRUTH: For one thing, pesticide residue can linger for years in the soil and water, and even longer when it's tracked indoors (see "Invisible Killers in Your Midst" on page 276). What's more—and this is really sobering, friends— even after a product has been removed from store shelves, you can bet your bottom dollar that it's still causing trouble. A case in point: Diazinon, one of the deadliest toxins of all, has been banned for use on residential lawns,

---

Why Your Doc Doesn't Diagnose Pesticide Poisoning

Jaw-Dropping DISCOVERY

If you've been exposed to pesticides, and you're having any of the classic telltale symptoms (see "Poisonous Words to the Wise" on page 312), don't be surprised if your doctor tells you that it's all in your head. In the first place, pesticide manufacturers are not required to release any health-related information to health-care professionals. Nor do medical schools include lawn-care dangers in their students' curricula. But perhaps more to the point, doctors who make a diagnosis of pesticide poisoning (which is all but impossible to prove beyond a shadow of a doubt) leave themselves wide open to lawsuits by the big chemical companies. And those proceedings could destroy their careers—and, therefore, their ability to perform their life-giving mission—in the blink of an eye!

---

golf courses, and sod farms; but it's perfectly okay for anyone who has a supply on hand to use it. (Can you say "stockpile"?) And pest-control professionals are still permitted to use diazinon in "extreme situations," whatever the heck that means!

Poisonous Words to the Wise

Aside from the infamous diazinon (see "The Lethal Lawn-Care Snow Job" on page 310), currently used poisons such as 2,4-D, Sevin®, MCPP, dicamba, and Roundup® (a.ka. glyphosate) stand ready to provide you with a pristine green lawn while potentially destroying your, your family's, and your neighbors' health. Pesticide poisoning can be the very dickens to diagnose because the symptoms mimic those of many other illnesses. But if you or a loved one has been exposed to lawn chemicals, and you experience any of the following signs with no other reasonable cause, get help *fast!*

- Asthma-like attacks
- Burning skin or ears
- Coughing
- Cramps
- Diarrhea
- Dizziness
- Excessive sweating or salivation
- Extreme depression
- Eye pain; blurred or dim vision
- Fever
- Numbness or tingling in hands or feet
- Sleep disturbances
- Sore nose, tongue, or throat
- Unexplained fever

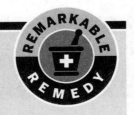

A Marvelous Milky Grub Destroyer

If grubs are demolishing your lawn, and their parents are trashing your flowers, shrubs, or vegetables, milky spore powder can save the day. It's a combination insecticide that consists of two bacteria, *Bacillus popilliae* and *B. lentimorbus*. Its big, and well-deserved, claim to fame is that it kills the grubs of Japanese beetles and several of their relatives, without doing a speck of harm to any other living things. This stuff doesn't come cheap, but if you've got a major problem on your hands, I say go for it—you'll be glad you did! You can find milky spore powder online and in many garden centers.

Know the Enemy

Destructive insects zero in on different parts of a grass plant, and the location of the damage gives you a good clue to the type of troublemaker you're dealing with—and, therefore, the best ways to send the pests packin' safely. Here's a roster of the perps that most often target turfgrass, and what's on the menu for each type:

Blades: Aphids, billbugs, chinch bugs, mites, scale

Crowns: Armyworms, cutworms, sod webworms

Roots: Mole crickets, pearl scale, white grubs

Two Terrific Tiny Hit Men

One of the safest, simplest ways to end your lawn-pest problems is to enlist a squad of either beneficial nematodes or Bt (*Bacillus thuringiensis*)—or both, depending on the nature of your turf's attackers. These organisms are deadly to destructive insects, but harmless to all other living things. You can find them in many garden centers and (of course) online. Bear in mind, though, that there are different species of nematodes and Bt, and it's crucial to get the one that's been bred to tackle your particular pests. You also need to launch the attack in exactly the right way at exactly the right time. The catalog description or package label should give you all those details, but here's how to figure out which general type of mini hero you need:

Beneficial nematodes are almost-microscopic critters that demolish amyworms, beetle grubs, cutworms, mole crickets, and sod webworms.

Bt is a beneficial bacterium that kills pests galore, but almost no beneficial insects. The prime lawn hit list includes armyworms, billbug larvae, mole crickets, and sod webworms. But there is one downside: Bt can't tell butterfly larvae from destructive caterpillars—so use it with caution.

5 Surprising Lawn Heroes

Simply by encouraging beneficial insects to set up housekeeping in your yard, you can polish off passels of insect pests without using a single drop of insecticide (be it chemical or otherwise). The handful of hungry helpers below all have huge appetites for some of the most common—and destructive—turfgrass terrors. You'll find the basic welcoming guidelines for these and other useful predators in "Deputize a Pest-Control Posse" (see page 314).

Assassin bugs go gunnin' for aphids, armyworms, beetles (a.k.a. grubs' parents), mole crickets, and sod webworms.

Big-eyed bugs hanker for aphids, armyworms, chinch bugs, and sod webworms.

Ground beetles gobble up ants, aphids, armyworms, cutworms, grubs, mites, and mole crickets.

Ladybugs love aphids, chinch bug larvae, mites, and scale.

Spined soldier beetles go bonkers for sod webworms.

Deputize a Pest-Control Posse

If you're using chemical pesticides in your yard because you're afraid that insects will destroy your lawn and gardens, I have one word to say to that notion: Hogwash! If you quit cold turkey, throngs of beneficial insects will show up and start devouring the plant trashers. Some of your most prolific allies are assassin bugs, ground beetles, minute pirate bugs, and—of course—ladybugs. These pest-control workers will quickly find their way to any flowers that are rich in pollen and nectar. But the secret to keeping them on the job is to follow this three-point plan:

1. Provide water. Just sink plant saucers into the ground, set some pebbles inside (letting some of the stones show above the surface), and pour in the H_2O.

2. Mix it up. The more kinds of plants you have, and the more menu and shelter options you provide, the more kinds of helpers you'll attract—and the more kinds of pests they'll polish off. It's especially important to plant a mixture of flowers so that *something* is in bloom throughout the growing season. You'll attract a variety of insects.

3. Go native. To enlist a first-class dream team, look for plants (especially trees and shrubs) that are native to your area. Local heroes will flock to your doorstep!

Beyond Beneficial Bugs

Many animals feast on destructive insects, but bats and toads have truly monumental appetites for "bad" bugs. Here's why:

- Every night, a single adult bat eats as many as 1,200 insects an hour, including mosquitoes, beetles, and the flying (and egg-laying) forms of cutworms, cabbage worms, and corn earworms. You can order ready-made houses from Bat Conservation International at www.batcon.org.

- The average toad consumes an astonishing 15,000 destructive insects a year—and almost no beneficial ones. Keep toads happy by providing some shallow water, like a birdbath sunk into the ground, and a place to hide from noise, predators, and the midday sun. You can buy "toad abodes" at garden centers, but an upside-down, clay flowerpot with a gap broken out of the rim works just fine.

3 Masterful Mole-Chasing Capers

Contrary to what a lot of folks think, moles do not eat plants. Unfortunately, though, as they tunnel through the soil in their quest for the worms, grubs, and other insects that they *do* eat, they damage plants' roots, leaving them vulnerable to drought, diseases, and other pests. What's more, rodents that *do* eat plants, such as mice and voles, take full advantage of the free-and-clear subway system.

Although moles dig a huge network of tunnels, many of them are used only once. To find the active ones, step lightly on every tunnel you can see (you want to disturb the underground opening, but not destroy it). Use sticks, rocks, or brightly colored golf tees to mark the tramped-on runs. Two or three days later, go back and see which tunnels have popped back up. Then employ one of these three tactics to make the little diggers scurry in a hurry:

Turn up the heat. Make a solution of 1½ tablespoons of hot-pepper sauce, 1 tablespoon of dishwashing liquid, and 1 teaspoon of chili powder per quart of water. Pour half a cup or so of the mixture into each tunnel entrance.

Offend their noses. Pop a few squirts of pine-based cleanser, several scoops of used cat litter, or a stick of Juicy Fruit® chewing gum and a partially crushed garlic clove into each hole. Whichever aromatic weapon you choose, you might have to repeat the delivery a few times, but eventually, the moles will give up and move on.

Sound em' out. Moles are super-sensitive to sounds and ground vibrations. To put that weakness to work, gather up a bunch of plastic toy pinwheels, and shove them into the active tunnels at regular intervals. The whooshing sound should solve your problem—and entertain the neighborhood kids, too.

The Big Mole-Poison Boondoggle

Jaw-Dropping DISCOVERY

In garden centers and online, you can buy poison-laced gummy worms, fake peanuts, and seeds that (their manufacturers claim) will kill moles. And it is true that the poison is lethal. The problem is, no mole will ever touch the stuff because they don't eat seeds, peanuts, or any other plant material. Nor do they eat what appear to be dead worms. A mole's diet consists solely of *living* worms, grubs, and other insects. So don't waste your time and money. You have plenty of other options to get rid of moles without filling your soil with poison.

The Devilish Turf Disease Deception

The folks who make and market "miracle" fungicides would have you believe your lawn is a sitting duck for every turf ailment that ever came down the pike. Baloney! These menaces most often target golf courses and similar playgrounds that are highly fertilized, closely mowed, and constantly bombarded with insecticides, herbicides, and (yes) fungicides. As long as you don't follow that egregious example, no lawn disease is likely to ever raise its ugly head in your yard. If parts of your grass begin dying off, what appears to be an illness is more likely to be the result of one of these factors:

- Buried objects (for example, stones or construction debris)
- Drought
- Fertilizer burn
- Freezing
- Gas, oil, or chemical spills
- Low light
- Meandering tree roots
- Road salt damage

Compost Conquers All!

Jaw-Dropping DISCOVERY

Earlier, I told you that simply spreading compost over your lawn is a terrific alternative to chemical (or even organic) fertilizers (see "2 Safer Ways to Feed Your Lawn" on page 308). But "black gold" can do a whole lot more than keep your turf well fed. Scientists at Cornell University and other top horticulture schools have discovered that this wonder drug works in three ways to keep your lawn (and all your other plants) strong and healthy: It produces chemicals that kill foul fungi and bad bacteria, feeds microorganisms that eat fungi, and provides essential nutrients in a safe, slow way.

When to Dial a Lawn "Doc"

Turf diseases do not generally strike home lawns, but it can happen, especially if you (or your home's previous owners) have routinely used synthetic chemicals on the grass—or if you have it cut by a lawn-care service, which brings fungal spores into your yard on its mowers. If you see brown, dying, or dead patches that you can't attribute to other causes (see "The Devilish Turf Disease Deception," above), don't waste your time trying to figure out which disease it is because most of them produce very similar symptoms. Frequently, the only way you can get a positive ID is to send a "biopsy" to your Cooperative Extension Service, or a specialist the service might recommend. Take your sample from an area where the trouble is just starting to take hold, with about half of it healthy turf and half showing early symptoms. Dig down about 2 inches, and try to lift up a section that's roughly 1 foot square. Then pack it up carefully (ask for instructions when you call the Extension Service), and send it off to the lawn docs with a cover note describing everything you know about the problem (see "10 Essentials for Getting a Positive Lawn Disease Diagnosis," below).

10 Essentials for Getting a Positive Lawn Disease Diagnosis

When you send off a turf sample to your Cooperative Extension Service or another soil lab, include a cover note telling everything you know about the problem, including these details:

- Age and overall appearance of the lawn
- Type and variety of grass
- Size, shape, and color of the affected areas
- Location of the damaged spots (for example, along your normal mowing path, at the base of your sprinkler heads, or on a slope)
- Appearance of individual grass blades (for example, streaked, spotted, or wilted)
- Root condition (for example, Does the turf pull up in a mat? Have the roots rotted?)
- When the problem first appeared, and weather conditions at the time
- Recent activity in your yard, such as construction or house painting
- Your mowing, watering, and feeding routine
- Any pesticides, herbicides, and/or fertilizers you've used

90% of **pesticides** in current use have **not** been **tested for safety**.

7 Fabulous Fundamentals for Foiling Foul Fungi

With the exception of one viral infection (St. Augustine decline, which strikes only in Texas and parts of the Deep South), all of the major lawn diseases are caused by fungi. And once they take hold, they can be the very dickens to get rid of. Fortunately—just like human health problems—you can avoid them by taking some simple commonsense measures. If you follow these seven safe and simple guidelines, you're all but guaranteed to keep fungi from fouling your favorite field of green.

1. Give it great groundwork. Whether you're starting a new lawn or reviving an existing one, your grass will only be as strong and healthy as the soil it's growing in. For an easy way to build world-class soil, see "Make a Super-Simple Soil Sandwich" on page 122.

2. Know your territory. Assess your climate and the growing conditions in your yard, including not only temperature and humidity, but also such factors as light level, soil type, and the amount of foot traffic your lawn gets. Then choose a type and variety of grass that's been bred to thrive (not merely survive) in that environment. The reason: Any grass planted on the edges of its comfort zone will be under constant stress. And stressed grass (much like a stressed-out person) is a sitting duck for diseases.

3. Know the enemy. Find out what lawn diseases are most prevalent in your area, and plant resistant varieties of grass. Your best sources of intelligence: your lawn-tending neighbors and the folks at your closest Cooperative Extension Service.

4. Water right. Water early in the day, so the grass can dry off before nightfall; and water deeply but infrequently, so the grass dries out between waterings.

Fix-It-Fast FORMULA

Fungus-Fighter Soil Drench

When a fungal disease strikes your lawn— or your flower garden—whatever you do, don't use a chemical fungicide. That will only make your situation worse because the fungi will come back with a vengeance. Instead, reach for this ultra-safe, but highly potent, potion.

4 garlic bulbs, crushed

½ cup of baking soda

1 gal. of water

Mix all of the ingredients in a big pot and bring them to a boil. Then turn off the heat, and let the mixture cool to room temperature. Strain the liquid into a watering can, and soak the ground in the problem areas (remove any dead grass first). Go *very* slowly, so the elixir penetrates deep into the soil. Then dump the strained-out garlic bits onto the ground and work them in gently.

---

5. Feed right. Many diseases target overfertilized lawns. Others prefer underfed turf. Follow the dietary guidelines that are right for your type of grass. (Your Cooperative Extension Service can help here, too.)

6. Mow right. Mow at the maximum recommended height for your type of grass, and keep your mower blades razor sharp. Cutting your grass too short weakens the plants, making them easy targets for diseases; and dull blades make ragged cuts, through which fungal spores swarm like ants at a picnic.

7. Don't take "cides." Never use chemical insecticides, herbicides, or fungicides. They kill off the earthworms, beneficial insects, and zillions of invisible organisms that keep diseases and pests in check.

Wily Ways to Whip Lawn Weeds

Believe it or not, botanically speaking, there is no such thing as a weed. But there *is* such a thing as a plant that's growing where it's not welcome, and unlike diseases, they can—and do—show up in even the best-tended lawns. As a result, Americans dump tons of highly toxic weed killers on their grass every year. Well, don't do that, my friends! You have plenty of options that are not only safer, but also more effective over the long haul. Which weed-wipeout routine you want to use depends on the kind(s) of unwelcome plants you're dealing with. Here's what you need to know:

Cornmeal Fights Fungi Fast

REMARKABLE REMEDY

No matter what felonious fungus has run roughshod through your lawn, here's a simple three-step plan to green it up again pronto.

1. Sprinkle cornmeal over the damaged area at a rate of 50 pounds per 2,500 square feet. Scientists have found that this common supermarket product makes a whole lot of fungal diseases vanish like magic. They haven't figured out exactly how it works, but it seems to attract and feed the beneficial organisms that devour the fungal spores. (Many websites and restaurant-supply stores sell cornmeal in 25- and 50-pound sacks, and in bulk by the pound.)

2. Buy the highest-quality grass seed you can find—preferably one that's resistant to the disease plaguing your lawn. Then sow it thickly so the seeds are almost, but not quite, touching each other.

3. Spread ¼ inch of good compost over the seedbed, and water well. And keep the seeds constantly moist until they sprout.

The Crafty Crabgrass Cover-Up

Here's a fast, easy, and effective way to get rid of crabgrass without tedious hand-weeding—and without using herbicides: Just cover the crabgrass with either black plastic or black paper mulch (available in most garden centers), and leave it in place for 10 days. When you pull it off, the ol' crabgrass should be dead as a doornail. Any grass that was also covered will be yellow, but it'll green up again fast once you take the mulch away and let the sun shine in.

Cool-season annuals (for example, chickweed, knotweed, mallow, shepherd's purse)

- If you live up north, avoid feeding your lawn in the spring; down south, hold the chow in the winter. That way, you'll deprive the wicked weeds of sustenance when they need it most.

- In the North, mow high in spring and fall, so the grass can shade the soil and keep seeds from germinating.

- In the South, mow high in late summer to deprive weed seeds of light. Then, in the fall, overseed your lawn with a cool-season grass like perennial ryegrass or Kentucky bluegrass, and keep it mowed high through the winter.

- When weeds do appear, pull them out by hand or with a garden rake.

Cool-season perennials (for example, broadleaf plantain, Canada thistle, clover, curly dock, ground ivy, wild violet)

- Early in the season, scrape the plants out of your lawn with a metal rake.

- Immediately after that, mow your lawn to its shortest recommended height, rake up the clippings, and get rid of them fast, before any remaining weed stems can root again.

Warm-season annuals (for example, carpetweed, crabgrass, foxtail, goosegrass, pigweed, prickly lettuce, purslane, sandbur, spurge, yellow wood sorrel)

- Mow at the maximum recommended height, and if you've hacked off a lot of seed heads in the process, remove the clippings.

- Avoid summer feeding, and always water slowly and deeply.

- Do everything you can to keep your lawn free of stress because these weeds *love* stressed-out turf.

- Aerate your soil, and do whatever else is necessary to reduce compaction.

Warm-season perennials (for example, bindweed, chicory, Dallisgrass, dandelion, yellow nutsedge)

- Dig out the clumps, toss some organic matter into the hole, and reseed.
- Mow high.
- Avoid summertime feeding.

96% of **fish** in rivers and streams **contain pesticide** residue.

2 Surprising Reasons to Mow High

By simply keeping your type of grass mowed at the maximum recommended height, you can wipe out a whole lot of worrisome weeds—and open up more time for health-giving endeavors for yourself, like hitting the gym or simply relaxing at the old fishin' hole. This easy trick works for a couple of reasons:

1. Tall grass shades and cools the soil, making it harder for weed seeds to get a toehold.

2. Mowing high makes for deep-rooted, healthier grass that's better able to crowd out any weeds that do develop.

High mowing is especially effective at controlling low-growing troublemakers, such as annual bluegrass, crabgrass, and witchgrass.

Poison-Packin' Posies

➡ It's probably safe to say that most folks rank flowers among the most beautiful living things on earth—which is why millions of Americans grow annuals, perennials, and bulbs in their yards and in containers on decks, porches, and balconies. Yet, ironically, these same lovers of beauty douse their lovely blooms with some of the deadliest substances in existence. Well, don't you do it! In this section, I'll let you in on some simple secrets for growing picture-perfect posies *without* using a speck of toxic chemicals.

The Naughty "Natural" Hoax

In Chapter 4, we looked at some of the ways the Big Food industry tricks you into thinking its edibles are made by Mother Nature rather than by scientists tinkering in laboratories. Well, some unscrupulous fertilizer makers hand you the same line of hooey. Whenever you're shopping for an organic fertilizer, read the label carefully, and avoid any products that claim to be "organic-based." These actually contain large percentages of synthetic chemicals, most of them by-products of petroleum refining. (Some of the ingredients in fine print may seem vaguely familiar from high school chemistry class.) A fertilizer that's truly organic will sport a label with simple, easy-to-understand wording. For example, here are some sources of The Big Three nutrients you might see listed on the package of an organic product:

Nitrogen: Alfalfa meal, cottonseed meal, fish emulsion

Phosphorus: Bonemeal, poultry manure, rock phosphate

Potassium: Cow manure, granite meal, kelp meal

Americans use
1.1 billion pounds
of **pesticides**
each **year**.

Fix-It-Fast
FORMULA

All-Purpose Organic Fertilizer

This balanced diet will keep every plant in your garden—flowers as well as vegetables—well fed and growing strong all season long.

5 parts seaweed meal

3 parts granite dust

1 part bonemeal

1 part dehydrated manure

Combine all of the ingredients* in a bucket, then side-dress your plants with a couple handfuls of the mixture, and water well. Repeat the process two or three times during the growing season.

NOTE: *Although this dosage is fine for most perennials, plant appetites can vary greatly, so just to be on the safe side, check the label, catalog description, or a comprehensive garden book before you serve up the food.*

* All available in most garden centers.

Don't Overdo It

Just as eating too much of even the healthiest foods can make you sick or fat (or both), overfeeding your plants can also cause trouble. Even with the best organic fertilizers, more is not better. An excess can trigger woes ranging from delayed maturity to malformed flowers and vegetables. Be especially careful to avoid an overdose of nitrogen. It will make your plants produce overly lush foliage, which will attract sap-sucking insects like aphids and scale (more on floral pests coming up). So whenever you feed your flowers (or vegetables), always err on the light side, blend any fertilizer thoroughly into the soil, and follow up with a long, cool drink of water.

The Phenomenal Feats of Compost

Earlier in this chapter, I sang the praises of compost for its almost-miraculous ability to keep your lawn well nourished and free of diseases. Well, it can work the same wonders for all the other plants in your yard, including trees and shrubs. What's more, with compost, there's no such thing as an overdose. And making your own supply is a snap. To get started, buy a commercial compost bin at a garden center or from a catalog. (I prefer the bins that look like big, fat black wheels, mounted on a turning mechanism.) Then throw in your raw ingredients, and give the wheel a spin every week or two to let air get into the mixture. The sides are perforated, so the more you twirl the wheel, the more oxygen gets in, and the faster the stuff inside breaks down. As for what to put inside, you want roughly three parts high-carbon ingredients, or "browns," for every one that's high in nitrogen, known as the "greens" (see "The Composting Menu," at right). If you have too much carbon, the compost could take years to cook. Too much nitrogen, and it'll give off an odor that'll make you hold your nose and run away—fast!

The Composting Menu

When you're making compost, it's important to use roughly three helpings of browns to each one of greens. Here's the lineup:

Browns

▶ Chipped twigs and branches

▶ Dead flower and vegetable stalks

▶ Dry leaves and plant stalks

▶ Hay

▶ Pine needles

▶ Shredded paper

▶ Sawdust

▶ Straw

Greens

▶ Coffee grounds

▶ Eggshells

▶ Flowers

▶ Fruit and vegetable scraps

▶ Grass clippings

▶ Green leaves or stems

▶ Hair (pet or human)

▶ Manure

▶ Tea bags

Compost Tea

One of the healthiest things you can do for your flowers, or your homegrown food plants (see "Grow Your Own" on page 120), is to serve up frequent drinks of compost tea. It delivers a well-balanced supply of all the nutrients—major and minor—that keep your plants looking their best and producing heaps of fruits, vegetables, or flowers. And it's far more than just a good fertilizer; applied every two to three weeks throughout the growing season, it's also one of your best defenses against diseases.

1 gal. of fresh compost*

4 gal. of warm water

Pour the water into a large bucket or tub. Scoop the compost into a square of cotton or burlap, or use a panty hose leg and tie it closed. Put the "tea bag" in the water, cover the container, and let the mixture steep for seven days. Pour some of the finished tea into a watering can, and sprinkle it around the base of your plants. Put the rest in a handheld spray bottle, and spritz it onto the leaves.

* To make manure tea—another garden-variety wonder drug—simply substitute 1 gallon of well-cured manure for the compost, and use the finished product in the same way.

The Secret to Fending Off Flower Fatalities

Like turfgrass diseases, flower maladies cause the most trouble in yards that are heavily treated with chemicals. But they can strike even the best-tended gardens. Fortunately, it's easy to stop many of them in their tracks—without resorting to potentially dangerous substances that can lead to more woe than you've got already. The secret is simple: Take a good look at each plant every day (or as close to it as you can), and if you spot any of the following symptoms, take action right away. Don't dawdle—even a short delay could spell the difference between a minor challenge for you and a fatal disaster for your plants.

• Spots on leaves. Pick off all the marked leaves and toss them in the trash—not in your compost bin!

• Mottled green-and-yellow leaves that are crinkled or curled up. These are signs of viruses at work. There is no cure, so pull up infected plants and throw them away immediately.

• Yellowed leaves, stunted plants, and/or wilting. These may be disease symptoms, or they could signify the presence of pests, cultural problems, or nutrient deficiencies. If a dose of a good all-purpose organic fertilizer doesn't solve the problem, call your local Cooperative Extension Service and ask for help.

3 Ways to Minimize Munching Marauders

By inviting a host of beneficial insects and other predators into your yard, you can head off the vast majority of your pest problems (see "Deputize a Pest-Control Posse" on page 314). Of course, in order to keep that army on the job, it is essential to provide food (a.k.a. "bad" bugs) for them to eat. But that doesn't mean you have to surrender your flowers or vegetables to hordes of hungry bugs. The key to stopping trouble early is to conduct regular inspections. This is especially important when you're just beginning to make your garden a no-spray zone, and the good guys are still building up their troop levels. Every day, or as often as you can, perform this three-step routine:

1. Brush your hand over each plant to see if any whiteflies, flea beetles, or wayward leafhoppers jump or fly away.

2. Look at the leaves. Large ragged holes usually indicate slugs, beetles, or caterpillars. Be sure to check the undersides of leaves, where many of these rascals like to hide.

3. Inspect the stems and buds carefully, because these are favorite feeding places for sucking insects like aphids and spider mites.

REMARKABLE REMEDY

Lethal Soap Spray

When beetles or other hard-bodied insects get so out of control that you need to take drastic action, mix 2 tablespoons of dishwashing liquid and 2 teaspoons of either citrus oil or peppermint oil in 1 gallon of warm water. Pour the solution into a handheld spray bottle, and squirt it directly on each target insect. Just be sure to aim carefully, so you don't accidentally kill any of your allies. The killing secret is the oil. It cuts right through a bug's waxy shell, so the soap can get in and work its fatal magic.

There are **55,000+** different **pesticides used** in the **U.S.**

6 Ultra-Safe Bug-Bashing Ploys

When you do find more unwanted diners than your predator pals can polish off, don't panic! Depending on the size and nature of the pests, go at 'em using one or more of these surefire methods:

Handpick them. This is the most effective way to deal with larger pests, such as slugs, snails, beetles, weevils, and caterpillars. Just pick

8 Glorious Rose Guardians

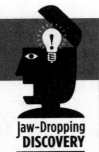

Jaw-Dropping DISCOVERY

Roses are gourmet fare for a whole lot of gluttonous insects—which is why the Queen of Flowers is generally bombarded with more chemical pesticides than any other plant on the planet. Well, friends, don't buy into that nonsense. The same nontoxic plant-care methods we've been talking about in this chapter work just as well for roses as they do for any other plants. What's more, simply by planting certain flowers and herbs around your rosebushes, you can close the buffet line, even to Frequent Diners Club members like Japanese beetles, aphids, and spider mites. Here are eight of the most potent bug chasers:

- ▶ Artemisia
- ▶ Catnip
- ▶ Chives
- ▶ Four-o'clocks*
- ▶ Garlic
- ▶ Nasturtiums
- ▶ Petunias
- ▶ White chrysanthemums (no other color)

NOTE: *Four-o'clocks are poisonous to Japanese beetles, and also to people and animals, so don't plant them if pets or small children play in your yard.*

them off the plants and drown them in a bucket of water laced with a cup of dishwashing liquid or rubbing alcohol. (Or hire a posse of neighborhood kids to do the honors.)

Dunk them. If you'd prefer a less hands-on approach, hold a bowl of soapy water under a bug-infested plant, and jostle the leaves; the pests will tumble into the drink and drown.

Hose them off. To get rid of aphids, thrips, whiteflies, and other tiny sucking insects, simply blast them off your plants with a strong spray from a garden hose.

Vacuum them. Put about 2 inches of soapy water into the reservoir of a wet/dry vacuum cleaner (a.k.a. Shop-Vac®), and suck the culprits up. Or use a regular handheld model and empty the contents into a bucket of soapy water. Vacuuming works especially well for insects that tend to scamper rather than fly—for example, lace bugs, harlequin bugs, rose chafers, and carrot weevils.

Clip them off. When you find a few leaves or stems covered with bugs, just cut off the afflicted plant parts. Put them into a plastic bag, tie it closed, and toss it into the trash can.

Pull them up. Sometimes, one plant will be seriously infested, while its neighbors are clean, or nearly so. In that case, simply throw an old sheet over the buggy plant, pull it up by the roots, and dump it into a tub of water laced with 2 cups or so of dishwashing liquid or rubbing alcohol. Leave it for a minute or two, then drop it in the trash. Handpick any stragglers.

6 Ways to Win the War on Weeds

A few weeds here and there won't hurt anything, but when they get out of control, they rob nutrients from your plants and give shelter to disease-spreading pests besides. How you get rid of the troublemakers depends on where they're growing, what you want to grow in their place, and how long they've been there. Here's my basic—and totally nontoxic—weed-management policy:

Each year in the U.S. **pesticides kill** up to **70 million birds**.

1. Smother them. If you're starting a new planting bed, or a whole series of them, see "Make a Super-Simple Soil Sandwich" on page 122. For unpaved walkways or paths between beds, use a variation on the theme: Just lay cardboard, brown paper bags, or newspapers over the soil, then spread on whatever kind of topping suits your fancy. Shredded bark, pea gravel, and pine needles, for instance, are all easy on the feet and the eyes.

2. Procrastinate. Don't rush to get warmth-craving plants into the ground. When heat lovers have to struggle to grow in cold soil, weeds can quickly do them in.

3. Seed heavily. Weeds pop up in any bare soil they find. When you're direct-sowing flowers, vegetables, or herbs, cover the space with the plants you want in your garden. Later, you can thin the seedlings to the right distance.

4. Use transplants. Young plants take off the minute you set them into the ground. That means they can start shading out weeds right from the get-go. Plus, when something green does appear, you'll know it's a weed, and you can pull it without worrying that you're ousting a future friend.

5. Mulch early and mulch often. A thick layer of organic mulch will stop weeds from sprouting among your plants. It will also keep disease-causing fungi in the soil from splashing up on stems and foliage.

6. Get 'em when they're down. Perennial weeds are at their weakest just before they flower. That's the time to give them a lethal dose of my Weed-Wipeout Tonic (on page 329).

Treacherous Trees and Shrubs

Just like any other plants, trees and shrubs attract their share of problems that need to be resolved. But they can also cause big and potentially fatal damage for two reasons:

Improper placement: Every year, during major storms, trees that are too big for their sites crash through the roofs of homes, sometimes killing folks inside. On a less lethal but still destructive note, an oversize tree or shrub can cause considerable damage to your bank account by sending its roots through your driveway or the sides of your swimming pool, dropping its leaves into your gutters, casting too much shade on your lawn and garden beds, and who knows what else! At the very least, a tree or shrub that's too big for its site will require constant pruning to keep it in bounds.

THE TAKEAWAY: Always buy a woody plant that will be the height and width you want when it reaches maturity, *not* when you see it in a pot.

Dangerous offerings: Many beautiful trees and shrubs produce slippery fruits that can stick to the soles of your shoes. Other types manufacture nuts that act like marbles under your feet. In either case, they could send you (or a visitor) crashing down—possibly with tragic results.
YOUR MISSION: Always site these "gift-giving" plants well away from places where people walk, play, or relax, including decks, patios, driveways, walkways, and stairs.

Stop Trouble in Its Tracks . . .

And stress, too. When woody plants have problems, they're usually big ones that can be stressful and expensive to deal with. The key to stopping them before they start: Go native. Trees and shrubs that are native to your region are much less susceptible to pests and diseases than any plant that's been brought in from somewhere else—even if the newcomer is a variety that can perform in your growing conditions. Don't worry: It won't take you much time to find top performers. In every part of the country, there are nurseries specializing in trees and shrubs that grow naturally in the area.

Tough Tactics for Tough Customers

When weeds are popping up among your flowers and vegetables, you know that if you start pulling or digging, you'll destroy some of your plants' roots in the process. But I've got a simple solution—just follow this four-step action plan:

Step 1. Cut each weed back to ground level.

Step 2. Slice the bottom off a 1-quart plastic bottle that has a screw-on cap. (You'll need one bottle for each troublesome weed.) Then set the bottle, with the cut side down, over the weed, and push it into the ground about 2 inches.

Step 3. Mix up a batch of my Weed-Wipeout Tonic (at right), remove the bottle's cap, then stick your sprayer head into the neck of the bottle and pull the trigger. Drench that weed until the potion is running off in streams, and screw the top on the bottle.

Step 4. Leave the bottle in place for a couple of weeks, and then check back. In the unlikely event that any of the weeds are still showing signs of life, give them another blast of the tonic. Before long, they too will be history!

> Fungicides **kill** more than **90%** of **earthworms** in the soil.

Attack of the Killer Weeds

Giant hogweed (*Heracleum mantegazzianum*) is almost a dead ringer for Queen Anne's lace, with umbrella-shaped clusters of delicate white flowers and deeply lobed dark green leaves—but it grows from 7 to 15 feet tall, its posy clusters can reach 2½ feet across, and the leaves can measure 5

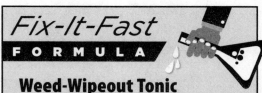

Fix-It-Fast FORMULA

Weed-Wipeout Tonic

When you've got weeds that just won't take no for an answer, knock 'em flat with this potent potion.

1 tbsp. of dishwashing liquid*
1 tbsp. of gin
1 tbsp. of vinegar
1 qt. of hot water

Mix all of the ingredients together, and pour the solution into a handheld spray bottle. Then drench the weeds to the point of runoff, taking care not to get any tonic on nearby plants.

Use a mild, unscented brand with no antibacterial ingredients.

feet or more in width. And, while "killer" is a slight exaggeration, this is one weed you don't want to mess with, in your yard or anyplace else! Its leaves and hollow, bamboo-like stems contain a toxic sap that can cause severe blistering burns, followed by skin discoloration and darkening that can last for years. And if it gets anywhere near your eyes, it can cause blindness. What's worse, merely brushing up against the plant is enough to release the sap.

The invasive species arrived on our shores in the early 1900s. Since then, the weed has spread across much of the northern United States and parts of southern Canada, and slowly but surely, its range is expanding. As you might expect, the invaded states and provinces are doing everything they can to get rid of the monster. If you see giant hogweed (or think you have), call your state's Department of Conservation or Natural Resources. They'll send a crew to make a positive ID and rout the menace from any public lands. If the troublemaker is in your yard, those folks can also recommend a contractor to safely remove it.

Wild Parsnip: A Second-Tier Terror

Wild parsnip (*Pastinaca sativa*), a kissin' cousin of giant hogweed, grows throughout the U.S. and Canada and causes similar trouble, but on a milder scale. Brief encounters mimic the effects of sunburn. In more severe cases, blisters appear a day or two later. Once they break, the affected skin begins to heal, but typically the burned areas retain a dark red or brownish discoloration for up to two years. Your best defense: Give a wide berth to patches of yellow flowers shaped like upside-down umbrellas, blooming on thick, three- to four-foot stems. If you do get zapped with the sap, wash the affected skin with soap and water ASAP, protect it from sunlight for at least 48 hours, and—just to be on the safe side—call your doctor.

Homeowners use **10 times** more **pesticide** than **farmers** do.

Outdoor Pitfalls

In previous chapters in this section, we've taken a cold, hard look at a lot of toxic substances and mischief-making invaders—living and otherwise—that may be lurking inside your home. We also explored alternatives to deadly yard and garden chemicals. Now we'll home in on how you can protect yourself and your family from three potent perils: potentially deadly insects (and snakes), the wrath of Old Man Winter, and treacherous travel travails.

Wicked Wildlife

➡ While the vast majority of the animal kingdom is perfectly harmless to humans, a few multilegged and slithering critters can deliver major, or even lethal, damage in the form of bites or stings. That's why, even in the tamest of suburbs, it pays to have some safe and savvy defensive tactics to call on.

The Great DEET Debate

Since its debut to the general public in 1957, DEET (*N,N*-diethyl-3-methylbenzamide in scientific lingo) has set the standard for insect repellents. So far at least, no other commercial product has come close to its effectiveness against disease-causing insects like mosquitoes, fleas, and ticks. That's why DEET-based liquids, lotions, sprays, wipes, and even wristbands fly

DEET Can Blast Your Brain

Jaw-Dropping DISCOVERY

In a study performed at Duke University to investigate the unexplained illnesses and neurological disorders suffered by U.S. soldiers during the First Gulf War, researchers exposed laboratory rats to insect repellent containing 70 percent DEET—the same concentration the troops had used in Iraq. The result: The rats experienced the same symptoms the veterans showed: cognition problems, muscle weakness, and difficulty walking. Brain examinations of the exposed rats discovered the reason: The DEET had killed cells in areas of the brain that control both cognition and muscle coordination.

Oust the "Ouch"—Fast!

REMARKABLE REMEDY

No matter how careful you are, sooner or later you're bound to wind up on the wrong end of some stinging insect. When that happens, remove the pain and itch by dabbing the bitten spot with one of these wonder "drugs": white vinegar, antiseptic mouthwash, white wine, vodka, or a thick paste made from baking soda and lukewarm water. Of course, if the perpetrator of the dirty deed was a bee, you'll need to remove the stinger first—and if you've ever had an allergic reaction to a bee sting or other insect bite, get to a doctor pronto!

off store shelves from coast to coast each summer. But is this stuff safe? The Environmental Protection Agency (EPA), the Centers for Disease Control and Prevention (CDC), and (of course) the folks who use it in their product formulations say yes—provided it's used as directed. Incorrect application can lead to skin irritation, disorientation, dizziness, seizures, tremors, and, on rare occasions, death. And some studies have linked regular use of DEET to birth defects and developmental problems, as well as damage to the kidneys, liver, and central nervous system.

4 Safer Skeeter Chasers

If you'd rather not take chances with DEET-based repellents, spread or spray one of these DIY formulas on your skin. They've all proven highly effective for folks who spend a lot of time in mosquito country:

- Straight rubbing alcohol
- A (gentler) half-and-half mixture of rubbing alcohol and Avon® Skin So Soft Original Bath Oil
- A half-and-half mixture of water and pure, clear vanilla (available online and in health-food stores—not to be confused with vanilla extract)
- Mentholated rub (also a terrific tick repellent)

Mosquitoes transmit more than 9 **deadly** human **diseases**.

Declare Victory over Vampires

To make sure that you and yours don't give blood when you're relaxing outdoors, set out oscillating fans to keep the air moving. And when you're barbecuing, toss a handful of sage, rosemary, or citrus peels on the coals. Both strategies will make mosquitoes keep their distance. But for long-term control, you need to eliminate the little devils' breeding grounds. And that's really not as hard as it may sound. Here's your six-item to-do list:

1. Get rid of any water-collecting debris, like old tires or discarded buckets.

2. Fill in holes and any low-lying areas in your yard where rainwater collects.

3. Change your pets' water at least once a day, and refill birdbaths every couple of days.

4. Empty portable wading pools as soon as the kids (or pets) are through using them. Then turn them upside down or take them indoors.

5. Keep rain barrels covered.

6. To make water gardens and other permanent water features off-limits, use either Laginex® or Bti (*Bacillus thuringiensis israelensis*). Both are available online and in many garden centers, and both kill mosquitoes without harming any other living things. Just one word of advice: If you go with Bti, make sure you look for slow-release tablets; some brands lose their effectiveness after about three days, so you'll have to add more.

Sobering Tick Talk

Ticks have gained nationwide infamy for spreading Lyme disease and the potentially fatal Rocky Mountain spotted

6 Signs of a Skeeter-Borne Disease

While mosquitoes do most of their deadly dirty work in tropical countries, they can spread a number of serious diseases in the United States, the most infamous being West Nile virus and several forms of encephalitis. But—and this'll get your attention, folks—just like bedbugs, which are thronging here from around the world (see "Beastly Bedbugs" on page 288), more kinds of skeeters are heading our way and bringing their sinister baggage with them. A recent case in point: two Caribbean species that transmit the crippling chikungunya virus, which was first diagnosed here in 2014.

Despite wide differences in both severity and damage, all mosquito-borne diseases share similar early warning signs. So if you're bitten by a skeeter and experience any of these symptoms, see your doctor ASAP:

▶ Chills

▶ Fever

▶ Headache

▶ Low blood pressure

▶ Malaise

▶ Nausea

fever, but that's just the beginning of the horror story. As of this writing, there are 14 different tick-borne diseases plaguing various parts of the United States, and new ones keep popping up with disturbing frequency. The specific ailments, as well as the exact kinds of ticks that carry them, differ from one part of the country to another. But all of the infections have similar symptoms. Both the severity and the time of onset can vary, but these are the most common signs:

DEET is used in **200+** insect **repellents**.

- Fatigue
- Fever and chills
- Headache
- Joint pain
- Muscle aches
- Rash

All tick-borne diseases are easily treated with antibiotics—but they can be very hard to diagnose. The key to fending off dangerous complications lies in fast action. If you've been bitten by a tick, and anywhere from a few days to several weeks later you experience any of the symptoms listed above, see your doctor *immediately*!

5 Alarming Reasons for the Rise in Tick-Borne Trouble

If you're wondering why the incidence of tick-spread diseases has been escalating over the past 10 years or so, you're not alone. Medical researchers and epidemiologists (a.k.a. the health community's number crunchers) have been searching hard for answers, too. Here's a handful of the major ones:

1. Increased travel opportunities. Just like bedbugs and mosquitoes, new species of disease-carrying ticks are arriving on our shores from other countries.

2. Pesticide resistance. For decades, ticks have been bombarded with ever-more-toxic control agents, with the result being that they've become immune to most of them.

3. Invasive vegetation. In many parts of the country, a drastic upping of the tick population is being blamed on the bush honeysuckle, a.k.a. Amur honeysuckle (*Lonicera maackii*). This beautiful plant was brought here from the temperate parts of Asia and promptly spread out of control. Deer just love Amur honeysuckle—and where deer go, deer ticks follow.

4. Habitat destruction. As more and more wild spaces fall to developers' bulldozers, deer and other critters are forced to move into or closer to populated areas—bringing ticks with them.

5. Medical progress. Because of increased awareness among physicians, and greatly improved diagnostic techniques, legions of people whose symptoms were initially blamed on scores of other ailments are now being accurately diagnosed and treated for tickborne maladies.

Tick Removal: A Review Course

Conventional wisdom once called for dabbing a tick with alcohol, oil, petroleum jelly, or some other substance before removing the foul thing. Well, forget that approach! Now we know that such pretreatment only causes the villainous varmint to regurgitate even more potentially deadly germs into the victim's skin. Instead, this is the routine to follow, whether you're de-ticking a human or a pet:

Step 1. Grasp the tick's head, as close to the patient's skin as possible, with curved forceps or tweezers. (If you must use your fingers, cover them with several layers of tissue or

---

Fix-It-Fast

F O R M U L A

Toodle-oo Tick Spray

Although ticks don't eat plants, they do perch on flowers, shrubs, and grasses (both ornamental and turf types) while they wait for "dinner" to saunter by in the form of a human or other red-blooded animal. If the germ-totin' terrors are hanging out in your flowers or ornamental grasses, cook their geese with this spray. (The alcohol is the secret weapon here: It penetrates the ticks' protective waxy covering so the soap can get in to do its lethal work.)

1 tbsp. of dishwashing liquid or liquid soap

1 gal. of rainwater or soft tap water

2 cups of rubbing alcohol

Mix the soap with the water in a 6 gallon hose-end sprayer jar, then add the alcohol. With the nozzle pressure turned on high, spray your plants from top to bottom—and make sure you get under all the leaves. Repeat whenever necessary. Just make sure you wait until evening to perform this maneuver; otherwise, the combination of sunshine and alcohol will burn your plants.

---

a handkerchief or, better yet, wear rubber gloves—*never* touch a tick with your bare hands.)

Step 2. Pull up with a smooth, steady motion. Jerking or twisting could cause pieces of the tick to break off and stay in the skin.

Step 3. Drop the tick into a container of alcohol, or flush it down the toilet. Don't crush it; you could spread disease organisms that may be present in the body fluids.

Step 4. Disinfect the wound with alcohol, then immediately wash the site (and then your hands) with soap and hot water.

Ticks transmit **14** different human **diseases**.

The Ultimate Tick Repellent

Legions of folks who live, work, and/or play in tick territory swear by old-fashioned pine tar soap as the most effective tick repellent that ever came down the pike. It also turns off many other kinds of insects, and it's perfectly safe to use on adults, children, and pets. Plus, it smells just like a Christmas tree. You can put this miraculous stuff to work in two ways:

1. Mix 1 tablespoon of pine tar soap (either liquid or shavings from a bar) per cup of warm water in a handheld spray bottle, and spritz your clothes, your skin, and Rover's fur. (Make sure you don't get any in his eyes; it won't do permanent harm, but it *will* sting.)

2. Simply use it in the shower, as you would any other soap, or bathe your pup with it.

Whichever method you choose, it'll keep you and yours free of ticks all day long. You can find pine tar soap, in both liquid and bar forms, online and in many brick-and-mortar stores that sell old-time country products.

Mow Your Way to a Tick-Less Summer

As a lawn guy from way back when, I know that giving your yard a crew cut is not the fastest way to a lush, healthy crop of turfgrass. But it *is* a surefire way to destroy a lot of ticks—and to keep more from moving in. And if tick-borne diseases are on the rise where you live, that's most likely higher on your priority list than a showstopping lawn. At least it *should* be! So move your mower blade to its lowest setting, and go for it!

Nix Ticks in the Nest

Throughout the country, many kinds of disease-spreading ticks spend their growing-up time on mice. And that gives you a great way to rub out the vile villains—and turn some potential trash into treasure at the same time. All you need is lint from your clothes dryer, empty toilet-paper rolls, and a pet shampoo that contains a flea-and-tick killer called permethrin. Once you've gathered your supplies, just soak the dryer lint in the shampoo and push a small wad into each cardboard tube. Then set the tubes out in brushy areas or other sheltered spots where the mice are likely to find them. The mice will take the fluffy stuff home to line their nests, and the freeloading ticks will be history.

> **CALL 911**
>
> In most cases, a sting by a bee or wasp is merely painful and annoying. But if you feel faint, your pulse is rapid, you have trouble breathing, your mouth and/or throat swell up, or you break out in hives, call 911 or have a pal rush you to the ER or the closest doctor *immediately*. Those are all signs of a potentially fatal allergic reaction.

3 Keys to Bee-Free Flowers

Bees are literally essential to life as we know it because they are the chief pollinators of many major food crops. They also perform that critical service for most of our flowering ornamental plants. But, life-giving heroes or not, you certainly don't want to entice them to your outdoor living areas if you or anyone in your family is allergic to bee venom. Does that mean you need to choose between safety and a yard filled with beautiful flowers? Not at all! Just make your plant selections based on these three criteria:

Color. Avoid flowers in bright shades of blue, purple, and yellow—they draw bees like magnets. Instead, go with blossoms that are white or red (which bees see as black).

Scent. Sweet-smelling flowers draw bees from far and wide. They generally steer clear of anything that has a musky, pungent, or faint aroma, like geraniums (*Pelargonium* spp.), marigolds, and feverfew (*Tanacetum parthenium*).

Shape. Bees love wide, flat daisy-like flowers that provide convenient landing fields on which to sit and sip. They usually bypass blooms that are tubular or dangling in shape, such as flowering tobacco (*Nicotiana* spp.), fuchsia, snapdragons, salvia, and columbine. Likewise, they tend to dodge double flowers, like dianthus, chrysanthemums, and most roses.

Open an After-Hours Garden

For a guaranteed bee-free deck or patio, plant flowers that bloom at twilight or later, when the bees are snoozing in their hives—which, most likely, is also when you have time to relax and enjoy the floral show. You have dozens of beautiful kinds to choose from, including these winners:

- Evening primrose (*Oenothera biennis*)
- Four-o'clocks (*Mirabilis jalapa*)
- Moonflower (*Ipomoea alba*)
- Night-blooming daylilies (*Hemerocallis* 'Moon Frolic' and *H.* 'Toltec Sundial')
- Night-blooming jasmine (*Cestrum nocturnum*)

NOTE: *Four-o'clocks are poisonous to people and other mammals, so don't plant them if small children or pets play in your yard.*

3 Need-to-Know Facts about Killer Bees

Contrary to what many folks think, killer-bee venom is no more potent than that of garden-variety honeybees. What makes these hybrid horrors so dangerous lies in these sobering facts:

1. While killer bees are not predatory, they are extremely aggressive when they're defending a hive. Dozens or even hundreds of them will swarm, chase, and viciously attack people or animals that inadvertently stray into their territory. And it doesn't take much to get them riled up. Even ground vibrations or simple sounds, like a barking dog or a lawn mower from as far as 100 feet away, can trigger an uprising, and the bees often chase their "invaders" for half a mile or more.

2. There's no telling where you might encounter trouble because killer bees are not picky about the places they set up housekeeping. They've been known to build hives in upturned flowerpots, old tires, cement blocks, and even empty soda pop cans.

3. Here's the crucial statistic: Although sensitivity to the venom varies from one person to the next, 8 to 10 stings per pound of body weight can generally deliver a fatal dose to a human or pet.

When Killer Bees Attack . . .

If you find yourself under siege by these nasty stingers, here's what to do:

- Run as fast as you can to the closest house, car, or other enclosure, and quickly close all doors and windows. Do *not* jump into a swimming pool or other body of water because the bees will hover just above the surface until you come up for air.

- Cover your head and face to prevent stings to your eyes, nose, and mouth (yes, ladies, even if it means removing your shirt). Stings to the face are much more dangerous than those to any other parts of your body. Also, killer bees are drawn to the carbon dioxide emitted from your nose and mouth.

- Stay calm, and if you do get stung, try to keep that stung body area below your heart.

- If you're fortunate enough to have gotten only a few stings, treat them as you would the results of a "regular" bee encounter.

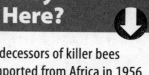

How the Heck Did They *Get* Here?

The predecessors of killer bees were imported from Africa in 1956 by Brazilian scientists hoping to develop a strain of honeybees that was better adapted to the tropical climate. Unfortunately, some of the "herd" escaped and began breeding with their local counterparts. Since then, their hybrid offspring, known as Africanized honeybees, have been multiplying and migrating. The first contingent to cross our southern border appeared in Hidalgo, Texas, in 1990. Since then, they've spread to parts of Florida, Georgia, across the Southwest, and into southern California and southern Nevada. On a hopeful note, the population is not likely to expand much beyond that range because (entomologists tell us) these bees cannot survive cold winters, and they seem to dislike prolonged or repeated periods of rainfall.

3 Plants That Keep Wasps at a Distance

There are more than 75,000 kinds of wasps in the world. Nearly all of them are not only harmless, but also highly beneficial because they prey on other insects, including disease-carrying mosquitoes and almost every crop-destroying garden pest you can name. But, zowie! Their stings really pack a punch. So plant any of this trio of repelling heroes wherever you want to keep wasps at a distance:

Citronella. This is most potent when you crush the leaves and rub them onto your skin (or use citronella oil, available in health-food stores). But dense groupings of the real deal also discourage wasp visits. **NOTE:** *Citronella cannot survive temperatures below 20° F, so if you live in cold-winter territory, plant it in containers, and move them indoors for the cold months.*

Mint. Both the oil and live plants repel wasps. Unlike citronella, mint will thrive in any climate. In fact, unless you grow it in pots, or confine the roots underground, you'll need to clip it back frequently—otherwise, it'll take over your whole yard before you know it.

Wormwood (*Artemisia absinthium*). If you want a great-looking border to enclose a wasp-free zone, this is the plant for you. It's a perennial with finely cut silvery-gray foliage. It's hardy in USDA Zones 4 to 8 and highly drought resistant. On the downside, the same aromatic chemicals that repel wasps (and scads of other insects) make wormwood poisonous to people and animals—so don't plant it if you have small children or pets on the scene.

Bug **bites & stings** send **500,000** people **to the ER** each year.

Attack of the Killer Ants

The southern part of our country is cursed with several species of imported fire ants. They all deliver a sting that would put any bee to shame, but the red devils have a couple of trump cards: a hearty appetite for any critter that moves, and a mean streak the size of Texas. What's worse, unlike most other stinging, biting bugs, fire ants are not solo performers. Nor are they one-shot wonders. They attack in droves and they sting repeatedly—sometimes with deadly results. Small children, elderly folks, and baby animals (both pets and livestock) are the most frequent fatality victims, but anyone can suffer a lethal reaction. And here's the really sobering part: Fire ants have stood up and said "boo" to just about every chemical pesticide known to man. In fact, like many other bugs, they've reacted to the poisonous onslaught by evolving into "superbugs" that can fend off anything the folks in white lab coats send their way.

Surprising Collateral Damage

Their methods of attack are not the only things that set fire ants apart from other potentially dangerous insects: Besides injecting their painful poison into your (or your pet's) skin, fire ants can deliver a piercing "bite" to your bank account. That's because a mature colony's mound—a rock-hard dome measuring up to 1½ feet high and 2 feet in diameter—is a disaster-in-waiting for any car or piece of machinery that runs over it.

A Penny for Your Sting

REMARKABLE REMEDY

If you spend much time outdoors in the summer, always keep a clean old penny and an adhesive bandage in your pocket. Then the minute you get stung by a wasp or bee, press the coin over the site, secure it with the bandage, and keep it on for 15 minutes. (If you don't have a bandage or tape on hand, hold the penny to the sting site.) The copper will neutralize the acid in the insect's venom, thereby helping to head off pain and swelling. There's just one caveat: You must use a penny that's dated 1982 or earlier. The ones minted from 1983 on are made almost entirely of zinc, with only a thin copper coating, and they aren't worth beans for sting relief.

Boots Can Save Your Life

If you must spend time in an area that's home to fire ants or poisonous snakes (or both), your best protection is a pair of high, sturdy boots. (Cowboys don't wear that footgear just because it looks snazzy.) To fend off fire ants, go with the tallest rubber boots you can find, and dust the outsides with talcum powder.

Call in the Pros

Don't be fooled by the visible part of a fire-ant mound—it's only the tip of the fireberg. The excavation often extends 3 feet or more below the surface, and flitting around inside there can be as many as a quarter of a million ill-tempered ants—including up to 3,000 egg-laying queens. And in order to destroy the colony, you need to kill off every single one of those mamas. So if you've got one of these "castles" in your yard, don't even think of trying to remove it yourself. Instead, call a pest-control professional, who will use one of these two weapons:

• An insect growth regulator such as abamectin

• Avermectin, a naturally occurring soil fungus that's lethal to fire ants

Whatever you do, don't let them talk you into anything more toxic—it'll only encourage the breeding of more super ants!

Americans spend **$200 million** per **year** on bug **repellents**.

Fire-Ant First Aid

When you've had a fire-ant encounter that resulted in only a few stings, quickly slather on either a half-and-half solution of chlorine bleach and water, or a paste made of meat tenderizer and water. Applied within 15 minutes of the sting, it'll ease the pain and swelling. Do not scratch any pustules that develop, or they may become infected. Eventually, they'll dry up and leave a temporary scar that should go away on its own.

If the pain is severe or spreads beyond the bitten spot—even if you have no other symptoms—get to a doctor *pronto*!

3 Dangerous Delusions about Treating Cuts

If you're still patching up garden-variety cuts the same way your grandma did, here's big news: Those time-tested techniques can actually do more harm than good.

Delusion #1: You should clean a cut thoroughly with hydrogen peroxide or rubbing alcohol.
FACT: Both of these cleansers can damage healthy tissue around the wound and delay healing.

Delusion #2: You should apply a topical medication, such as iodine, Mercurochrome®, or Merthiolate® to fight germs.
FACT: These and other ultra-strong antiseptics can interfere with your body's natural healing mechanisms. Instead, look for a product that contains natural ingredients, such as St. John's wort, calendula, or vitamin E oil.

Delusion #3: You should keep the cut dry and let air get to it so that a scab can form.
FACT: Keeping wounds moist and scab-free helps them heal more efficiently and minimizes scarring.

Cutting-Edge Cut Care

Medical gurus recommend this four-step plan for treating cuts:

1. Stop the bleeding. Cover the injury with clean padding, and apply firm, even pressure.

2. Clean it right. Rinse the cut under running water, or wipe dirt away with a wet cotton ball or pad, moving from the center of the wound outward.

3. Apply a natural antiseptic. Cover it with a nonsticking bandage.

4. Keep it clean. Every few days, clean the wound with a mild saline solution (2 teaspoons of salt per quart of boiling water, cooled to room temperature).

When *Not* to Try This at Home

If any of the conditions below describes your gash, forget DIY treatments—get to the ER *fast*!

• Blood is spurting out of the wound and/or doesn't stop within 10 minutes.

• You can see yellow fat or red muscle tissue.

• It's wide and/or jagged; and gravel or other debris is embedded in the wound.

• The cut is on a joint or your face.

Snakebite-Survival Strategies

First, the good news: In the unlikely event that you find yourself among the 7,000 to 8,000 people in the United States who get bitten by poisonous snakes each year, it's a good bet you'll survive. The reason is, for every type of snake venom, there is a highly effective antivenom to counteract it—that is, provided you react in exactly the right way and get to the ER fast. The key is to keep calm, and forget all those snakebite scenes in old cowboy movies. Here's your real-life game plan:

Do:

- Dial 911, or call the nearest hospital and tell the staff you're headed their way.

- Take a digital picture of the snake if you can, so the docs can choose the right antivenom.

- Remove rings, watches, or anything else that constricts blood flow.

- Wash the wound with soap and water, and keep it below heart level.

- Immobilize the affected limb during evacuation.

Do *not*:

- Try to capture or kill the snake.

- Apply ice or a tourniquet. (Constricting blood vessels concentrates the poison in one area, which could lead to amputation of the bitten limb.)

- Cut into the wound with a knife.

- Try to suck out the venom.

- Drink alcohol or caffeinated beverages.

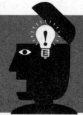

The Real Lowdown on Repelling Snakes

Jaw-Dropping DISCOVERY

You'll find this bit of advice all over the Internet: Scattering sulfur or mothballs around your yard will keep snakes out. Hogwash! Neither one is effective at deterring snakes. Nor are commercial snake repellents, which, aside from not working well, are arguably more dangerous than snakes are. The key ingredient in most of them is naphthalene, which causes liver damage, anemia, and possibly (according to the EPA) cancer. If you're receiving regular visits from snakes—whether poisonous or otherwise—it's a good bet that you've inadvertently laid out a great big welcome mat for them in the form of ample food (especially rodents) and plenty of safe, cozy cover. So do yourself a favor: Before you call a snake-removal contractor, who could only provide a temporary solution anyway, follow the rodent-riddance guidelines in Chapter 11 (see "Wretched Rodents" on page 292).

- Take any medications.
- Drive yourself to the hospital, unless you have no other choice, because snakebite impairs motor function.

If you follow those guidelines—thanks to anti-venom—the odds are about 400 to 1 that you'll live. But be forewarned: For a few days, you may not want to.

A **severed snake head** can **bite** for up to **1 hour**.

Winter—The Deadliest Season of Them All

➡ Winter's cold, gray days and long nights are notorious for triggering seasonal affective disorder (SAD) in millions of people (see "'Tis the Season to Be SAD" on page 47). But wintertime also packs a potent passel of physical perils. Here are some terrific timely tips for keeping you and your family safe and sound.

2 Freaky Ways Winter Can Wipe You Out

The cold, crisp days of winter can trigger a couple of conditions that can range in severity from painful and debilitating to fatal. Here's the dastardly duo:

Chilblains (a.k.a. pernio) is the inflammation of small blood vessels in your skin that occurs in response to sudden warming after exposure to cold temperatures. Signs that you've been struck include itchy red patches, swelling, and sometimes blistering, most often on your fingers, toes, ears, and nose. Chilblains generally clear up within a few weeks if you follow these guidelines:

- Use mild skin lotions to alleviate swelling and itching.
- Clean the affected skin daily with a natural antiseptic, and cover it to prevent infection.

CALL 911

If you develop chilblains, and you have diabetes or poor circulation, see a doctor immediately to prevent potentially fatal complications. Even if you're in the pink of health overall, get to a doc if your skin color changes from red to dark blue, accompanied by swelling and burning pain; blisters develop; or the affected skin appears to be infected.

- Keep the afflicted area(s) warm but away from heat sources.
- Don't scratch!

To prevent trouble, stay warm at all times, especially if you've suffered chilblains in the past.

Raynaud's disease is a disorder in which the blood vessels narrow in response to cold air, thereby reducing blood flow to the fingers, toes, and sometimes the ears, lips, and nose. The affected body parts turn white, blue, and then red, generally accompanied by burning pain when the blood begins flowing back to the stricken areas. There is no cure and, so far at least, no known prevention. If your extremities begin to feel tingly or numb and start to lose color, suspect the onset of Raynaud's. Hightail it to a warm place where you can quickly raise your body's core temperature and get your blood flowing normally again. If you already have the disease, do everything you can to protect yourself from the cold, whether that entails bundling up to the nth degree or, if possible, moving to a warmer climate.

The Christmas Coronary Conundrum

Study after study has shown that more deaths occur by heart attack and stroke during the winter months than at any other time of the year. And that's not counting the tens of thousands of folks who get rushed to the hospital for cardiovascular events (as they're known in scientific lingo) and live to tell about the experience. The medical crowd has dubbed this seasonal increase in heart-related woes the "Christmas Coronary Phenomenon." So why do all these diabolical disasters happen during the season of joy and light? For these reasons:

Winter cold kills twice as many people as summer heat does.

Cold weather: Exposure to low temperatures leads to a loss of body heat, quickly followed by a rise in metabolic rate and narrowing of the blood vessels—all of which can contribute to cardiovascular problems, especially in people who are already at high risk for them (see "Heart Disease—Give It the Heave-Ho!" on page 158).

YOUR BEST DEFENSE: If you're on the high-risk list, don't venture outdoors in extremely cold weather unless it's absolutely necessary. And whenever you do go out, bundle up!

Sloppy habits: During the winter months—and especially between Thanksgiving and New Year's Day—most people eat more and exercise less than they normally do.

YOUR BEST DEFENSE: By all means, enjoy the holiday season. Unless you're on a very strict doctor-ordered regimen, a little more food and drink than usual won't hurt you. But don't overdo it. And make sure you get in some exercise, even if it's only strolling around your neighborhood admiring the Christmas decorations.

Unaccustomed exertion: When snow piles up on sidewalks and driveways, people (primarily middle-aged men) who rarely move a muscle except to start the car or click the TV remote, charge outdoors to clear snow from their sidewalks and driveways.

YOUR BEST DEFENSE: Don't put your life at risk—hire a teenager or a snow-removal service to uncover your buried surfaces. And when you have no choice but to do the job yourself, follow the commonsense guidelines in "6 Slick Tricks for Safe Shoveling" (below).

You're Allergic to *What*?!

Jaw-Dropping DISCOVERY

Lots of folks find cold weather uncomfortable, but for those who suffer from an allergic condition called cold urticaria, exposure to cold weather or cold substances sets off the flow of histamines and other chemicals into the bloodstream, with results ranging from itchy red welts to lethal anaphylactic shock. No one knows what causes cold urticaria, and there is no cure. But more health professionals are waking up to the dangers of this kooky-sounding, but very real, problem. See your doctor if you break out in hives shortly after exposure to cold, or your hands swell up when you're holding a cold object. And get medical help *immediately* if you feel dizzy, you have trouble breathing, or your tongue or throat begins to swell. To learn more, visit the website of the Cold Urticaria Foundation at www.coldurticaria.info.

6 Slick Tricks for Safe Shoveling

The next time you look out the window and see your driveway covered with a thick white blanket, consider this fact: Shoveling snow or pushing a heavy snowblower is more strenuous than running on a treadmill set at full throttle. For that reason, clearing away several inches of snow is a dandy way to get some first-class exercise—but only if you're healthy and fit. Otherwise, you could find yourself being rushed to the ER with a heart attack or severe back injury, as tens of thousands of folks are each winter. Even if you are (or think you are) in pretty good shape, following these half-dozen guidelines can literally spell the difference between life and death:

1. Warm up. Do some light exercises and stretches in the house before you head outdoors.

2. Dress for success. Wear warm, slip-resistant boots, and dress in layers, so you can peel one off while you're working, then put it back on during breaks.

3. Work smart. Whenever possible, push the snow out of the way instead of lifting it. When hoisting is necessary, shovel many light loads instead of fewer heavy ones. And never throw the snow over your shoulder or off to the side because the twisting motion can wrench your back. Instead, turn, slowly and gently, so you can toss the load forward. And always be sure to bend your knees, and lift with your legs—not with your back!

4. Pace yourself. Take frequent breaks, drink plenty of water, and don't try to do the whole job in one stint. Especially if you're not used to exercising or you've had previous back problems, shovel (or snow-blow) for 5 to 10 minutes, then go back inside for 10 to 20 minutes.

5. Forget perfectionism. Don't try to remove every speck of white from your snow-covered surfaces. Instead, tackle the areas that could pose problems for cars or pedestrians, and let Mother Nature take care of the rest in her own good time.

6. Know when to quit. Head indoors immediately if you feel light-headed or short of breath, your heart begins to race, your chest starts hurting, or you feel any other alarming physical sensation. And (of course!) if you even suspect that you're having a heart attack, call 911.

When to Shun the Shovel

If you're out of shape, or have a history of back injuries or heart disease, don't even think about getting out there to shovel snow. Likewise, farm the job out to someone who's strong and fit if you're obese, are diabetic, or have high blood pressure—all of which put you at ultra-high risk for a heart attack or stroke.

Heart-related **deaths increase 22%** in the week **following** a **snowstorm**.

A Wintertime Driving Quiz

So you think you know all there is to know about driving in the winter? Well, maybe you do. Or maybe these answers will come as a surprise—and possibly save your life.

True or false? In the winter, you should always carry a big, heavy sack of sand or cat litter in the trunk of your car because the added weight will give you better traction on snowy or icy roads.

SOMETIMES TRUE, BUT USUALLY FALSE. Here's the deal: If your car has front-wheel drive, adding weight over the back wheels will actually make a rear-end skid *more* likely. In the case of a model with rear-wheel drive, that extra weight may help you get started from a standstill on a slick road surface. But once you're under way, it will increase the distance you need for stopping—and that could get you in *big* trouble. As for the "sometimes true" part of the answer, if you have a rear-wheel-drive pickup truck or a similar vehicle that has very little built-in weight in the back, then it is a good idea to toss in some ballast when Old Man Winter arrives on the scene.

True or false? If you have a four-wheel-drive vehicle, you can go anywhere without a concern in the world.

ABSOLUTELY FALSE! When you're on an icy road, four wheels slip and slide just as readily as two wheels do. And if you cling to that false sense of security, it can lead to deadly mistakes during dicey travel conditions.

 If you're one of those intrepid travelers who jumps in the car and takes off regardless of poor driving conditions—even when you don't really need to go anywhere—consider these sobering stats from a recent study at the University of California Berkeley School of Public Health: Every year in the United States, inclement weather is associated with more than 1.5 million car crashes that result in about 800,000 injuries and 7,000 deaths. The associated financial damage: at least $42 million.

3 Deadly Winter Driving Blunders

There's an old riddle that asks, "What's the most dangerous part of a car?" The answer is, "The nut behind the wheel." Unfortunately, that riddle is no joke. The vast majority of accidents are caused not by any vehicular problems, but by careless, lazy, or deliberately daredevil drivers. It's especially true in winter, when hordes of otherwise sensible people seem to think all roads are created equal—whether they and the skies above are travel-brochure pristine or covered in snow and ice with visibility near zero. Here are three common driving habits that could cost you your life or kill innocent victims—or both:

Driving too fast. Ignore speed-limit signs. They're set for normal road conditions. Instead, take it slow and easy until you know how much traction you can expect from your tires. And *never* use cruise control on a wet surface. If you even touch the brake pedal, it can send you into a tailspin in a heartbeat.

Following too closely. On a dry summer road, staying a count of three seconds behind the car ahead of you may provide ample time to stop, but in poor conditions, double or triple that figure. When you're driving on ice, don't stop at all if you can help it, or you could have a dickens of a time getting going again. Also, allow 200 to 300 feet between your vehicle and snow-removal equipment, which needs plenty of maneuvering room.

Driving when you're tired. It's every bit as dangerous as driving when you're drunk, especially in rain, snow, or dark of night. Get a good 40 winks before you start off on a road trip, and allow yourself more time than you think you'll need to reach your destination. If your energy starts to lag, switch drivers, pull over and take a break—or, if necessary, find a nearby motel and crash for the night. (For more on the dangers of drowsy driving, see the Yikes! box on page 18.)

3 Timely Tips for Safe Winter Driving

REMARKABLE REMEDY

While it is true that you can't control the behavior of other drivers, there is plenty you can do to ensure you and your passengers are less likely to become accident statistics. Here's your three-part game plan:

1. Have your car thoroughly checked and winterized, inside and out, before cold weather arrives.

2. Stock your vehicle with emergency supplies, including warm jackets, blankets, flares, a spare tire, matches, a first-aid kit, an ice scraper, a shovel, chains or sand for traction, nonperishable snacks, water, and a fully charged cell phone.

3. Take a specialized course to brush up your skills, especially if you're new to cold-winter territory. To find a class near you, do a quick Internet search for "winter driving course."

Words to the Wise about Watches and Warnings

Confused about the difference between winter storm watches and warnings? Both terms describe identical weather conditions: at least 6 inches of snow, with visibility less than a quarter mile, and winds gusting at 35 miles per hour or more. The difference lies in the timing. A winter storm watch means the trouble could arrive in the next 12 to 36 hours. When a winter storm warning goes out, it means you can expect heavy going sometime within the next 12 hours.

69% of **deaths** in the U.S. **occur** in the **winter**.

The Secret to a Safe and Sane Winter Is . . .

Be prepared! If you wait for the 24-hour weather channels to announce a winter storm warning—or even a watch—and then join the panicked crowds at the local supermarket, you may not be able to get all the supplies you need to survive. At best, you'll send your stress and anxiety levels sailing off the charts. So do yourself and your family a favor: If you live in an area that gets even occasional snow and ice storms, gear up long before the season's first flakes begin to fall. Here's what you need:

- Basic cleaning and first-aid supplies
- Battery-powered radio and/or television
- Candles and matches

Being Cozy-Warm Could Kill You!

Jaw-Dropping DISCOVERY

Each winter, thousands of people die from carbon monoxide poisoning and from fires caused by fireplaces and home-heating systems. So in early fall, have your furnace inspected by an HVAC pro, and get your fireplace professionally cleaned and your chimney linings checked. Make sure your carbon monoxide and smoke detectors are in good working order, and put fire extinguishers in the kitchen and every room that has a fireplace or woodstove. And burn only thoroughly dried hardwoods like oak or maple. Avoid soft, sappy, or creosote-treated woods, and never toss cardboard, paper, or trash of any kind into either a woodstove or an open fireplace. (For more on CO poisoning, see "Carbon Monoxide: A Silent Killer" on page 301).

- Emergency heating source

- Flashlights with extra batteries

- Food, water, and medications—both prescription and OTC—for all people and pets in your household (FEMA recommends you have a two-week supply.)

- Heating fuel, such as oil for your furnace and extra wood for your fireplace or woodstove

- Home-entertainment options that don't require electric power, such as books, board games, playing cards, and jigsaw puzzles

Travelin' Trouble and Woe

➡ In the previous section, I clued you in on the dangers of wintertime driving and the steps you can take to keep you and your passengers safe on the road. Now we'll slam the brakes on some driving habits that can do you in at any time of the year—as well as some potentially life-threatening risks of flying the sometimes-not-so-friendly skies.

2 Malevolent Myths about Cell Phones and Driving

Cell **phone use** while **driving** makes you **4 times** more likely to **crash**.

Every year, thousands of people are killed and hundreds of thousands are injured because they, or other drivers, were chatting or texting from behind the wheel of an automobile. And the toll continues to rise, despite laws that place restrictions on the practice. Part of the reason lies in these two major misconceptions, among lawmakers and drivers alike, about the true nature of the problem:

Misconception #1: It's safe to talk on a cell phone as long as it's in hands-free mode.

BALONEY! Study after study has shown that keeping both hands on the wheel while talking does not reduce your accident risk one iota. That's because (contrary to what dedicated "multitaskers" would have you believe) the human brain simply is not capable of fully concentrating on two things at the same time. Your gray cells have what scientists call a finite "cognitive load." When you're chatting on a phone, you're using up a full 37 percent of your brain's capacity to gather and process the kind of data you should be using to drive safely—regardless of what your hands are doing.

Misconception #2: Talking on a cell phone while driving is no different from conversing with a passenger in your car.

HORSEFEATHERS! In fact, passengers can actually increase your degree of road safety (unless you are a teenager). The reason, researchers tell us, is that when other adults are in the car, conversation tends to flow according to the demands placed on the driver. Unlike people on the other end of a phone line, passengers can point out road conditions the driver might not notice. Plus, when the going gets dicey, drivers generally suspend chatter in a vehicle, but (studies show) they do not tend to put callers on hold in similar situations.

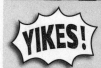 When it comes to dangerous distracted-driving habits, texting tops the list. The folks who study automotive stats tell us that reading or writing a text message while you're at the wheel increases your accident risk 23 times—or, to put it in more graphic terms, by 2,300 percent. That's because, not only does it use at least as much of your brain's cognitive load as a phone chat does, but it also takes your eyes away from the road. And if your peepers leave your driving path for just five seconds when you're going 55 miles an hour, you travel the length of a football field without seeing where you're going—or what may be coming at you.

6 Deadly Dangers of Distracted Driving

It's not just talking and texting that can put your life—and the lives of others—at high risk on the road. Snacking on a bag of chips or swigging your morning coffee can also divert your attention long enough to cause major trouble. Even if you don't indulge in this seemingly innocent habit, you need to be on the lookout for other drivers who do. A recent Harris Interactive/Health Day poll found that 86 percent of respondents admitted to eating or drinking (non-alcoholic beverages) while driving, which more than doubles their chance of causing an accident. But that's not all! A great many of these same "responsible" folks freely owned up to indulging in a half-dozen other extracurricular drive-time activities that have been proven to cause fatal accidents galore, including:

- Applying makeup
- Reading paper road maps
- Setting or adjusting their GPS devices
- Styling their hair
- Surfing the Internet
- Watching videos on handheld devices or dashboard DVD players

On an even more sobering note, this list does not include the hundreds of thousands of drivers who hit the road when they're stressed out, sleepy, or drunk (see Chapter 1 for the lowdown on the dangers of driving after too much booze or too little sleep).

A Killer of an Excuse

Police reports consistently show that about half of the fatalities from auto accidents could have been prevented if the victims had been wearing seat belts. If you've heard that alarming figure already, but you don't buckle up consistently, chances are it's because you're fooling yourself with one of these potentially fatal excuses:

Excuse #1: I'm only going a few miles down a local road.
FACT: At least 80 percent of traffic fatalities occur within 25 miles of home, when the vehicles are traveling under 40 miles an hour.

Excuse #2: I've got an air bag, so I don't need a belt.
FACT: While an air bag increases the effectiveness of a seat belt in a front-end collision, it won't provide one iota of protection against side impacts.

Excuse #3: If there's a crash, I can brace myself.
FACT: Even if you have the split-second reaction time to pull this stunt off, the force of the impact will shatter the limb(s) you used for the purpose.

Excuse #4: The belt will trap me in the car.
FACT: In the event of a crash, that's exactly where you want to be. According to statistics, if you're thrown out of a vehicle, you're 25 times more likely to be killed than you are if you remain inside.

The Truth about "Germy" Airplane Air

True or false? When you're traveling in an airplane, you can easily get sick from breathing in the recycled, germ-laden air.
ABSOLUTELY FALSE: In fact, the air in a plane is one heck of a lot cleaner than the air in a typical office building. That's because during a flight, the plane's engines continuously pull in cool, thin air from the outside,

in the process heating and compressing it to make it breathable. Some of the existing cabin air is vented outside, while the rest is mixed with the incoming supply and run through high-tech filters. These filters remove 99.97 percent of particles, including whatever disease germs the passengers and crew members may be exhaling.

The "Yes, But" Factor

While it is true that the cabin air of a modern jetliner is virtually germ-free, it can still raise your odds of contracting a serious illness. How so? Here's the deal: By necessity, the same filtration system used to clear disease-causing organisms from the air also happens to drastically lower its humidity. Otherwise, the moisture accumulating from passengers' breath could cause the plane's electronic gear to malfunction. But that arid atmosphere also ups your chance of contracting a potentially fatal disease in two ways:

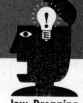

Your Seat-Back Tray Could Kill You

Jaw-Dropping DISCOVERY

So could the seat-back pocket. Or the armrest. Researchers at the University of Arizona found the frequently fatal bacteria methicillin-resistant *Staphylococcus aureus* (MRSA) on 60 percent of flip-down trays it tested. And in a recent study presented at the annual meeting of the American Society for Microbiology, Auburn University researchers found that MRSA can survive for 168 hours on the seat-back pocket. Furthermore, other studies show that the only slightly less dangerous *E. coli* bacteria last for 96 hours on the armrest material. Surfaces on trains and in highway rest stops pose similar hazards. The exact degree of danger varies on any given day, depending on the nature of the materials, as well as when and how thoroughly they were last cleaned. So don't take chances: Whenever you're traveling by plane, train, or car, wash your hands as often as possible, use a hand sanitizer between washings, and avoid touching your face.

It dries out the mucous membranes in your eyes and nose, which all but guarantees you'll rub those body parts. When you touch your face, you transfer whatever germs you've picked up from any surfaces you've touched (see "Your Seat-Back Tray Could Kill You," above).

Dehydration can set in and weaken your immune system in a flash. And a compromised immune system makes you a sitting duck for every ailment under the sun. Fortunately, there's a simple solution to this problem: Drink plenty of water or other nonalcoholic beverages while you're airborne.

The Cheap Seat Delusion

If you spend much time in the air, for business or pleasure, you're no doubt well aware of a condition called deep-vein thrombosis (DVT), in which blood clots in your legs can travel through your bloodstream to your lungs and cause a pulmonary embolism. You may have heard that these potentially deadly clots are brought on by the cramped legroom in the economy-class section. Well, according to new findings by the American College of Chest Physicians, it just ain't so. What causes blood clots to form is not lack of space—it's lack of movement. Here's what the docs recommend when you're on a flight of four to six hours or longer:

- Whenever possible, opt for an aisle seat, which gives you increased mobility over a window location.

- Stand up frequently at your seat, and walk around the cabin at least once an hour—every 20 to 30 minutes is better. Stretch your calves as you go, and do a few waist bends and arm circles if you can.

CALL 911

If you have a heart condition or circulation problems, consult with your doctor before you take a long flight. After you reach your destination, even if you're in the pink of health, watch for signs of a blood clot in your legs. Get medical help if you notice pain or tenderness, warmth, redness, or swelling in your calf. And if you experience shortness of breath, rapid heart rate, stabbing pain in your chest, or an unexplained cough, hightail it to the ER—those are all symptoms of a pulmonary embolism.

- When you can't leave your seat, at least move your feet and legs every 20 to 30 minutes. Flex your feet and ankles, and lift your knees toward your chest so that your feet rise slightly off the floor.

- If you're at high risk for DVT*, wear below-the-knee graduated compression stockings (available online and in most pharmacies and medical-supply stores).

Disease-causing **bacteria linger** on **airplane surfaces** for up to **1 week**.

* Advanced age, recent surgery, obesity, heart disease, or other circulation disorders all increase your risk of developing DVT during air travel. So do pregnancy and the use of oral contraceptives or other forms of estrogen.

Index

Anxiety
    color and, 38–39
    drugs for, 36–37, 40
    formulas for reducing,
        39, 40
    GAD, 36
    health basics and, 38
    health risks, 184
    prevalence, 38
    remedies, 39–40
    signs of, 36
    vs. worry, 35
Aphids, 313, 326
Apitherapy, 180–181
Apple cider vinegar uses.
    See also Vinegar uses
    headache relief, 192
    psoriasis relief, 243,
        244
    shingles relief, 223
    strep throat relief,
        227–229
    tonic recipe, 164
    type to use, 229
Apple juice, 3
Apples
    for conjunctivitis relief,
        84
    health benefits, 83,
        151, 175
    for joint pain relief, 86
    pesticides in, 85–86,
        112
    salad recipe, 200
    storing, 114
Armyworms, 313
Arnica oil, 187
Aromatherapy
    for anxiety relief, 40
    for CFS/FM relief,
        199

for stress reduction,
    43, 45
for weight loss,
    135–136
Artemisia, 326
Artemisia absinthium
    (wormwood), 340
Arteriosclerosis, 170
Arthritis
    causes, 176, 179
    formula for relieving,
        182
    hazards to avoid, 178
    myths, 176–178
    prevalence, 181
    remedies, 73, 180–183
    types, 177
Artichoke Cholesterol-
    Control Tonic, 168
Artificial sweeteners,
    64–66, 68
Asbestos, 303–304
Asparagus, 112
Aspartame, 66, 95
Aspirin, 178
Assassin bugs, 313, 314
Asthma
    causes, 9, 172–174
    remedies, 85,
        174–175
    signs of, 205
Athlete's foot, 34, 84
Ativan®, 36
Autoimmune diseases.
    See also specific types
    facts, 231
    genetic factor, 230
    prevalence, 231, 233
    signs of, 234
    toxins and, 231–234
    types, 232

Avocados
    for blood pressure
        reduction, 86
    for heart health, 162
    pesticides in, 112, 114
Avocado seeds, 86
Avon® bath oil, 332

B

Bacillus thuringiensis (Bt),
    313
Back pain
    emergencies, 184
    formula for relieving,
        186
    myths, 183–184,
        187–188
    risk factors, 184–186
    treatments, 185–187,
        188
Baking soda uses
    cleaning, 253–255
    cold and flu relief,
        215–216, 218
    insect sting relief, 332
    laundry, 251
    lawn care, 318
    pest control, 282, 296
    psoriasis relief, 244
    shingles relief, 223
Ballroom dancing, 54
Bananas, 64, 81
Banana-Walnut Smoothie,
    156
Bariatric surgery,
    126–127
Basil, 43, 209
Bath treatments
    bronchitis, 208
    flu, 218
    headaches, 192

freshness test, 113
health benefits, 167
labels, 101
production of,
  100–101
for skin care, 30–31
Elderberries, 216
Emergency preparedness,
  351–352
Emphysema, 9
Endocrine system, 249,
  252
Energy bars, 143
Energy drinks, 97
English plantain, 207
Enlist™, 107
Environmental Working
  Group (EWG), 111–112,
  250
Epidemics, 217
Epsom salts, 73, 223, 244
Ergonomics, 189
Essential oil uses. *See also*
  specific oils
  anxiety reduction, 40
  carpet deodorizer, 255
  mood booster, 48, 49
  psoriasis relief, 243
  smoking cessation, 17
  stress reduction, 43, 44
Ethanol, 251
Ethyl acetate, 251
Eucalyptus oil, 45, 208
EWG (Environmental
  Working Group),
  111–112, 250
Exercise. *See also*
  Inactivity
  brain function and, 52
  calories burned, 147
  cancer prevention, 149

cautions, 43, 203, 212
  eating after, 142–143
  energy bar recipe, 143
  immunity and, 225
  SAD and, 50
  skin health and, 30
  weight control and,
    143–147
Expiration dates,
  112–113
Extreme-Relief Muscle
  Massage Oil, 186

F
Fabrics, 251, 267–269
Fabric softeners, 250–251
Fabulous Fat-Burning
  Smoothie, 135
Faith, 60
Fast food, 63
Fats and oils, 96, 135, 183
Fennel oil, 48
Fennel seed, 207
Fermented foods, 196
Fertilizers
  chemical, 306–308
  formula for, 322
  organic, 308–309,
    321–322
  runoff from, 308
Feverfew, 196
Fiber, 134
Fibromyalgia. *See* Chronic
  fatigue syndrome/
  fibromyalgia
Fight-or-flight, 41–42
Financial costs
  clutter, 273
  smoking, 5–6, 10, 11
Fipronil, 277
Fire ants, 340–342

Fish and seafood,
  103–105, 224, 321
Fish aquariums, 37
Fish oil, 100
Flame retardants, 256,
  257–258
Flaxseed, 64, 151
Flaxseed oil, 49
Fleas, 284–285, 293, 295
Floor cleaner, 266
Flooring, 257, 260–261,
  264–267
Flounder, 224
Flow, 57
Flower gardens
  bee-free, 337–338
  disease control, 324
  fertilizers, 321–323
  pest control, 325–327
  weed control, 327–330
Flu. *See* Colds and flu
Flu shots, 211
Flypaper, 283
Fly traps, 283–284
Folate, 64
Food. *See* Nutrition;
  Organic foods;
  Processed foods; *specific*
  foods
Food additives
  in processed food, 93,
    94, 97–99, 102
  in supplements, 100
Food allergies, 90, 105,
  235
Food coloring, 264
Food cravings, 50, 85
Food labels
  on eggs, 101
  expiration dates,
    112–113

Hormone disrupters
(*continued*)
   phthalates, 256–257
   Roundup®, 106–109
Hormone-replacement
  therapy (HRT), 54,
  173–174
Horseradish, 79, 210
Hot Healing Liniment,
  182
Hot-pepper sauce, 134,
  315
House fires, 292–293
Houseflies, 282–284
Housekeeping, 146–147.
  See also Cleaning
  products
Houseplants, 252
HRT (hormone-
  replacement therapy),
  54, 173–174
Hugs, 60
Hydration. *See* Water
  intake
Hydrion® paper, 233
Hydrogenation, 93–94
Hydrogen peroxide, 216,
  343
Hypertension. *See* High
  blood pressure
Hypothyroidism, 141

I

IBD. *See* Inflammatory
  bowel disease
IBS (irritable bowel
  syndrome), 236
Immune system. *See also*
  Autoimmune diseases
   air travel and, 355
   boosting, 85, 225

   chronic pain and, 176,
    184
   happiness and, 55
   nutrition and, 62, 68,
    73
   smoking and, 9
   stress and, 42
Inactivity
   arthritis and, 178, 179
   diabetes risk, 154, 156
   immunity and, 225
   sitting disease, 25, 26
Inflammatory bowel
  disease (IBD)
   cause, 41, 236–237
   food and, 235,
    237–239
   formula for relieving,
    237
   vs. IBS, 236
   natural remedies, 238
   signs of, 236
   types, 235
Insect repellents,
  331–332, 342
Insects, in food, 99
Insect stings, 332, 337,
  340
Insurance costs, 5–6, 10
Intentional inefficiency,
  25
Interphone study, 22–23
Iron overload, 92, 160
Irritable bowel syndrome
  (IBS), 236
Ischemic stroke, 169

J

Japanese beetles, 326
Jasmine oil, 44
Jaw-bone loss, 11

Joint pain, 86. *See also*
  Arthritis
Juicy Fruit® gum, 315
Juniper oil, 40

K

Ketchup, 108
Ketoacidosis, 157
Ketosis, 71
Kidney disease, 124
Kidney stones, 73, 85
Killer bees, 338–339,
  340
Kindness, 57
Kitchens, 137
Kiwi, 112
Klonopin®, 36
Knotweed, 320
Knuckle cracking,
  177–178

L

Lace bugs, 326
Lactose intolerance, 90,
  238–239
Ladybugs, 313, 314
Laminate countertops,
  264
Landlines, 24, 305
Laptop computers, 24
Laughter, 60, 174, 225
Laundry products,
  250–251, 269
Lavender uses
   back pain relief, 187
   migraine relief, 197
   pest control, 287
   skin care, 151, 223
   sleep aid, 21
   stress reduction, 43,
    44, 45

Pesticides and herbicides
(continued)
    safety testing, 317
    statistics, 322, 325,
      327, 330
PETE (polyethylene
  terephthalate), 262
Pets. *See* Cats; Dogs
Petunias, 326
PFCs (perfluorochemicals),
  256, 268
PFOA (perfluorooctanoic
  acid), 256
pH balance, 233
PHN (postherpetic
  neuralgia), 221–222
Phosphates, 97–98
Phosphorus, in fertilizer,
  322
Phthalates, 256–257
Phytates, 98
Phytic acid, 98
Phytonutrients, 72–73
Pigweed, 320
Pineapples, 112
Pine-based cleaner, 315
Pine tar soap, 336
Pinwheels, 315
Piperonyl butoxide (PBO),
  277
Plaster of paris, 293
Plastic bags, 270
Plastics
  diabetes and, 154, 155
  toxins in, 118–119
  types by number, 262
PMS, 86
Pneumonia, 9, 205
Polycarbonates, 262
Polychlorinated biphenyls
  (PCBs), 225

Polyester fabric, 267, 268
Polyethylene, 262
Polyethylene terephthalate
  (PETE), 262
Polypropylene, 262
Polystyrene, 119, 262
Polyurethane, 258–259
Polyvinyl chloride. *See*
  PVC
Popcorn, 117–118
Pork, 86
Portable generators, 301
Postherpetic neuralgia
  (PHN), 221–222
Posture, 189
Potassium
  in fertilizer, 322
  nutrient, 50, 92,
    164–165
Potatoes
  arthritis and, 178
  for blood pressure
    reduction, 165
  health benefits, 88
  pesticides in, 112
  as rat bait, 293
  storing, 115
Potpourri, 155
Poultry, 103. *See also*
  Eggs
Prediabetes, 153, 155
Prescription drugs
  alcohol and, 4
  anti-anxiety, 36–37, 40
  antidepressants, 58
  dangers of, 161
  dementia and, 52
  headaches and, 193
  psoriasis and, 241–242
  stevia and, 67
Prickly lettuce, 320

Processed foods
  additives and chemicals
    in, 93, 94, 97–99, 102
  GMOs in, 66, 94–97,
    100
  hydrogenation, 93–94
  intake of, 63, 94
  labels, 96, 97
  pesticides and
    herbicides in, 108
Promensil®, 174
Prostate cancer, 148
Psoriasis
  cause, 239, 242–243
  formula for relieving,
    242
  health risks, 239–240
  prevalence, 239
  remedies, 242–244
  risk factors, 240–241
  triggers, 241–242
Psoriatic arthritis, 177,
  240, 244
Pulmonary embolism,
  356
Purslane, 320
PVC, 118–119, 140–141,
  256–257, 262

R

RA (rheumatoid arthritis),
  177
Race, and diabetes, 154
Radiation, 22–24, 26
Radon, 299–300
Raised-bed gardens,
  120–122
Raspberries, 81
Raspberry blossoms, 223
Raspberry leaves, 166
Rats. *See* Rodents